AF840173

Critical Perspectives in Public Health Feminisms

Critical Perspectives in Public Health Feminisms

Edited by Renée Monchalin

CANADIAN SCHOLARS
Toronto | Vancouver

Critical Perspectives in Public Health Feminisms
Edited by Renée Monchalin

First published in 2023 by
Canadian Scholars, an imprint of CSP Books Inc.
180 Bloor Street West, Suite 1401
Toronto, Ontario
M5S 2V6

www.canadianscholars.ca

Copyright © 2023 Renée Monchalin, the contributing authors, and Canadian Scholars.

All rights reserved. No part of this publication may be reproduced, stored in a retrieval system, or transmitted, in any form or by any means, without the prior written permission of Canadian Scholars, under licence or terms from the appropriate reproduction rights organization, or as expressly permitted by law.

Every reasonable effort has been made to identify copyright holders. Canadian Scholars would be pleased to have any errors or omissions brought to its attention.

Library and Archives Canada Cataloguing in Publication

Title: Critical perspectives in public health feminisms / edited by Renée Monchalin.
Names: Monchalin, Renée, editor.
Description: Includes bibliographical references.
Identifiers: Canadiana (print) 20230228526 | Canadiana (ebook) 20230228607 |
ISBN 9781773383569 (softcover) | ISBN 9781773383583 (EPUB) | ISBN 9781773383576 (PDF)
Subjects: LCSH: Health and race—Canada. | LCSH: Women—Health and hygiene—Canada. |
LCSH: Health—Sex differences—Canada. | LCSH: Social status—Health aspects—Canada. |
LCSH: Equality—Health aspects—Canada. | LCSH: Discrimination in medical care—Canada. |
LCSH: Public health—Canada.
Classification: LCC RA450.3 .C75 2023 | DDC 362.1089—dc23

Cover art by Matsuko Friedland
Cover design by Rafael Chimicatti
Page layout by S4Carlisle Publishing Services
Printed and bound by CPI Group (UK) Ltd, Croydon, CR0 4YY

EU Authorized Representative: Mare Nostrum Group B.V., Mauritskade 21D, 1091 GC
Amsterdam, The Netherlands, gpsr@mare-nostrum.co.uk.

Canada

Contents

Acknowledgements

I want to acknowledge all of the public health feminist authors for their chapter contributions that made this text possible. I also want to acknowledge the University of Victoria, which has provided a subvention through the Book and Creative Works Subvention Fund. Lastly, I wish to acknowledge Lizzie Di Giacomo at Canadian Scholars, who supported me in bringing this text to completion while I welcomed baby Yima Rhéal into the world in January 2023.

Cover Art

By Matsuko Friedland

INTRODUCTION

Hajimemashite! This is a Japanese phrase used when meeting someone for the first time, before introducing oneself, and to signify the beginning of a relationship. I would like to begin our relationship with an introduction of myself and my artwork, which is featured on the cover of this book.

My name is Matsuko Friedland and I use they and she pronouns interchangeably. Aspects of my identity are continually evolving, but some things are innate. I was born on the traditional and unceded Coast Salish territory of the lək̓ʷəŋən (Lekwungen/Songhees) and W̱SÁNEĆ (Saanich) peoples, colonially known as Victoria, BC. This land is where I was born and have spent the majority of my life so far. It was where I was raised by several strong women, including an educated, immigrant single mother, an older and wiser sister, and a variety of makeshift aunties. I reside on this land and study at the University of Victoria (UVic), where I am about to graduate with a BA Health and Community Services in the school of Public Health and Social Policy (PHSP). As I share my story, I am reminded of the privilege I have in accessing an education that, like other colonial institutions, is so valued in our society while being so harmful to many marginalized folks, including the First Peoples of this land. Even in my limited time in post-secondary education, I have witnessed growth in the recognition and integration of Indigenous ways of knowing and am hopeful for safer education for all in the future.

My art piece was created for the final assignment, an art project, in Renée Monchalin's inaugural Public Health Feminisms course at the University of Victoria. It synthesizes many of the topics explored in the course, as well as in this book. The following sections have been adapted from my assignment and further describe the art piece and its relationship to public health feminisms. I am so honoured and grateful to be able to share my artwork with all of you reading this book. Yoroshiku onegaishimasu—the ending to a good beginning: please take care of me, and I will take care of you.

EMBROIDERY AS ART

The medium of this piece, embroidery, was chosen with intention.

While this is an "art" project, I deliberately chose a medium that is largely considered a "craft." I did this as an act of rejection of the art/craft hierarchy. The art/craft hierarchy suggests that there is a distinction between arts and crafts and that crafts are less artistically significant than arts (Parker, 1989). In fact, the real difference between the two is not material, skill, or purpose but rather where they are made (i.e., at home versus at work) and who tends to make them (i.e., lower-class women versus upper-class men) (Parker, 1989). Much like patriarchy, the art/craft hierarchy is a construct rooted in sexist and capitalist values. By submitting a "craft" as "art," I purposefully chose to conflate the two, thereby renouncing the art/craft hierarchy.

Embroidery is a method of sewing images or patterns onto fabric with thread, and it can be decorative or functional (e.g., to reinforce weak fabric) (Day & Buckle, 1907). It is a slow, intentional, and therapeutic form of creativity that is present worldwide (Segalo & Fine, 2017).

Embroidery is often thought of as "women's work" and considered "light and easy" (Wharry, 2021). In fact, embroidery—like much of "women's work," particularly care work—is incredibly labour intensive, time consuming, and underappreciated (Segalo & Fine, 2017; Wharry, 2021). Indeed, the relatively simple piece I created for this project took several hours to complete.

In some cultures and times, embroidery marked a girl's path into womanhood and kept them from actively participating in politics (Segalo & Fine, 2017). Despite this, women have used embroidery for communication when they otherwise were unable to, creating journals, propaganda, and more (Segalo & Fine, 2017; Wharry, 2021).

This craft has a long relationship with politics, power, and resistance: for example, embroidery was used by slavery abolitionists and suffragettes (Wharry, 2021). The relationship between craft and politics continues to this day with the concept of "craftivism," first coined by Betsy Greer in 2003 and defined as "a form of activism based on practices of craft, such as knitting, sewing, and other 'domestic arts'" (Pratt Institute, 2021). Craftivism can be included alongside more general feminist activism in advancing sexual and reproductive rights and gender equality (Fulu et al., 2021).

DESIGNING PUBLIC HEALTH FEMINISMS

As I discussed, embroidery was intentionally chosen due to its relationship to feminism and communication. While the resulting piece is visually quite simple, it represents significantly more complex ideas. I incorporated many of the topics explored throughout the course, including intersectionality, knowledge sharing, reciprocity, the social determinants of health (SDOH), and feminism. The creation of this piece was itself a practice of public health feminisms—with each stitch, I reflected on many of these topics and how they could be actualized.

The background material of the piece is a white fabric remnant cut from an old towel. While this was mainly chosen out of practicality, the fabric can also represent the existing foundation of public health on which we build public health futures: predominantly white, timeworn, and in desperate need of replacement or repair.

The design of the piece consists of embroidered dots in a variety of sizes and colours. The colours were intentionally pulled from the Philadelphia pride flag, which includes the standard seven rainbow colours (red, orange, yellow, green, blue, indigo, and violet) as well as black and brown (Queer in the World, n.d.). The flag's black and brown stripes represent queer black and brown people and their unique experiences (Queer in the World, n.d.). This was the first version of the pride flag to incorporate black and brown stripes and intersectionality. In my piece, the colours represent diverse populations and also serve to recognize some of the groups who continue to be disproportionately affected by negative health outcomes (e.g., 2SLGBTQIA+, BIPOC, and/or disabled people [Kielsgard & Brown, 2021]).

The sizes of the coloured dots vary to represent variegated levels of power, including SDOH such as gender, race, disability, and income (Raphael et al., 2020).

The dots are arranged to loosely form three overlapping circles. The number three is significant in that it represents strength (triangles, with three points and sides, are the strongest geometric shape) and is literally "beyond the binary" (more than two). These circles represent different types of groups, such as communities, sectors, generations, and identities. When the circles are viewed as identities, their convergences represent intersectionality, acknowledging that individuals experience unique oppressions based on the sum of their identities (Crenshaw, 1989).

A light beige thread, almost the colour of the background, forms connections both within and between the dots. This represents communities, sectors, and generations working together and sharing knowledge, which is necessary for improving population health—for example, trans, BIPOC, and disabled communities making space for each other in their communities (Kielsgard & Brown, 2021); public health sectors and urban planning sectors collaborating to improve housing and transportation (Galea, 2021); and Métis kokums (grandmothers) and iskwêsisisak (girls) sharing health knowledge intergenerationally (Jones et al., 2020).

It is my hope that the resulting art piece will be used as a tool to explain many of the complex topics to newcomers and ignite their interest in public health feminisms.

Contributing Authors

Ifrah Abdillahi is a PhD candidate in the Social and Behavioural Health Sciences division at the Dalla Lana School of Public Health (DLSPH). Her dissertation poses critical questions at the intersection of racism, public health, the social determinants of health, and health equity through examining the emergence of the City of Toronto's Action Plan to Confront Anti-Black Racism and the role of the COVID-19 pandemic in interfering with, disrupting, or galvanizing focus on addressing anti-Black racism through policy action. Having worked extensively on social justice projects in Canada, Europe, and East Africa, her research is situated within broader critical reflection on regional, national, and international reckoning on racial inequality and social transformation in contemporary times. She holds a master's in gender and political science and is a fellow in the Collaborative Doctoral Specialization in Global Health at DLSPH. In addition to her dissertation work, Ifrah is also a senior policy analyst at the Public Health Agency of Canada.

Maren B. Akyürek (she, her, they, them) was born and grew up on the traditional, ancestral, and unceded territories of the səl̓ilwətaʔɬ təməxʷ (Tsleil-Waututh), šxʷməθkʷəy̓əmaʔɬ təməxʷ (Musqueam), Skwxwú7mesh-ulh Temíx̱w (Squamish), and S'ólh Téméxw (Stó:lō) or what is known as Vancouver. Maren identifies as a queer person with several (dis)abilities. Maren is a graduate student in the Social Dimensions of Health program at the University of Victoria. Maren strives to bridge different disciplines, with research interests that include 2SLGBTQIA+ issues, reproductive rights, (dis)ability, Indigenous health, the social determinants of health, and equitable access to healthcare.

Michelle Amri, MPA, PhD (she/her), is a cisgender woman and a daughter of refugees to Canada. She is a Takemi fellow 2021–2023 at Harvard University and a Social Sciences and Humanities Research Council (SSHRC) postdoctoral fellow. Michelle's scholarship is in the field of politics of health, largely at the intersection of global public health, policy, and governance. Some of her research includes investigating how health equity is conceptualized and operationalized by the World Health Organization and high-level policymakers, enablers and barriers to intersectoral and multisectoral health policy, how equity can be better considered by policymakers globally, and decolonizing global health through assessing colonial discourses and the modus operandi of global health. Michelle consults for the World Health Organization, sits on the board of directors for the

Canadian Association for Global Health, and was named to the list of Canadian Women in Global Health.

Falan Bennett is an MD–PhD candidate at the University of Toronto's medical school. She is a Master of Public Health graduate from the Dalla Lana School of Public Health, University of Toronto. She also holds two undergraduate degrees from York University in biology and psychology. Her interests broadly span the structural determinants of health, health equity, Black reproductive justice, and social policy as a fundamental causative of reproductive health disparities. Her research is grounded in Black feminist thought.

Celeste Bilbao-Joseph (she/her) is an Argentinian-Canadian mental health clinician with a master's degree in adult clinical psychology and a master's degree in psychology education. She has worked in the mental health field for over 20 years, including the HIV/AIDS Prevention Program at the Centre for the Spanish Speaking Peoples and at the Department of Psychiatry at Mount Sinai Hospital, both in Toronto. She currently provides individual, group, and couples therapy to a variety of underserved populations. For the last 16 years she has been serving migrants and refugees from over 20 Spanish-speaking countries. She specializes in crisis and trauma counselling, including substance use disorders, and she provides education and training on request to various agencies and organizations throughout Ontario. Celeste is the founder of Trans Latinas Ontario (TLO), the first group in Canada of its kind, supporting the mental health of Latina Trans Women. She is also an active member of the Global Migration and Health Initiative (GloMHI) and has participated in several national and international ethno-racial community-based research projects. Her research interests are global mental health; the relationship between social justice, power imbalance, and ethno-privilege; the right to health equity of migrants and refugees; community-based participatory interventions; and initiatives that have a real impact on the lives of vulnerable populations. Celeste continually uses her clinical and research work as a tool for health equity.

Ivy Lynn Bourgeault, PhD (she/her), is a cisgender white settler of European descent, born in Prince Albert, Saskatchewan, and raised in rural farming communities in Saskatchewan and Alberta. She is currently a professor in the School of Sociological and Anthropological Studies at the University of Ottawa and the university research chair in gender, diversity and the professions. She leads the Canadian Health Workforce Network and the Empowering Women Leaders in

Health initiative. Dr. Bourgeault has garnered an international reputation for her research on the health workforce, particularly from a gender lens, and was named on the Canadian Women in Global Health list. She is a member of the Canadian Academy of Health Sciences.

Bianca Carducci is a white cisgender woman raised in Toronto, Ontario. She is currently a CIHR Banting postdoctoral fellow at the Bloomberg School of Public Health and the Berman Institute of Bioethics, Johns Hopkins University. Her current research interests lie in the nexus of food system transformation and climate resiliency and sustainability, especially gender inequities within food system governance and nutrition outcomes.

Erica Di Ruggiero, PhD (she/her), is a cisgender white settler of European descent, born in French-colonized Guadeloupe. She is currently an associate professor of global health, social and behavioural health sciences division, and the director of the Centre for Global Health, Dalla Lana School of Public Health, University of Toronto. Dr. Di Ruggiero's research examines the gender, health, and equity impacts of different policies at global and national levels and explores different conceptualizations of work and gender as social determinants of health equity and the implications for policy uptake. She was named on the Canadian Women in Global Health list.

Astrid Escrig-Pinol is an associate professor and head of research at the Mar Nursing School (Barcelona, Spain) who received her PhD from the Social and Behavioural Health Sciences division at the Dalla Lana School of Public Health, University of Toronto (2020). Astrid has an MA in critical international development studies (York University, 2012) and a BA in journalism (Universitat Pompeu Fabra, 2008). She is a researcher in the Social Determinants and Health Education Research Group at Hospital del Mar Medical Research Institute (Barcelona) and an associate researcher at KITE Research Institute, Toronto Rehabilitation Institute—University Health Network (Canada). Her research follows three lines of inquiry: health systems and the older adult population; health inequalities and work; and the intersection of gender, migration, and health. She uses research as a tool to promote social justice and health equity and has extensive experience in qualitative research and knowledge translation and mobilization.

Natalie Frandsen is an assistant teaching professor at the University of Victoria (School of Public Health and Social Policy) and holds a PhD from Simon Fraser

University (Educational Technology and Learning Design). Natalie's career brings together practice experience in public health, mental health, and post-secondary teaching. Her area of research focuses on accessible and inclusive education for students with mental health–related disabilities who are studying online. Natalie is a SSHRC, Joseph-Armand Bombardier scholarship (2020–2023) recipient.

Mikaela D. Gabriel (Italian and Mi'kmaw of Ktaqmkuk) has a PhD in Clinical and Counselling Psychology from the Ontario Institute for Studies in Education at the University of Toronto. She is presently a postdoctoral fellow at the Waakebiness Institute for Indigenous Health at the DLSPH. Her research explores how traditional knowledge and Elder connections can support Indigenous Peoples' mental health across life transitions. Together with her research team, community partners, and mentors, Mikaela has explored life transition needs in collaboration with community partners in culturally safe methods in urban settings. She has clinical training and experience across inpatient, outpatient, and community mental health treatment settings, focusing on Indigenous cultural approaches to mental health, trauma-centred approaches, and narrative therapeutic strategies. She is a writer when able, a traveller when possible, and an auntie always.

Nicola Gailits, PhD, completed her doctorate in public health sciences at the Dalla Lana School of Public Health, University of Toronto. She holds an MSc in global health from McMaster University, during which time she conducted a qualitative study in northern India with women in community-led mental health support groups. In 2017, she began working in partnership with the Centre for Spanish Speaking Peoples (CSSP) in Toronto, conducting narrative and arts-based research. She worked with the CSSP on a community-based project with trans immigrant women from Latin America. For her PhD, she worked alongside the CSSP to conduct a qualitative study with immigrant women from Latin America. Using postcolonial narrative methodology, her study used a series of community-based story circles in order to critically explore how migration impacts women's mental health and how their stories may challenge mental health approaches that are dominated by a colonialist biomedical ideology.

Denise Gastaldo, PhD, is an associate professor at the Bloomberg Faculty of Nursing and the former director of the Centre for Critical Qualitative Health Research, University of Toronto. She is also a member of the Global Migration and Health Initiative. Dr. Gastaldo's academic work explores health as a social phenomenon. She focuses on how health is produced through social, political, and economic processes, exploring migration and gender as social determinants of health both in Canada and internationally.

Karima Joy (she/her) is a registered social worker and PhD candidate at the Dalla School of Public Health, University of Toronto. She works with people in private practice and is passionate about addressing systemic issues through research, education, and advocacy. She has been working in mental health since 2006, specializing in grief and bereavement since 2008. She redeveloped and launched the Grief Education Program at the Ontario Institute for Studies in Education's Continuing and Professional Learning, University of Toronto, where she currently teaches.

Leanne Poitras Kelly, a Métis/Cree cisgender woman originally from Saskatchewan's Qu'appelle Valley, currently lives and works on the unceded and occupied territory of the Coast Salish people of Vancouver Island. She has worked in First Nations community and public health for over 30 years in various communities in Saskatchewan and British Columbia. Currently she is an assistant teaching professor with the University of Victoria's School of Nursing and a PhD candidate in the Social Dimensions of Health Program, in Public Health and Social Policy. According to Leanne, "My work continues to be informed by my strong relationships with local First Nations communities, anti-racist pedagogy and intersectionality of complex gendered community systems which influence health outcomes."

Nakia Lee-Foon holds a PhD in the Social and Behavioural Health Sciences stream of the Dalla Lana School of Public Health, University of Toronto. Her award-winning doctoral research explored the state of young, self-identified African, Caribbean, and Black gay and other young men who have sex with men's sexual health literacy in Toronto, Ontario. Nakia completed her master's of health sciences, specializing in community health, from Ontario Tech University. Her master's thesis explored the state of Black-Canadian parent-youth sexual health communication in Toronto. She has also conducted work focused on mental health in Black communities and increasing breast and cervical cancer awareness among Black women. She has taught various aspects of public health at the community, graduate, and undergraduate levels. Nakia is currently a health equity postdoctoral fellow at Dalla Lana.

Miranda Lesperance (she/her) is an Anishinaabekwe (Ojibwe woman) from Opwaaganisiniing (Red Rock First Nation) in Ontario. She holds a PhD from the Dalla Lana School of Public Health, University of Toronto. Her research interests include Indigenous Peoples' health equity, health labels and behaviours, and the social determinants of health. She had worked with the Public Health Agency of Canada for over 14 years and her most recent research contract is with the Bruyère Research Institute and the STROBE-Equity study. After 15 years in Toronto, Miranda recently returned home to the Thunder Bay region to complete her PhD research, titled "We Are Stories, Not Labels: Anishinaabekweg Child-Rearing Experiences." She is now the vice-president of Indigenous Collaboration, Equity, and Inclusion at the Thunder Bay Regional Health Sciences Centre, and when not lecturing at Lakehead University, she spends as much time as possible at her home on Oliver Lake with her partner and her two children, Nodin and Waseya.

Muriel Mac-Seing (she/her) is of Chinese descent, born in Madagascar, and grew up in French-speaking Montréal. She is a CIHR postdoctoral fellow at the Centre for Global Health, Dalla Lana School of Public Health, University of Toronto. Adopting an intersectionality-based policy analysis framework, she completed her doctoral degree examining the relationships among legislation, health policy, and the utilization of sexual and reproductive health services by people with disabilities in post-conflict Northern Uganda. She is currently conducting a study on COVID-19–related global health governance and how it is redefining population health research priorities in Canada through an intersectionality-focused equity lens. She was named on the Canadian Women in Global Health list.

Tola Mbulaheni is a PhD candidate in the Social and Behavioural Health Sciences program at the Dalla Lana School of Public Health, University of Toronto. She holds a master's in anthropology from the University of the Witwatersrand in Johannesburg, South Africa, and a bachelor's in anthropology from the University of Waterloo. Her doctoral research focuses on critically examining structural forms of racism shaping HIV services accessed by Black women in the Greater Toronto Area and how their experiences influence their prevention and treatment decision making. Tola is a scholar of critical theories of race and racism and Black feminist thought. She also pursues scholarly work on the ways genealogies of scientific discourses concerning Black women are taken up in present-day medical and public health responses.

Corey McAuliffe, PhD (she/her), is a white, cisgender disabled settler of European descent, born in Portland, Oregon, US. She is currently a health system impact postdoctoral fellow with the Canadian Mental Health Association, BC Division, and the School of Nursing, University of British Columbia in Vancouver. Corey has over 15 years of experience in global and public health practice.

Her research focuses on researcher and student mental health and well-being, safe work environments, trauma and distress, embodiment, disability, and critical global health. Her work explores the harm of work precarity to students, experiences of sexual and gender-based violence and misconduct at the university and in the workplace, as well as the impact of globalization on the health and well-being of incoming and outgoing students. She has a multidisciplinary theoretical and methodological focus on critical, social, holistic, phenomenological, and community-oriented responses. Corey's research likewise explores the structural and systemic barriers that prevent learners from reaching their full potential, with an aim to impact policy and oriented toward a process of social change and equity through heightened attention to contextual and cultural differences.

Renée Monchalin is an assistant professor in the School of Public Health and Social Policy at the University of Victoria and a Michael Smith Health Research BC scholar. She holds a PhD in public health science from the Dalla Lana School of Public Health. Renée is an affiliate scientist with the Well Living House, situated within the Li Ka Shing Knowledge Institute of St. Michael's Hospital, and an assistant professor (status only) at the Dalla Lana School of Public Health, University of Toronto. Born and raised in Fort Erie, Ontario, Renée is a citizen of the Métis Nation of Ontario from the historic community of Sault Ste. Marie and is of both settler and Indigenous background, carrying Métis/Anishinaabe, Scottish, and French ancestries.

Patricia O'Campo is a professor at the Dalla Lana School of Public Health at the University of Toronto and is the chair of Intersectoral Solutions to Urban Health Problems. Dr. O'Campo has an active research program that focuses on understanding the health impacts of complex urban social problems experienced by low-income populations. Through her scholarship over the past 25 years, dedicated partnerships with affected communities, and scientific leadership, she has collaborated globally to generate strong evidence to improve the lives of low-income urban populations.

Apondi J. Odhiambo is a critical qualitative and community-engaged global health scholar. She has years of experience in applied research, public service, policy, and community environments to advance equity, social justice, implementation science, and innovative community-based participatory research and teaching approaches. Dr. Odhiambo has a PhD in public health from the Dalla Lana School of Public Health, University of Toronto. She also holds a master's of law specializing in health law from Osgoode Hall Law School, a master's of science specializing in organizational psychology and development from Walden University, and an undergraduate degree majoring in sociology and communication from University of Nairobi, Kenya. Currently, Dr. Odhiambo is a senior policy analyst at Public Health Agency of Canada. Dr. Odhiambo is an innovator in using intersectional, anticolonial, and critical race theoretical insights and materialist research strategies, including institutional ethnography, to develop and implement research to understand health systems, social justice, health equity, access, and the social determinants of health. Her research currently explores how legislative frameworks, policies, and institutional practices at the nexus of health, immigration, social welfare, and criminal justice systems interface to impact the health and well-being of marginalized and racialized communities, particularly Black communities. She unmasks structural violence within these systems and the resultant effects of systemic and anti-Black racism, inequities, and social exclusion on Black communities.

Melissa Perri, MPH (she/her), is a PhD candidate in Social and Behavioural Health Sciences at the Dalla Lana School of Public Health (DLSPH) at the University of Toronto and a SSHRC doctoral fellow. Melissa is a cisgender woman and a settler born on the traditional lands of the Huron-Wendat, the Seneca, the Haudenosaunee, and the Mississaugas of the Credit. She also completed her master's of public health in Social and Behavioural Health Sciences at the DLSPH. She has strong research interests in the areas of harm reduction, housing, and gender and assessing how gendered ideologies shape health and social outcomes for women and gender-diverse people. Melissa is a research coordinator at the University of Toronto and the MAP Centre for Urban Health Solutions based at St. Michael's Hospital in Toronto, Ontario.

Katrina M. Plamondon (she/her) is an assistant professor and Michael Smith Health Research BC scholar at the School of Nursing at the University of British Columbia Okanagan, and she lives on the traditional and unceded territory of the Syilx People. As an Indigenous woman scholar of Cree and settler ancestry and a registered nurse, Katrina grounds her work as an equity scholar in critical anti-oppressive pedagogy and relational theory and practices. Her research focuses on critical questions about how to facilitate integration of equity-centred principles and practices across sectors and settings, equipping people to engage in methods, partnerships, policy, and society in ways that contribute to more equitable futures. She plays a national leadership role in advancing health equity.

Kimberly Robinson is a second-year PhD student in the Social and Behavioural Health Sciences program at the Dalla Lana School of Public Health, University of Toronto. She holds master's and bachelor's degrees in nursing from Toronto Metropolitan University (previously Ryerson University) and a bachelor's degree in political science from Carleton University. Her professional background is in community nursing and case management. She has also worked in program and policy development in Indigenous communities. Her research interests include African, Caribbean, and Black (ACB) communities and mental health, particularly men and depression, and the social determinants of HIV vulnerabilities for ACB communities.

Arie Ross is a grateful uninvited guest of mixed European Jewish, and western, northern, and central European descent on the traditional territory of the Lekwungen, Songhees, and W̱SÁNEĆ Peoples. She is completing her master's of public health and social policy at the University of Victoria and holds a bachelor's of arts in philosophy from the University of British Columbia. She received the James & Phillippa Kerr scholarship (2022) and a patient-oriented research fellowship (2021–2022) with the BC SUPPORT Unit for her graduate work on abortion access. She is writing her thesis on abortion stigma based on interviews from a pilot study exploring access to abortion for Indigenous Peoples in Canada. Her professional background is in environmental advocacy, with experience as a campaigner, community organizer, and communications coordinator. She is a proud dog-mom to Eclipse.

Lori E. Ross is an associate professor in the Social and Behavioural Health Sciences Division of the Dalla Lana School of Public Health, University of Toronto. She leads the Re:searching for LGBTQ2S+ Health Team. Lori uses a combination of quantitative and qualitative approaches in her work, with a strong focus on integrating the principles of community-based research. Much of her research focuses on understanding the mental health and service needs of marginalized populations, including 2SLGBTQ+ people, in order to improve services for these communities.

Izumi Sakamoto, PhD, is an associate professor at the Factor-Inwentash Faculty of Social Work and an academic fellow with the Centre for Critical Qualitative Health Research. She is also a core faculty member of the Asian Institute, Munk School of Global Affairs. Her research focuses on immigration, anti-oppressive practice, gender, empowerment, critical consciousness, community organizing, and the arts. She has methodological expertise in qualitative, community-based, and arts-informed research methodologies.

Christina Salmon (elle/she/her) is a multiracial (Black, White, Native American), able-bodied, straight, middle-class cisgender woman and mother raised in

Toronto, Ontario. She is the research program manager of the Knowledge Translation Program of the Li Ka Shing Knowledge Institute at St. Michael's Hospital. She was asked to sit on Unity Health Toronto Council for Anti-Racism, Equity and Social Accountability, the Patient and Community Engagement in Research Committee and is the co-chair of the EDI Community of Practice. Christina is also an expert consultant in concept mapping methodology and has worked for over 17 years in low-income, racialized communities. Christina is dedicated to social justice, anti-racism, and anti-oppression.

Mylène Shankland (elle/she/her) is a French-Canadian raised in Salaberry-de-Valleyfield, Québec. She is a white and queer woman enrolled in a PhD program in the Institute of Feminist and Gender Studies at the University of Ottawa. She is currently a SSHRC doctoral fellow (2022–2025). She completed a master's in sociology at the Université du Québec à Montréal and a graduate diploma in bioethics at the Université de Montréal. Her research focuses on the sociology of sexual and reproductive health and clinical ethics in obstetrics and gynecology, particularly through a queer lens.

Jeannie Shoveller (she/her) is a white settler of Nordic and European descent, currently a professor in the Department of Community Health and Epidemiology at Dalhousie University.

Michelle W. Y. Tam is a PhD Candidate at the Dalla Lana School of Public Health, University of Toronto. Michelle holds a master's in gender studies from Queen's University. Her work is at the intersections of critical race theory, queer theory, and reproductive justice, and her doctoral research focuses on assisted reproductive technologies and access for racialized 2SLGBTQIA+ folks. She is also a member of the Re:searching for LGBTQ2S+ Health Team.

Andrea Tricco (PhD, MSc) is a white, straight, middle-class, cisgender woman and mother raised in Sudbury, Ontario. She is a scientist and director of the Knowledge Synthesis Team in the Knowledge Translation Program of the Li Ka Shing Knowledge Institute, St. Michael's Hospital. She is an associate professor at the University of Toronto in the Dalla Lana School of Public Health and Institute of Health Policy, Management, and Evaluation. She is also a co-director and adjunct associate professor for the Queen's Collaboration for Health Care Quality Joanna Briggs Institute (JBI) Centre of Excellence at Queen's University. She is passionate about gender equity and holds peer-reviewed funding examining the impact of gender on academic medicine and public health. She is a member of the Research Equity, Diversity, and Inclusion committee at Unity Health Toronto.

Giselle Vazquez works at the Centre for Spanish Speaking Peoples and has been there since 2012. She is a mental health counsellor for the Women's Program, particularly for newcomer Latina women who have experienced domestic abuse or are in distress. She is also a group facilitator for the Wellbeing Project for Spanish Speaking Women with Culturelink, in partnership with the Canadian Mental Health Association.

Fiqir Worku is a Canada Graduate Scholarship—master's (CGS-M) recipient and master's student in Health Services Research at the University of Toronto's Institute for Health Policy, Management and Evaluation. Her master's thesis will explore knowledge, attitudes, and practices related to COVID-19 among the Black community of the Greater Toronto Area. Prior to her graduate studies, Fiqir worked as a constituency assistant under the Ontario Legislative Assembly and has a passion for implementing health-focused public policy. Fiqir is also the recipient of the 2019 Lincoln M. Alexander community award—a prestigious provincial award given to one young person who shows strong leadership and has done significant work in addressing racial discrimination. Currently, Fiqir is actively involved in various community-based initiatives and research projects.

4theRecord Research Team is an international, interdisciplinary, and intergenerational feminist research group exploring how COVID-19 has impacted ideas about risk among young queer and racialized women and non-binary folx in Toronto (Canada), Melbourne (Australia), and New York (United States). The chapter authorship team is listed below:

Kezia Arinka is a 4theRecord youth peer researcher and undergraduate student in communications and global gender studies at the University at Buffalo (New York).

Caitlin Arizala is a 4theRecord youth peer researcher and undergraduate student in the Department of Health and Society at the University of Toronto Scarborough (Toronto).

Nadia Bevan is a graduate research assistant with the 4theRecord project and a PhD candidate in the Faculty of Arts at Monash University (Melbourne).

Kethmi Egodage is a 4theRecord youth peer researcher and undergraduate student in the Psychology and Criminology program at the University of Toronto (Toronto).

Julia Ferguson is a 4theRecord youth peer researcher and recent graduate of the Psychology and Biology program at the University of Toronto Mississauga (Toronto).

Jessica Fields, PhD, is a co-principal investigator of the 4theRecord project. She is a professor in the Department of Health and Society at the University of Toronto Scarborough (Toronto).

Sarah Flicker, PhD, is a co-principal investigator of the 4theRecord project. She is a York research chair in community-based participatory research and a full professor in the Faculty of Environmental and Urban Change at York University (Toronto).

Amanda Galusha is a 4theRecord youth peer researcher and undergraduate student in the Faculty of Environment and Urban Change at York University (Toronto).

Seventy Hall is a graduate research assistant with the 4theRecord project and a PhD candidate in the School of Social Work at the University at Buffalo (New York).

Nadha Hassen is a graduate research assistant with the 4theRecord project and a PhD candidate in the Faculty of Environmental and Urban Change, York University (Toronto).

Jessica J. Mencia is a graduate research assistant with the 4theRecord project and a PhD candidate in the School of Social Work at the University at Buffalo (New York).

Vaishnavy Puvipalan is a 4theRecord youth peer researcher and undergraduate student in psychology and English at the University of Toronto (Toronto).

Reece Rabanal is a 4theRecord youth peer researcher and undergraduate student in psychology at York University (Toronto).

Anjalee Srinivasan is a 4theRecord youth peer researcher and undergraduate student in the Faculty of Education at York University (Toronto).

Emily Sutton is a 4theRecord youth peer researcher and undergraduate student in psychology and law at the University at Buffalo (New York).

Zarin Tasnim is a graduate research assistant with the 4theRecord project and a PhD candidate in the Department of Anthropology at the University of Toronto (Toronto).

CHAPTER 1

Public Health Feminisms, An Introduction

Renée Monchalin

LEARNING OBJECTIVES

1. Understand the core concepts and background of public health feminisms.
2. Explore the waves of feminism in Canada.
3. Learn about the significance of social justice in public health and the role of public health in feminist movements.

INTRODUCTION

Public health in Canada is defined as "the organized effort of society to keep people healthy and prevent injury, illness and premature death. It is a combination of programs, services and policies that protect and promote the health of all Canadians" (Canadian Public Health Association, 2020b). But one must ask: who is considered "people" within this definition? Why is it that—despite being overrepresented in most, if not all, social determinants of health categories—Black, Indigenous, racialized, refugee, immigrant, neurodiverse, disabled, two-spirit, non-binary, trans and/or gender-diverse, and/or other marginalized/oppressed groups of women in Canada still lack programs, services, and policies that protect and promote their health?

Following a bachelor's degree and PhD in public health at two different Canadian universities in the early 2000s, and now having begun a faculty position in public health at another Canadian university, I have come to realize these marginalized and oppressed groups of women's voices and perspectives were often missing from course syllabi. Rather, they were just presented as a statistic. In fact, in my undergraduate public health degree, I had a professor tell me that the correct way to write an academic paper was to begin with writing the negative statistics about marginalized/oppressed groups of people (this perspective was thankfully later flipped from the guidance of my master's supervisor). Further, as a young urban Métis woman coming from a working-class family, I never saw myself within my course materials, had little in common with my peers or professors, and struggled to understand mainstream public health approaches.

The first memory I have of learning about public health is when I was about 19 or 20 years old, sitting in a large university lecture hall. The professor spoke to public health's "origins," giving credit to John Snow and the Broad Street Pump in mid-19th-century London, United Kingdom. For those of you who may not be familiar with the Broad Street Pump story, between 1831 and 1854, tens of thousands of people in England died of cholera. In August of 1854 in particular, Soho, a suburb of London, was hit hard by an outbreak of the bacterial disease. Dr. John Snow, an obstetrician, lived near Soho at the time and was determined to figure out what had led to the outbreak (Tulchinsky, 2018). Most homes and businesses dumped their untreated sewage directly into the nearby Thames River or into open pits called cesspools. The Broad Street Pump, located within Soho, had direct access to these dumping sites. Water companies often bottled water from the Broad Street Pump and delivered it to pubs, breweries, homes, and businesses. Snow found that the sewage that was dumped into the Thames River and cesspools near town wells had contaminated the water supply, leading to the rapid spread of cholera. With this theory, Snow was able to trace the Soho cholera outbreak to the now infamous Broad Street Pump. While many doctors and city officials at the time believed that the spread was due to cholera being airborne, and others thought it was "God's will," they listened to Snow and removed the handle from the Broad Street Pump as a trial, only to find the outbreak of cholera almost immediately stopped (Tulchinsky, 2018).

While Snow is no doubt a pioneer in the world of public health, being young and ignorant in my late teens and early 20s, I never thought to question why I was only being taught Western colonial public health models and examples from the United Kingdom, and nothing was said about the intergenerational public health knowledges that were (and continue to be) here in the Indigenous communities of Turtle Island and among which our universities sit. Another example I was taught during my public health bachelor's degree was the Walkerton case, located in the municipality of Brockton, Ontario. In the year 2000, a water contamination outbreak occurred after *Escherichia coli* (*E. coli*) and *Campylobacter jejuni* were discovered in the community's drinking water. Heavy rainfall had contributed to excess runoff of livestock fecal contaminants from agricultural fields into a shallow municipal well. This resulted in many accounts of illness and death among the population of 4,800 (Lisnyj & Dickson-Anderson, 2018). While Walkerton was both a tragic and important public health event, I wonder why we did not learn about the countless drinking water advisories in First Nations communities across the country? While the Canadian government has been working to reduce the number of drinking water advisories, approximately one in eight First Nations communities are under a boil water advisory issued by public health at any one time (Baijius & Patrick, 2019). Never was I taught this country's true history, current experiences of the First Peoples on the land which we refer to today as Canada, and the role that public health has, and continues to play, in perpetuating a colonial agenda. Today I ask myself: why were we only being taught one perspective in public health? These are a few of the *many* reasons I thought there was a need for public health feminisms in the classroom. The goal of public health feminisms is to learn from those in public health who are often silenced and ignored, while providing an analytical tool that supports students and researchers alike to reveal and unpack how public health in Canada is a direct reflection of the country's very own beginnings—that of patriarchy and colonialism. Canada is a country that, when it was formed, did not consider women as persons (Loreto, 2020). This edited collection is an effort to convene voices that are not often heard or listened to in the realm of public health and to highlight the critical importance of moving beyond colonial public health models.

My perspective and understanding of public health began to shift during my master's and PhD—not in the classroom, but rather due to working as a research assistant for an Indigenous-led action research centre focused on Indigenous infant, child, and family health and well-being in Toronto called the Well Living House. The Well Living House, led by Métis physician Dr. Janet Smylie and guided by a committee of Indigenous Elders called the Counsel of Grandparents, engages in bridging mainstream public health with Indigenous ways of knowing and doing. It was the first time in my public health journey that I learned that communities outside of the mainstream held effective and locally tailored public health knowledges and methods that worked, while prioritizing the health of this land's First Peoples.

Following this role, I began a faculty position in public health at a Canadian university. I was given the freedom to create my course syllabi from scratch. As many of my students are either working within or planning to enter the field of public health following graduation, I felt it was my responsibility to expose students to public health methods, strategies, and practices that are beyond the mainstream while teaching them about the often "hidden," or silenced, public health experiences and events in Canada. I aim to facilitate a classroom space that has students asking critical questions about the materials, seeing themselves and their identities represented in the syllabi, and understanding the subtle—and, at times, not so subtle—roles that colonialism and patriarchy play within public health decision making.

One example is the COVID-19 pandemic and incorporating into the syllabus examples of the effectiveness of community-led responses. I speak to how Indigenous communities on Turtle Island held and continue to hold locally relevant and effective pandemic public health strategies. With the Yellowhead Institute nestled within Toronto Metropolitan University, Isaac Murdoch (Ojibwe), along with Travis Porter (Mohawk) and Fallon Simard (Anishinaabe-Métis), co-developed a film titled *COVID-19: Anishinaabe Pandemic Prophecies* that illustrates Anishinaabe pandemic knowledge and experience. Accompanying the film, Murdoch states,

> We felt it was important to get the message out that traditional knowledge plays an important role in ensuring safety and security from COVID-19. Together when we use the teachings of the past along with current strategies, we can make a difference and make our families and communities safe. (Yellowhead Institute, 2020, para. 2)

Public health responses that go beyond the mainstream and are community-led and locally relevant are vital for community well-being and survival. The COVID-19 pandemic was a clear example of the many failures of mainstream public health within Canada and around the world, particularly for women of colour (Berkhout & Richardson, 2020). As highlighted by the United Nations (UN) (2020), "Across every sphere, from health to the economy, security to social protection, the impacts of COVID-19 are exacerbated for women and girls simply by virtue of their sex" (p. 2). In speaking specifically to the Métis community experience, Métis social worker Carly Jones and colleagues (2020) build on the above example by Isaac Murdoch:

> The pandemic public health protocols such as physical distancing and stay-at-home measures also stand in sharp contrast to matrilineal social kinship and intergenerational knowledge exchange systems that Métis young women and girls rely on for their health and wellness. This is worrisome since Métis survival relies on the transmission of cultural knowledge from the Kokums [grandmas] to the Iskwêsisisak [girls].

> It is because of this rich matrilineal knowledge base and the strengths of our knowledge exchange systems that Métis communities have resisted and survived colonial attempts to erase our ways of knowing, being, and doing. (pp. 116–117)

Public health measures meant for "all" Canadians are largely tailored to middle- and upper-class nuclear families and ignore the diversity and lived experiences of those who fall outside of this category (Jones et al., 2020). To demonstrate the failure of a one-size-fits-all pandemic public health response, the Native Women's Association of Canada (2020) conducted a study to learn about Indigenous women, two-spirit, and gender-diverse experiences of COVID-19 in Canada. Of the 750 participants who filled out the survey, results indicated that 64% were more worried about domestic violence than they were about the COVID-19 virus itself. In a 2021 report, the UN proposed 17 Sustainable Development Goals (SDGs), which are intended to be achieved by the year 2030 (United Nations, 2021). SDG 5 declared that one in three women worldwide have been subjected to physical and/or sexual violence, and this has been exacerbated by COVID-19; women's equal participation in decision making is thus fundamental for pandemic response and recovery. In order to achieve this, public health programming, services, policies, and education must acknowledge the colonial and patriarchal underpinnings of public health to understand why marginalized/oppressed groups of women fall through the cracks, while taking a community-led approach to ensure that the intersectional experiences of those at the centre of public health issues are recognized and met. This calls for a public health feminisms lens.

To better understand and explore public health in Canada, this edited collection aims to act as a toolbox for public health students and scholars to reveal and unpack how public health in Canada is embedded within patriarchal and colonial ways of knowing and doing. *Critical Perspectives in Public Health Feminisms* brings together voices from Canadian public health disciplines that are often silenced: Black, Indigenous, racialized, refugee, immigrant, neurodiverse, disabled, two-spirit, non-binary, trans and/or gender-diverse, and/or other marginalized/oppressed women. Through reading about firsthand experiences and issues commonly "swept under the rug" in Canada, this volume interrogates why things are the way they are in public health practice, policy, programming, and education. What are public health decisions rooted in, and who do they actually serve? What are the implications for marginalized and/or oppressed groups of women and their communities? In the next sections in this chapter, I will explore feminism and its role in public health, followed by the need for intersectionality in public health feminisms. I then conclude with an overview of each chapter, demonstrating the diversity of perspectives within public health feminisms.

PUBLIC HEALTH AND FEMINISM

bell hooks, world-renowned professor, author, poet, and feminist, defines feminism as "a movement to end sexism, sexist exploitation, and oppression" (hooks, 2015, p. 1). Gloria Steinem, writer, lecturer, political activist, and feminist organizer, defines a feminist as "someone who believes in the full humanity of all people. That's it" (Master Class, 2022). Feminism is a layered movement that is constantly evolving, as the origins of mainstream feminism were "white, upper class, ableist and racist" (Loreto, 2021, p. 14). Mainstream feminism has largely argued that all "women should unite on the basis of their gender alone to fight the patriarchy" (Loreto, 2021, p. 28). However, as Loreto (2020) points out, this idea is flawed, as it overlooks how patriarchy oppresses women in very specific ways. Notably, in feminist movements in Canada and globally, public health issues have long been at the centre of many struggles. Despite this, the two fields are not often brought together. Below, I will briefly walk through the waves of feminism to set context for this book, while demonstrating how public health has shown up in each wave.

It is often argued that there have been four waves of feminism in North America. The first wave, beginning mid-19th century and going until the early 20th century, focused on the women's suffrage movement; the most important goal for feminists at this time was to give women the right to vote. However, feminists during this first wave campaigned against allowing Indigenous, Black, or Asian women the right to vote (Eidinger, 2022). At the same time, the provinces of Alberta (1928) and British Columbia (1933) passed Sexual Sterilization Acts, which were not repealed until the 1970s and largely targeted Indigenous women and women of colour (Stote, 2022). Further, in the 1892 Canadian Criminal Code, a federal law passed that made it illegal to sell or advertise birth control in Canada (Eidinger, 2022). Residential schools were also introduced during this first wave, operating from 1831 to 1996 (Kelly, 2008), and in 1920, the federal government made it mandatory for all Indigenous children ages 7 to 15 to attend (L. Monchalin, 2016). Given these injustices, the first feminist wave was exclusionary and racist, led by settler white women.

The second wave of feminism, beginning in the 1960s and continuing until the 1980s, largely centred on ending gender discrimination, gaining equal work opportunities for equal pay, as well as improving access to abortion and contraception

(Eidinger, 2022). It was not until 1969 that contraception was decriminalized and abortion access was made legal, albeit with restrictions. The latter could only be performed in a hospital and only if three doctors on a hospital committee agreed the pregnant person's life was in danger (Ackerman & Stettner, 2019). In response, in 1970, 17 women drove from Vancouver to Ottawa forming the "Abortion Caravan," gathering supporters as they went and making history as the first time the House of Commons was shut down by an act of resistance (Eidinger, 2022). However, it was not until 1988 that the Supreme Court of Canada struck down Canada's abortion law. While Canada is often praised for having no access restrictions surrounding abortion, many groups across Canada continue to face barriers due to geographic constraints, a lack of knowledge, cost, racism, and colonialism (Monchalin, 2020; Shaw & Norman, 2020). Abortion access is further explored in chapter 5. Alongside these struggles, maternity leave was introduced in Canada in 1971. While originally limited to only 15 weeks, maternity, parental, and other family leaves continue to evolve as the family unit changes with our society thanks to public health feminist activism. Despite these advancements, this second wave has been critiqued by many working-class women along with Indigenous, Black, and racialized women; queer, trans, gender-nonconforming, and non-binary people; and women with disabilities, as the movement was dominated by white middle-class women (Eidinger, 2022).

Activism, Social Movements, and Public Health

Activism and social movements are fundamental to the progress of public health. Ananya Banerjee (2021), who is an assistant professor in the School of Global and Population Health and the Equity, Diversity, Inclusion and Anti-Racism (EDIAR) lead at McGill University, states that "social justice is the view that everyone deserves equal rights and opportunities—this includes the right to good health" (para. 2) and reminds us that "public health is the place where science, policy, politics and activism converge" (Banerjee, 2021, para. 4). Acknowledging that social justice is a pillar of public health, the Canadian Public Health Association (2017) states that "social justice ensures that the population as a whole has equitable access to all public health initiatives implemented to minimize preventable death and disability" (p. 5).

The third wave of feminism, largely taking place from the 1990s to the early 2000s, emerged from the gaps of the second wave. The goals of the third wave fought for justice for all people who experience gender discrimination, including cis women and trans, non-binary, two-spirit, and gender-diverse people (Eidinger, 2022). The third wave also focused more on including racialized and marginalized individuals, with the term *intersectionality* being coined by scholar Kimberlé Crenshaw (1989, 1991) to address the ways in which mainstream feminism had ignored the intersections of race and patriarchy. Intersectionality posits that socially constructed categories of oppression and privilege interact on multiple levels (Collins, 1998; Crenshaw, 1991). For example, rather than arguing that either racism or sexism is the cause of one's oppression, intersectionality emphasizes that both racism and sexism could contribute to the oppression of individuals and groups (Crenshaw, 1989). Carbado and colleagues (2013) contend that intersectionality has moved beyond its original origins, has broadened in scope, and is not a contained entity. They state that intersectionality is a work in progress, moves across disciplines (including public health), and acts as a social movement (Carbado et al., 2013).

The fourth wave of feminism has been referred to as the "digital wave," owing to the rise of the internet. Beginning in 2008 and up to the present, this wave has been credited with being more inclusive and with supporting and empowering sexual violence survivors to come forward with their stories (Eidinger, 2022). For example, Tarana Burke founded the #MeToo movement in 2006, and in 2017 it went viral, bringing attention to the magnitude of the problem of sexual violence (me too, 2022). A pressing public health issue facing women, girls, two-spirit, trans, and gender-diverse people globally, violence is a violation of human rights (Harper, 2018). While impacting groups differently based on their intersectional identities, research has determined that one third of women and girls will experience physical or sexual violence in their lifetime, usually from an intimate partner (Harper, 2018). The #MeToo movement, which grew exponentially through the hashtag, has blossomed into programming, opportunities, and policy change to tackle violence against women throughout North America and globally. Critiques continue surrounding the fourth wave, however, including a disregard for sex workers' struggles and exclusion on the basis of class, race, gender, and disability (Eidinger, 2022). Some have argued that the fourth wave is "hashtag activism"; with the success of the movement started by Tarana Burke, however, the internet and social media platforms can be seen rather as a tool to mobilize. Other examples include the #BlackLivesMatter movement, founded by Alicia Garza, Patrisse Cullors, and Opal Tometi in 2013. Black Lives Matter arose out of a mission to eradicate white supremacy and to intervene in violence inflicted on Black communities by law enforcement. Another movement is #IdleNoMore, launched by Jessica Gordon, Sylvia McAdam, Sheelah McLean, and Nina Wilson. Idle No More emerged in November 2012 as a response to the injustices faced by Indigenous Peoples in Canada. As the movement began online, it has been attributed to connecting the most remote communities with urban Indigenous people and non-Indigenous people.

In each of the four waves, public health issues were often at the centre of feminist movements, whether it was abortion, maternity leave, or violence. Despite this, as mentioned, the two fields are not often brought together. The first published literature around feminism in public health was in a 1999 edited collection in the *Scandinavian Journal of Public Health*. The guest editor, Anne Hammarström (1999), stated that "feminist public health could ... be defined as an interdisciplinary field in which basic questions about the meaning of gender constructions in health matters are highlighted as well as the importance of gendered power relations for the uneven distribution of health in any given population" (p. 242). Over 20 years later, though, feminist perspectives have remained largely absent from public health policy and practice.

Available literature has examined public health through gendered power relations, but it has not acknowledged intersectional and gendered experiences in regard to race, colonialism, identity, and class—and it has yet to explore conversations beyond the gender binary. There is also a vast body of literature that brings together gender, health, and healthcare that has made visible the connections between inequalities and women's health. Yet there remains an analytical gap in recognizing the patriarchal and colonial underpinnings of public health research, policy, and practice. These patriarchal and colonial underpinnings may be subtle in the 21st century, but they are the root of why Black, Indigenous, women of colour, refugee, immigrant, two-spirit, non-binary, trans women and/or gender-diverse, and/or other marginalized/oppressed people in Canada are overrepresented in all social determinants of health categories. Further, there is no literature around the role of feminism in public health from these marginalized voices across Canada, and we are only just beginning to see space given to marginalized voices that name the injustices faced by them within public health policies, programming, and services.

Given this knowledge, the goal of this edited collection is to learn from those in public health who are often silenced, while providing students and researchers alike with analytical tools to help reveal and unpack how public health in Canada is embedded within patriarchy and colonialism. The goal of public health feminisms (PHF) is to give space to Black, Indigenous, racialized, refugee, immigrant,

Social Determinants of Health

The Canadian Public Health Association (2020b) defines the social determinants of health as "the social and economic factors that influence people's health. These are apparent in the living and working conditions that people experience every day. The SDH influence health in many positive and negative ways" (para. 1). Examples of social determinants of health include, but are not limited to, income, education, employment, food insecurity, housing, health services, gender, disability, racism, and colonialism (Allan & Smylie, 2015; Canadian Public Health Association, 2020a).

disabled, two-spirit, non-binary, trans and/or gender-diverse, and/or other marginalized/oppressed women's perspectives in Canada who are public health scholars, policymakers, and/or front-line workers and who are experts in their fields and in their communities' experiences and public health needs. By exposing the ways that patriarchy and colonialism are embedded in public health services, policies, and programming, *Critical Perspectives in Public Health Feminisms* provides an innovative approach that aims to explore what it means to protect and promote the health of *all* Canadians.

OVERVIEW OF CHAPTERS

Public health feminisms is a relatively new and unexplored concept. When putting a call out for chapters for this edited collection, it was quite broad, asking authors to define what public health feminism really meant to them, or what it could mean. By having authors who belonged to Black, Indigenous, racialized, refugee, immigrant, two-spirit, non-binary, trans and/or gender-diverse, neurodiverse, disabled, and other marginalized/oppressed groups of women in Canada, this book was an opportunity to begin conversations on what public health feminism looks like and/or possible futures for public health feminism, and, most importantly, bringing forward experiences and issues commonly ignored in mainstream public health. Our aim was to bring forward perspectives with(in) public health discourse that we do not often hear in the mainstream, as public health conversations are largely centred on white, upper-class, ableist, and often racist perspectives. This edited collection is an effort to bring "marginalized" and/or "oppressed" voices into public health classrooms, because while we may often be labelled as the minority, we are actually the majority.

The contributing authors to this volume all approach the concept of public health feminisms in their individual ways, whether utilizing it as an analytical lens, sharing possibilities of what it could offer, or reflecting on different feminisms such as Black feminism or Indigenous feminism within the realm of public health and what these various feminisms can offer. While the chapters are each unique, they are woven together with the recognition that public health services, policy, and programming in Canada have neglected to prioritize the unique and intersecting challenges and experiences faced by women across the country. This edited collection carves out space in public health for women who are at the intersections. As Salmon and Tricco remind us in chapter 11, "Through their lived experience, Black and Indigenous women who carry various intersections are the experts to overhaul the current public health system due to centuries of their lived experience of being at the bottom."

Chapter 2, titled "A Really Good Brown Nurse," speaks to reflections of being a Métis public health nurse and (re)claiming space in public health nursing discourse. Through the lens of Indigenous feminism, this chapter explores being an "outsider" as a Métis public health nurse on the west coast, away from one's homelands, tacitly participating in oppressive systems, and the legacies of Indian hospitals and vaccines in Canada.

Chapter 3, "Exploring Gender Equality and Equity in Canadian Global Health Institutions," outlines how gender inequity is perpetuated in the global health ecosystem, provides broader insights and discussions drawing from a critical intersectional lens, and discusses future research directions for gender inclusion. This chapter aims to raise awareness of gender inequity in Canadian global health research, practice, and policy organizations and address it together through better data and evidence about gender-transformative policies.

Chapter 4, "Stuck in a High Wire Act: Ways of Understanding Immigrant Women's Mental Health beyond Biomedicine," demonstrates how colonialism, capitalism, and patriarchy work collectively to create migratory distress. It explores ways of understanding immigrant women's mental health beyond biomedicine: this includes holding on [*aguantando*] as a reaction to structural instability, migratory grief as reaction to community loss, and performing strength as a reaction to gendered expectations.

Chapter 5, titled "Spurring the Witch Hunt: Abortion, Colonialism, Stigma, and Indigenous Knowledges in Canada," applies a public health feminist lens that acknowledges that traditional reproductive knowledges and practices surrounding bodily autonomy and self-determination exist(ed) in Indigenous communities on Turtle Island prior to settler contact. This chapter acknowledges and honours these knowledges and practices to reduce abortion stigma in Canada today, providing examples of community-led initiatives that are tackling the abortion access gap.

Chapter 6, "Deconstructing Ableism in Healthcare," demonstrates how ableism in healthcare education leads to structural violence for all people with disabilities. The authors state that public health feminism can be used to work towards identifying, naming, and decreasing barriers rooted in ableism and oppression, improving representation of and health outcomes for persons with disabilities through the education and training of more healthcare providers with disabilities.

Chapter 7, "Queer and Trans Perspectives on Obstetric and Gynecological Violence: Centring Those at the Margins to Capture the Intersectional Effects of the Phenomenon," speaks to how obstetric and gynecological violence (OGV) has been documented and discussed predominantly from a cisgender women's perspective, excluding genderqueer people's experiences. The chapter illustrates how reproductive healthcare and services are described and experienced as discriminatory and abusive among those beyond the gender binary. The authors demonstrate how this occurs at individual, structural, and policy levels, and they cite the need for queer and trans perspectives in reproductive health services.

Chapter 8, "Black Feminism in Critical Public Health Research, Policy, and Programming: Theory and Practice for Promoting the Health and Well-being of Black Women," aims to reconceptualize how we think about the health disparities Black women face and to reposition how they are constructed in public health discourses. The authors demonstrate how a Black feminist approach is critical to understanding health disparities Black women experience, as it requires a recovery of Canada's histories of enslavement and colonization and the structural continuities that make Black women more vulnerable to poverty as a social determinant of health.

Chapter 9, "Taking a Reproductive Justice Lens in Public Health Policy: A Case Study on Family Law for LGBTQ2S+ Parents and Families," describes ways in which LGBTQ2S+ people in Canada encounter formal legal and political barriers to family expansion. Through a reproductive justice framework, the authors examine why and how family expansion is regulated in Canada and how it can be changed.

Chapter 10, "Strangers in Our Homeland: The Impact of Racism across Healthcare Policy and Delivery for Indigenous Peoples in Canada," provides an overview of Indigenous health policy and procedures while demonstrating the negative impacts of the colonial government in Canada and its implications on Indigenous Peoples' health and access today. The chapter shares voices of Indigenous Elders, youth, and service providers in searching for representation, safety, and a way forward in access to healthcare in Canada.

Chapter 11, "The Critical Importance of Addressing Gender and Racial Inequities in the Public Health System," interrogates barriers and social constructs that Black and Indigenous women face in public health settings and illustrates how patriarchy and systemic racism are embedded in public health, requiring drastic overhaul. The authors suggest critical system improvements; due to lived experience, Black and Indigenous women who carry various intersections are the experts to overhaul the current public health system.

Chapter 12, "Reclamation of Matriarchy and Kinship Systems," examines how early settlers of Canada brought over patriarchal archetypes that discounted the essential roles of mothers, caregivers, and kinship systems, impacting the perception of these roles in early Canadian history and today. Although the chapter includes historical examples of genocide, like residential and Indian day schools, and policies that continue today, like forced sterilization and child apprehension, it also cites examples of how mothers and caregivers reclaim their ancestral matriarchal knowledge and kinship systems. Feminist thought and female kinship systems are paramount in most traditional First Nation societal systems. The author argues that public health practitioners and policymakers must recognize and promote these practices to avoid perpetuating harmful colonial stereotypes and truly address the service gaps in public health policy and services.

Chapter 13, "Engendering a Feminist Ethic of Care to Training a New Generation of Public Health Researchers: Reflecting on 4theRecord," speaks to enacting and threading a feminist ethic of care though an international, interdisciplinary, and intergenerational research team. Written collaboratively and including investigators and graduate and undergraduate student research assistants, this chapter reflects on their process and paradigm for how public health research can be done from a standpoint that strives to confront sexism and racism in its implementation.

Chapter 14, "Chronicles of Public Health Doctoral Students: Overcoming the Ivory Tower through a Revolution of 'Self-Care' for a Better Future," speaks to how universities continue to be places of colonialism and how this shows up in Canadian academic public health programs. Through personal accounts from each of the authors, the chapter argues that university public health programs must create authentically safe and supportive spaces for students who represent marginalized/oppressed groups. In conceptualizing "self-care," the chapter demonstrates the need for a feminist ethics of care on imagining paths forward in academia.

Chapter 15, "Public Health Feminism and Housing: Status Quo or Transformational?," demonstrates how public health has historically neglected the unique challenges faced by women of all backgrounds, such as housing insecurity, and how feminism and its myriad movements facilitate a comprehensive analysis of public health issues and inform the design of effective and inclusive solutions.

The authors identify how forms of feminism that focus on assessing and dismantling forms of oppression can benefit the development of public health feminism while informing strong solutions for mending gendered inequities.

The concluding chapter 16, "Public Health Feminist Futures and Moving Forward," speaks on how each of the chapters in this edited collection are interwoven for a public health feminist future. Drawing on critical perspectives shared throughout this volume, the chapter offers the concept of public health feminism as praxis to transform the field of public health.

CRITICAL THINKING QUESTIONS

1. How would you define public health feminism? Has your view changed after reading this chapter?
2. What would you describe as an example of a public health feminist movement?
3. Who would you describe as a public health feminist leader?

KEY TERMS

public health education
social justice
feminist movements

SUGGESTED FURTHER READINGS

1. Kielsgard, R., & Brown, L. (2021). Trans, autistic and BIPOC: Living at the intersections of autism, race, and gender diversity. In M. Kourti (Ed.), *Working with autistic transgender and non-binary people: Research, practice, and experience*, pp. 71–88. Jessica Kingsley Publishers.
2. Jones, C., Monchalin, R., Bourgeois, C., & Smylie, J. (2020). Kokums to the Iskwêsisisak: COVID-19 and urban Métis girls and young women. *Girlhood Studies, 13*(3), 116–132. https://doi.org/10.3167/GHS.2020.130309
3. Loreto, N. (2020). *Take back the fight: Organizing feminism for the digital age.* Fernwood Publishing.

CHAPTER 2

A Really Good Brown Nurse

Leanne Poitras Kelly

LEARNING OBJECTIVES

1. Reflect on personal positionality and your own social location.
2. Explore the ways and the whys in which we tacitly participate in oppressive systems.
3. Explore social constructs that influence our life experience and the ways in which we engage with each other.

I'm young, brown and wrought
By an approval seeking ethic
Torn down by whiteness; formidable and firm.
My vision obscured by oppression and fear.

I'm a brown woman
Mutating for others
Infiltrate the language I need to blend in
Coded in color that washes me out

I'm a brown nurse walking
paths constructed by whiteness
bade to join once I wear the right shoes

I'm a brown nurse unsettled by
Awareness but silent,
Thoughts lurk and stay muted
As the white nurse speaks loud.

I'm old brown and wrought
By an ethic for wisdom
Built up by my sisters and aunties and friends
My vision less blurry, my voice finding purchase
White clouds dissolving
My brown face is seen.

I want to raise my hands, in the way I have been taught by the Coast Salish people, to Métis poet and disruptor Marilyn Dumont. Marilyn's book *A Really Good Brown Girl* (1996) revolutionized my thinking, my voice, and my sense of self. It is a powerful experience to see oneself in the words of another and to feel validated and materialized. My verse is my own brittle attempt to communicate my thoughts in this way and is built on courage I have discovered through the writings of powerful Indigenous women. Hiy Hiy to Marilyn, my hands are raised high.

Although my verse implies a binary between white and brown, I want to be clear that binaries are neither helpful nor do they truly exist. Their expression simply illustrates the polar ends of division within systems used to assert power. My use of the word *white* illustrates the powerful mainstream societal influences that made me afraid. At the same time, I acknowledge that I have had many close allies and supporters who are white and who see me. My verse, however, reflects the scars of a thousand paper cuts made by the microaggressions of being undermined, minimized, questioned, set aside, and patronized by white healthcare providers, administrators, educators, and clients. As uncomfortable as I am with this statement, for me it is my truth.

A *Really Good Brown Nurse* is a reflection on being a public health nurse while finding and becoming myself. My story is both a claiming and reclaiming of my place in public health nursing discourse. I finally feel confident to reflect and comment on my role within systems that both support and frustrate me. I am simultaneously a participant and disruptor in oppressive public health actions. Coming to understand and see this truth is part of my own journey to see and understand myself.

WHO AM I?

My name is Leanne Poitras Kelly. I am the daughter of Rose Amyotte (born in 1926) and the late Alex Poitras (born in 1918). My mother's family is from the Katepwa Road Allowance community in the Qu'Appelle Valley, Saskatchewan.

My father's family migrated to the Qu'Appelle area from the Turtle Mountain Ojibway and Métis settlements in North Dakota in the late 1800s.

My parents lived in a time where Métis exclusion from accepted white society was commonplace. Métis families relied on each other for social connection, cultural cohesion, and economic stability. Their time was also one of profound racial discrimination and social exclusion. Settler ideology and land dominance relegated Métis families to tracts of land allocated for municipal infrastructure development and road allowances on the fringes of towns and cities. This was also a time of great pressure to assimilate and conform to the demands of being "white" and acceptable. Survival depended on finding ways to "fit," and in most cases that meant adopting the ways of settler society.

My Métis identity flows from this experience, which is deeply rooted within the blood memory of my parents' generation. We hid our cultural roots from white eyes, the Michif language was not passed to the children, and only when we were with other Métis families could we let down our guard and revel in our own identity. It is no accident that my nursing career has been in First Nations communities in Canada. I took refuge in the context of other brown people while wanting to learn more about myself. I tell you this as a statement of my positionality and as the starting point for my personal narrative.

PERSONAL NARRATIVES AND FEMINISMS

Asserting my voice within a feminist-named space is intimidating and creates expectation on the part of the reader. Damn ... it creates expectations on the part of the writer. Lee Maracle writes in her book *I Am Woman* (1996) that "until March 1982, feminism, indeed womanhood itself was meaningless to me. Racist ideology had defined womanhood for the Native woman as non-existent, therefore neither the woman question nor the European rebel's response held any meaning for me" (p. 15). I cling to this quote as it illustrates not only my own trajectory of understanding feminist assertions; it aligns with the divergence of Indigenous experience with European/settler women's evolutionary story of claiming feminine space.

How does my story fit within the umbrella of "feminisms"? I think that, like other contentious "isms" such as ageism or racism, feminism suggests a certain ideology or state of being where values held fall into a lane that somehow predicts behaviours, social positions, or beliefs. As a young woman growing up in the prairies in the 1970s and 1980s, I was superficially aware of the "feminists" that emerged from the 1960s revolution and white women's experience. I distinctly remember seeing a film entitled *Killing Us Softly* (Lazarus & Wunderlich, 1979) in the early 1980s that examined the ways advertising influenced women's identity and stereotyping. This was my first foray into unpacking systemic influences on my personal understanding and for many reasons, this film stuck with me. The idea that powers beyond personal choice have direct impact on my experience was a new concept. Although I did not see my image reflected back in those women being killed softly, I did understand that one could push back against the stories being told about you by others. I recall thinking that the ways in which white prairie settler society enacted racism, social policy, and exclusionary tactics were in fact *killing me harshly* ... and perhaps they could be contested and ultimately resisted. My exploration and disruption of definitions of identity shaped by systems of patriarchy, sexism, and Eurocentrism was just beginning.

Writing about my public health nursing experience from a feminist perspective, then, flows from my understanding of what Indigenous feminism looks like and my journey to embody that insight and perspective in my work. What I know now is that exploration through disruptive critique of status quo narratives is a strength in developing solid public health practice. It may seem obvious to students of today that the social construction of our lived realities is influenced by so much more than individual choice. The "woke" demographic will all be nodding their heads in agreement. But for me, the internal tension to fit in, and become a really good brown girl, excluded thoughts of disruption.

A few years ago, I discovered a book entitled *Making Space for Indigenous Feminism*, edited by Joyce Green (2007). This book was full of Indigenous voices articulating their journeys to understand and make space for their experiences. Many of the contributors expressed their own complex journey of coming to understand feminism and its place in the spectrum of Indigenous experience. Verna St. Denis (2007) writes how she learned that although "feminism may be generally categorised as the struggle to increase women's access to equality in a male dominated culture, there has never been a universally agreed agenda for feminism" (Gamble, 2000, as cited in Green, 2007, p. 35). Somehow, this lack of agreement on a singular definition makes sense to me. The fluidity with which we learn and develop our understanding is not static. It is always moving. We must also factor in the trajectory of how knowledge is articulated and by whom. The voices, thoughts, and opinions of people of colour have largely been ignored in most Western fields of discourse until very recently. To have a feminist definition that is inclusive of all gendered and racialized experience is impractical. As I think back on my own evolution with this concept, I understand that it is informed by my personal and contextual access to the perspectives of those early writers who demonstrated resistance and my own willingness to reject or conform to dominant social rules of conduct.

When I was completing my master's of nursing in the mid-1990s, I read bell hooks' *Teaching to Transgress* (1994) as well as *I, Rigoberta Menchu, An Indian Woman in Guatemala* (1983). These works were new to me and somewhat difficult to process. The voices spoke of asserting one's own knowledge and experience as valid feminist discourse beyond white women's experience. hooks describes the articulation of racism with the feminist movement as necessary but that it also meant "not concentrating our energies on creating a climate where we could focus intensively on creating a body of scholarship that would look at black experience from a feminist standpoint" (p. 122). Rigoberta Menchu's work describes the experience of being "Indian" within a Spanish-colonized state with layers of identity and hierarchies, which position and silence oppressed persons such as herself. She makes the statement, "I am an *Indianist*, not just an Indian. I'm an Indianist to my fingertips and I defend everything to do with my ancestors" (p. 166). Her story weaves the role of Indian women within colonized spaces and the struggle to assert both her ancestral knowledge and current social currency as a method of activism. Though she doesn't use the word *feminism*, her narrative positions her experience firmly within the spectrum of feminist struggle. When reading these works and their uncovering of a racialized experience, I was both drawn to and eschewed their words. My own need to hide, conform to, and minimize the pain of rejection inhibited my uptake of these writings in an overt way. They were, however, ovular in creating a silent and intense internal process that framed my own reflections on my experience.

Thus, my personal narrative encompasses a feminism that is built on newly acquired courage and intersectionality. I seek to embrace a wider approach of examining colonialism and patriarchal systems that intentionally exclude Indigeneity. The exclusionary practices within our public health systems that suppress anything other than cisgender, heterosexual, white, able-bodied, neurotypical experience require our commitment to uncover and disrupt.

The telling of one's story under any heading is an act of resistance and an assertion of one's life. What I have learned as an Indigenous nurse-academic is to rely on my strengths, build on what I know, and believe that the ways we have been taught to "tell" our stories are valid. Cree-Métis scholar Cora Weber-Pillwax (2021) writes so effortlessly about the value of personal narrative in reaching the reader:

> I call upon personal narratives of my own experiences in order to demonstrate the manner and means by which the simultaneous layering and fusion of narrative and multi-dimensional experience constitutes the ancient flow of Indigenous knowledge from one generation to the next. The constancy of this knowledge flow upholds

> the integrally coherent and evidentiary continuity of Indigenous being, and Indigenous expressions of that being. In this knowledge flow, personal narrative represents a form of communion, enlivening Indigenous being engaged through and in the narrative. (p. 1)

For me, this means that our stories are the method through which we give evidence of our experience and our knowledge. Stories, which contextualize us among our ancestors, provide strength to resist assimilation. Personal narrative is my data and as such, it demonstrates my existence and insight while lengthening my ties to our genealogy and ancestral knowledge. Personal narrative upholds the way in which our identity and perspective reflects our complex intersections and helps us find context and meaning in our experience. I am also reminded that my words carry the responsibility to represent my ancestors in honourable ways. My personal reflections represent *my* story and do not implicate all Métis nurses in a similar journey. They illustrate my experience of being a Métis public health nurse within a system fraught with complex barriers and supports that both enabled and restricted Indigenous pathways to wellness.

THE FEDS

I was hired shortly after I graduated from the University of Saskatchewan. I had no other nursing experience except what I had learned in school. I believe I was hired because I was Métis and there was an impetus to "hire Native nurses" to work in Native communities. My first job was in the Qu'appelle Valley, near my ancestral home, working for Health Canada's Medical Services Branch. This arm of the federal government was responsible for making good on the "medicine chest clause" from the Numbered Treaties and provided health programming for reserves all over Canada. I drove an old Ford Fairmont wagon with a federal government logo and arrived in a community every day with my bag of supplies, logbooks, and binders. Many people that I met were happy to see a brown nurse driving the government car and, of course, everyone wanted to know "where I was from." The importance of knowing your roots and establishing relationships cannot be overstated. Sadly, despite being brown, I had virtually no knowledge or understanding about reserves and only slightly more about public health systems.

I can say that even though I experienced racism in my daily life, as a Métis person, I had no knowledge of what reserve life was like or the systemic implications of the Indian Act. My great Granny Skipper (Emmerance Bellegarde) was from Little Black Bear First Nation and attended residential school in Lebret, but that was never spoken of. She married a Métis man (Charles Racette) and left the reserve.

My Gran (Emma Racette) never attended residential school because she was not a "status Indian." My mother also did not attend, as their family lived in the Métis Road Allowance community of Katepwa. My mother, like other Métis children, attended a small country school run by the Oblates just for Métis families. I did not have the stories of residential school prior to working in communities, nor was I provided with any information about this national phenomenon by my employer.

I first heard about residential schools in whispers. I worked for George Gordon First Nation. I would go to the school to provide vaccines to the students and hold health-focused workshops and sometimes have coffee with the staff in the kitchen. The school itself was a big red brick building with an old smell and hollow-sounding hallways. I worked for Gordon's from 1989 until 1994 and learned that this was one of the last residential schools in the country to close, in 1996. During my time there, students still attended from the surrounding communities, but it was no longer a school policed by federal agents or with mandatory attendance. It was more of a residential "option" for families in the area to send their children. The decision to have your children attend was influenced by the family's past experience with the schools, the expectation that this was what was done, the desire to have your child with other Indigenous children, and in response to racism experienced at the "town school" or as a measure taken due to circumstances in the family home. There were complex reasons why the school was still functioning at this time. I did not know any of this and did not realize that every time I entered that school, I was walking through hallways and dorms where aggressions, racism, violence, and abuse toward children had occurred.

I recall a conversation with a community member telling me little bits about another member who had charged a former school administrator with abuse and got a money settlement. She looked at me knowingly and said, "you know what I mean." This was long before the Truth and Reconciliation Commission (TRC), or any of the Common Experience payouts.[1] I remember being so shocked and disturbed by this. I did not fully understand what she meant but I wanted to find out more, yet I could feel the cloak of silence that surrounded this and the reluctance to talk. I asked the zone nurse manager about this and was told that "things that happened in the past don't change what we have to do today, nor is it any of our business." Case closed. Thirty years ago, I wasn't equipped with knowledge of colonization, the Indian Act, residential schools, or Indian hospitals. The idea of critical approaches that interrogate the social determinants of health were not part of my education process. I think that people in the community assumed I had a common understanding of their experience, but I didn't. What I had to learn about, I had to do on my own.

I attended a workshop sometime in the early 1990s where I heard researcher Roland Chrisjohn (Chrisjohn & Young, 1994) present survivor stories of residential schools and federal government policy. This was the first time I heard publicly about abuse and a national cover-up and systemic oppression. It was hard to hear and hard to understand what role I had in supporting and disrupting these systems. I felt ignorant about all of this and in collusion with white people for covering this up. I also felt like an imposter in that somehow my version of being Native wasn't anything like the people I worked with. The story of residential schools explained a whole other level of colonization that I knew nothing about. Had I known more or been taught to interrogate and dissect patriarchy and racism, my reflections here today might have been different. But then again ... perhaps not; thinking back the overriding motivation was to be a really good brown nurse.

SIGN ON THE BOTTOM LINE

My first five years as a nurse, I worked *for* the federal government but *in* First Nations communities. This was a big distinction. I was accountable to the Government of Canada, not the people of the community I served. There was a very structured system for both clinical and administrative duties. I had to submit my planned schedule a month in advance, fill out triplicate forms for everything from a day off to ordering supplies. I had two supervisors above me—the nurse in charge and the zone nurse officer. Programming requirements, outputs, and developments were laid out in binders with core responsibilities. In many ways, this was great support for a new grad. I learned a lot about public health, statistical collection, program management, and reporting. Like a good girl, seeking approval, I fell into line with this. I understood that this was the way we needed to be and did all my documentation accordingly.

The complexity was that I had to deliver all this programming within a unique community setting, which had its own rhythms and ways of managing people, programs, workflows, and priorities—but what did I know of that? Add to this the unspoken expectation that because I was Métis, I would be accepted and welcomed into all First Nation communities with open arms. There was a lot of pressure to succeed on all fronts.

At that time, the government employed a community member in the position of "community health representative" or CHR. This position required the employee to be a member of that particular First Nation and act as facilitator/liaison for the nurse to engage with community members. This position was and remains an essential part of all community health programming. Without insider community knowledge of events, relationships, and histories, the work of health providers cannot be done in a way that matters. The CHR is essential, whereas the nurse will come and go. Despite this, I was the supervisor of the CHR because of my Western education and the hierarchy of the federal government. The CHR "reported" to me. I was responsible for her time sheet, monthly calendars, activity reports, and so on. You can see where this is going.

The particular CHR that I worked with at Gordon's was a long-time employee, very knowledgeable, a residential school survivor, highly respected in the community, and—initially—very happy to have me aboard. She laughed as she said, "well, it's good we've got a little Michif girl here now and not a great white savior." I was 24 years old, had no reserve life experience, barely understood the ramifications of residential schools, and did not have insight into the importance of nuances within key relationships. One incident remains with me all these years later. It taught me the value of understanding my own place and the complexity and importance of community knowledge and priorities.

An Elder died in another First Nation community about two hours away. The CHR told me she was going to attend. I agreed and brought her the paperwork to fill out for her "leave" to be approved. This act of power assertion and authoritarian structure on that day opened a can of worms that coloured our working relationship for the remainder of my time there. Without knowing it, I had asked her to categorize her crucial community-to-community relationship work as "vacation time." Time not spent in public health work, as defined by white societal systems, was not considered work. Honouring Elders and families in their final passage was deemed "vacation time." Or so I had implicitly asserted.

In the days that followed, there were hard feelings, silence, avoidance, and I felt completely lost. One of the CHR's friends called me an "apple"; another stated that I looked like an Indian but, really, I was white. The injury I had caused by insisting on regulating cultural currency was palpable. I knew I had fucked up. I consulted my nurse in charge and the zone nurse officer. They both told me that I had to have those documents signed to account for her time. "We weren't paying her to drive all over the country." Ultimately, I let the form languish and the issue was "resolved" through non-resolution. I avoided talking about it and so did she. I realize now I had breached community protocol and undermined the importance of her role and standing as a respected community member and knowledge holder as well as her relationship to the Elder who had passed.

It is so obvious now, that processes created within larger systems need to be applied with nuance, understanding, and adapting to the context. This situation demanded that recognition be given for the priorities of community history and cultural standing. For an outsider to be effective in supporting members of any community, relationships are contingent on implicit agreements built on recognition of one's use of power and the invitation to express priorities openly. Public health initiatives work much better when there is a mutual understanding of context and the realities of community priorities. The CHR and I never really got there. We did our best to fit a round peg in a square hole, but it never really worked.

WEAR YOUR SCAR ON YOUR SLEEVE

As I write this chapter, we are in the middle of a global pandemic where public health measures like immunization are being held up as our way forward. This past year I worked at many vaccination clinics, administering the Pfizer and Moderna vaccines to First Nation community members in hopes of turning the tides. When many of the adults born before the year 2000 roll up their sleeves, I see the evidence on their bodies of public health measures felt only by First Nations people. I am referring to the use of the Bacillus Calmette–Guérin (BCG) vaccine and tuberculosis (TB) public health programs.

From the 1900s to the 1960s, TB was a spectre in many First Nation communities (Lux, 2016; Kelm, 1998). Poor housing, poverty, and restrictions introduced by the Indian Act profoundly changed the lifeways and patterns for Indigenous Peoples all over Canada. The resultant overcrowding, food insecurity, and lack of access to sound medical care led to the proliferation of TB infections. In response to the impending "danger" of infection spreading beyond reserve borders and into settler populations, the government created "Indian hospitals" with wards of beds and filled them with First Nations people removed from their communities and held hostage for years in order to confine the infection to an institution (Lux, 2016). TB has left an imprint on First Nations experience and memory. Relocation, segregation, and stigma frame the ways many First Nations families think about infection and ultimately treatment and prevention measures.

For me, working as a public health nurse meant delivering TB services in the 1990s. By then, the epidemic was largely over. Sanatoriums closed, as did many Indian hospitals, but the scars, policies, and directives from Ottawa remained. Reserve nurses were expected to do TB screening via skin testing and vaccinate infants with the notorious BCG vaccine until 2003, despite the rest of the country discontinuing this practice in the 1970s (Cook & Elwood, 2004).

BCG was given to infants just under the skin. I would explain to parents that they should expect this vaccination to blister up, ooze, scab over, and then leave a scar. This would take a couple of months. So many parents were hesitant and to be honest, I don't think they really would have chosen to have this done if they felt free to make a decision. It was impressed on me when I started my job that my main function as a public health nurse was to deliver communicable disease control programming. The prevention of infectious diseases was in my hands. Woah. I had to produce monthly reports on my immunization statistics. I had to demonstrate that all infants were given BCG. I had to go to the reserve schools and test and vaccinate the grade school children who had somehow missed out on this BCG opportunity as an infant. I did not realize that provincially employed public health nurses in cities were not doing BCG. It was only mandated on reserves.

By the early 2000s I was working for a First Nations community on Vancouver Island. Typically, we would try to give the BCG as soon after birth as feasible, usually within the first couple of weeks. The last BCG that I ever administered was to an infant that remained in hospital for postnatal support for a couple of weeks. It was common for First Nation community nurses to go to hospitals and administer the vaccine there. I remember bringing the vaccine in my cooler, getting set up, and talking with the mom. She knew what the vaccine was and laughingly showed me her BCG vaccine scar. She said: "I guess this scar means I'm a real Indian, eh?" We both smirked as "insiders" who see and understand the gravity of this. A white nurse who was in the same room asked about the BCG: "What is that? Why is this baby getting it? Do you have TB? Why don't my babies get this?" I explained about on-reserve health programming, but I know it sounded unconvincing and racist. I felt pathetic. I was hyper-aware of how this mom's scar was a record of health policy gone awry. I decided that this was the last time I would give this vaccine.

BCG reliability as a sound method of preventing TB was suspect when the case numbers were so low or zero (Cook & Elwood, 2004). This was exacerbated by the fact that we continued to offer tuberculin skin testing and were seeing false positive responses (related to prior BCG administration), which would then trigger a series of other investigations and often result in mandatory prophylactic anti-TB medication that meant hardcore antibiotics administered daily for up to a year. To be clear, the client usually didn't have TB or hadn't come into contact with a TB case but had been given BCG as a child. Thankfully, by 2003, the province of BC had discontinued use of the BCG vaccine for First Nations people (Cook & Elwood, 2004).

AN IDENTITY UNDER REVIEW

When I began to work directly for Cowichan Tribes in the 1990s, I was told very clearly that I was to mind my place—keep my prairie culture within myself. I was to be mindful to not interrupt or influence the cultural ways of the people with whom I would be working. I am a visibly Indigenous woman but cloaked by an unspoken agreement that Métis/Cree teachings would not displace Coast Salish community ways. I understood this as the community asserting cultural sovereignty and prioritizing how knowledge is sustained. What I didn't realize was that working within a community, which was working to resist overarching colonial oppression, somehow silenced my voice and rendered my own Indigeneity invisible. To be more explicit, working for a Coast Salish First Nation community that was pushing back against white Eurocentric normativity meant a centring of their own community cultural priorities. This, of course, is valid and imperative. What is less obvious is the way in which my solidarity with the Cowichan people and my shared experience of being Othered in mainstream white society became invisible. As a migrant from the prairies, I was not a member of the Cowichan community, nor did I have social or familial connection or standing. Ironically, space created for white nurses came with tacit status within the powerful hierarchy of societal structure. White voices asserted authority and were allocated positions despite the community desire to break free from dominant white discourse and white policy directives. The white voice is something known and deeply embedded in our constructed realities. Being Métis bound me to the community through a general definition of being Othered by white society, but at the same time it excluded me from cultural membership. Ultimately, the decision I made to move to the west coast removed me from my own ancestral cultural roots and the day-to-day evolution of our extended family culture, placing me in a bubble twice enforced. Not white. Not Coast Salish. Indigenous, but *Other.* I had to come to understand this before I could feel completely at ease in my skin. Knowing is freedom and releases you from having anything to "prove." It is important to understand the matrix of intersections that influence one's position in society. Knowing who you are and where you are located is the starting block for critical interrogation.

DEFICIT DISCOURSE YIELDS DEFICIT SOLUTIONS

Looking back, I see how First Nations communities and reserves in particular were/are generally analyzed through a pathologizing lens. A history of TB does not confirm current TB. Being First Nations should not be an "at-risk" criteria for TB or any other condition. The tendency for public health to create categories of people defined by statistical narratives, imagined or real, makes for tenuous relationships with the healthcare system. Scores of research papers and reports define First Nations people as having higher rates of everything bad in life and lower rates of everything good. I know I am being facetious here. The point I am making is that framing reserve life as a risk factor perpetuates the perception that all people on reserves live in deficit spaces only and have little capacity to thrive. I recall being on a region-wide conference call in the early 2000s as the pneumococcal vaccine was being introduced for children in BC. The "high risk" dosage series (four doses) was being recommended for all Indigenous children without consideration of family circumstance, while the standard series was three for the "rest of the population." It was difficult work to push back against medical health "experts" advocating for "more is better," not "appropriate is better." Never mind the abilities of public health nurses to assist in decision making for administration in response to actual health assessments.

AND SO IT GOES ...

So, here I am, having been a nurse for over 30 years and only now coming to find my voice. My early days were built on strategies and approaches to "re-educate" people, offer behavioural changes in hopes of addressing deficit measures, never realizing that I was oblivious to the real issues of systemic oppression. What I know now is that people need validation of their experience and strength. Statistics reflect the method of collection and not the people being measured. Pathologizing communities perpetuates deficit discourse and propagates erroneous beliefs. Imposition of Eurocentric and white societal standards of measuring what's "good" only fragments Indigenous community and family processes. Checklists are designed as shortcuts and are often devoid of contextual knowledge and the ability to be flexible. I know that the "public" in public health initiatives has for years referred to the white middle-class public unless otherwise stated. Garnering all this insight takes intention, time, and knowledgeable teachers who support disruption. It also takes courage on the part of a really good brown nurse, raised to be invisible, attuned to defined rules of behaviour, acquiescent to authority, and a member of a profession with a complex history of complicity within colonial healthcare delivery.

It's the stories that help us see. These personal narratives give evidence that rules need to be questioned and systems interrogated. As I approach my sixth decade of life and my fourth decade of nursing, my voice is finally my own. I no longer look to be a really good brown nurse. But I do so very much love being brown.

CRITICAL THINKING QUESTIONS

1. What are some of the implicit agreements that you make as a member of a profession or within the public health system?
2. Consider where you fit within health and wellness indicators. Do you see yourself represented?
3. How does your participation within public health systems align with your values and how is it contested?

KEY TERMS

public health nursing
Métis
Indigenous
personal narrative
colonization

SUGGESTED FURTHER READINGS

1. McCallum, M. J. L. (2014). *Indigenous women, work, and history: 1940–1980* (Vol. 16). University of Manitoba Press.
2. Richmond, C. A. M., & Cook, C. (2016). Creating conditions for Canadian aboriginal health equity: The promise of healthy public policy. *Public Health Review*, *37*(2). https://doi.org/10.1186/s40985-016-0016-5
3. CIHI Canada. (2022, September). *Addressing anti-Indigenous racism in Canada's health care systems through measurement and Indigenous data governance* [Video]. YouTube. https://www.youtube.com/watch?v=glVy7Rc6hxA

NOTE

1. The Common Experience Payment (CEP) is a lump-sum payment that recognizes the experience of living at an Indian residential school and its impacts. All former students who resided at a recognized Indian residential school and were alive on May 30, 2005, were eligible for the CEP. This includes First Nations, Métis, and Inuit former students (Government of Canada, 2013).

CHAPTER 3

Exploring Gender Equality and Equity in Canadian Global Health Institutions

Michelle Amri, Bianca Carducci, Katrina M. Plamondon, Muriel Mac-Seing, Jeannie Shoveller, and Erica Di Ruggiero

LEARNING OBJECTIVES

1. Understand gender inequities and inequalities in Canadian global health research, practice, and policy organizations.
2. Explore systemic disadvantages faced by cis women, transgender people, non-binary people, and gender-nonconforming people, particularly those with marginalized or disadvantaged intersectional identities, in global health career advancement and leadership.
3. Understand how a critical intersectional lens can be applied to gender equity and equality in global health research, practice, and policy.
4. Explore future research directions and actions to address gender inequities in the global health ecosystem, such as generating better data and evidence on gender transformative practices and policies.

INTRODUCTION

Despite greater awareness about the importance of gender and its intersections and increased educational attainment by women in higher education (surpassing men in some fields, such as medicine [Canadian Medical Association, n.d.] and other healthcare provider fields [Porter & Bourgeault, 2017] in Canada), gender inequities[1] persist in Canada's global health ecosystem. In this global health ecosystem, we include academia, non-governmental organizations, and research funders. Although 70% of the global public health workforce is comprised of women, women only occupy 25% of senior leadership positions (World Health

Organization, 2019). A Global Health 50/50 (2020) study of two hundred global health organizations reported that 73% of executive heads and 68% of board chairs are men. Gender inequities in global health leadership positions are present at all career stages (Global Health 50/50, 2020) and these disparities are even greater in certain geographical regions (Jones et al., 2018) and for those who are primarily French-speaking (Ouédraogo et al., 2019).

Although the majority of global public health academic programs include women, gender-related obstacles cause many women to leave the global health leadership career pipeline early in their career trajectories. Women also are underrepresented as senior authors in academic publishing (Dimitris et al., 2021; Merriman et al., 2021). For instance, in assessing publications from *The Lancet Global Health* between June 2013 and November 2018, Canadian women only constituted 34% of all Canadian authorship lists[2] and articles authored by women received fewer citations than those authored by men. The disproportionately low representation of women in senior leadership roles in general is also present in the global public health academic sector (Larivière et al., 2013; Shannon et al., 2019; Tricco et al., 2021). In the face of these gender inequities, many nation-states have developed policy directives to address this in multiple realms, including by governments, civil society, and the private sector. A few are outlined below.

CANADIAN EFFORTS ON GENDER EQUITY AND EQUALITY

In 2015, 193 member countries, including Canada, ratified 17 Sustainable Development Goals (SDGs). Among the targets of SDG 5, to achieve gender equality and empower all women and girls, is "women's full and effective participation and equal opportunities for leadership at all levels of decision-making in political, economic and public life" (United Nations, 2015). As has been documented elsewhere, the COVID-19 pandemic has exacerbated shortcomings in health, social, and economic systems (Amri & Drummond, 2021) and has had disproportionate impacts on women's health and economic well-being (United Nations, 2020). Similar patterns have been observed within academia. For example, a study examining gendered differences in publication and service found that the first wave of the COVID-19 pandemic created cumulative advantages for men (Squazzoni et al., 2021). According to the 2022 World Economic Forum Global Gender Gap Index, which benchmarks 156 countries on global parity, Canada ranks above the global average at 25th. However, Canada has fallen six spots since 2020. This drop is primarily due to poor performance in two of four sub-indices: (1) political empowerment and (2) economic participation and opportunity. These metrics reveal widening gaps in participation, advancement, and remuneration between men and women (World Economic Forum, 2022).

In 2017, the Canadian government launched its Feminist International Assistance Policy (FIAP) to reduce poverty and build a more peaceful, inclusive, and prosperous world. It includes work in the following areas to support their priorities: "gender equality and the empowerment of women and girls," "promote human dignity," "foster growth that works for everyone," "promote environment and climate action," "support inclusive governance," and "help strengthen global peace and security" (Government of Canada, 2017). While the FIAP is a key feature of Canada's foreign policy, gender inequality remains a major systemic issue domestically (Cadesky, 2020).

There have been other efforts to build global health research and policy capacity through the work of funding agencies together with partners within and outside of Canada. Two key research funders recently published their strategic plans. First, the International Development Research Centre (IDRC) renewed its commitment to gender equality in their recently released 10-year strategy. And second, the Canadian Institutes of Health Research (CIHR)'s strategic plan includes a strong focus on the social determinants of health and health equity, including gender equity. These commitments are also reflected in the CIHR's Framework for Action on Global Health Research (Canadian Institutes of Health Research, 2021). The CIHR, particularly through the leadership of its Institute of Gender and Health, has also been championing the meaningful integration of sex and gender in health research and conducting regular analyses of sex and gender differences in funding success rates (Canadian Institutes of Health Research, 2017, 2018, 2021; International Development Research Centre, 2021). Whether and how these aspirations will be meaningfully operationalized into actions that promote genuine transformative and lasting change remains an open question.

There are also many Canadian-based non-governmental organizations actively working in global health with partners and communities around the globe, some of whom have explicitly recognized gender equity as a priority, such as the Canadian Association for Global Health (CAGH). The CAGH was established in 2021 through the amalgamation of the Canadian Coalition for Global Health Research (CCGHR) and the Canadian Society for International Health (CSIH). The CCGHR Principles for Global Health Research emphasize inclusion, responsiveness to the causes of inequities, humility, and authentic partnering (Plamondon & Bisung, 2019)—all of which align with and support the goals of gender equity. While visibility and recognition of these issues is important, these principles need to be formally adopted and integrated to result in transformation. For instance, these principles have been mainstreamed in CIHR research funding mechanisms, including in peer review guidance. In 2018, the CSIH partnered with *The Lancet* to launch the Canadian Women in Global Health list to increase the visibility and recognition of Canadian women leaders in global health (Canadian Association for Global Health, 2021).

As noted above, the Canadian government's FIAP has identified inclusive governance as a priority. Despite this favourable context, including potential windows of opportunity for influencing institutional policies (Coe et al., 2019), less is known about how and how well global health organizations in Canada are addressing gender and its intersections in their governance, policies, and/or practices. Canadian women, particularly women with multiple intersecting identities, are at risk of being delegitimized and less meaningfully engaged in the global health workforce (Kapilashrami & Hankivsky, 2018). Women continue to face barriers in career advancement to leadership, management, and governance positions (Downs et al., 2016; Moyer et al., 2018). Gender-related gaps in data manifest in both global health research and at the institutional level. The lack of both empirical accounts of women's lived experiences and gender-disaggregated data—particularly relating to gender and its intersections—makes identifying issues and assessing changes over time even more challenging (Diehl et al., 2020). Furthermore, in COVID-19 recovery efforts, planning, implementation, and evaluation should be data-informed and gender-transformative to ensure that key areas affecting women and their intersections are financially and materially resourced and sustained (Rosser et al., 2021). There is a need for collaborative co-production approaches to research to serve as a safe "buffer" or platform for generating both knowledge and transformation that accounts for and informs action on promoting gender equity in science and science leadership (Plamondon et al., 2022).

APPLYING AN INTERSECTIONAL LENS TO GENDER EQUITY AND EQUALITY IN GLOBAL HEALTH

By definition, *gender* refers to the non-binary social construct of characteristics, experiences, and expressions of individuals, inter alia, the manifestation and evolution of roles, behaviours, and attributes (Global Health 50/50, 2020). However, beyond gender, multiple systems of power intersect to generate systemic discrimination and structures of privilege that impact individuals and societies. In other words, one must also consider the intersections of gender (Kapilashrami & Hankivsky, 2018). In 1989, Kimberlé W. Crenshaw defined *intersectionality* as a lens to understand how aspects of an individual's social and political identities (e.g., gender, sex, caste, class, religion, disability, physical appearance, sexual orientation, and other social categories), when combined, create different axes of systemic discrimination and privilege (Crenshaw, 1989).

Rooted in a long and deep history of Black, Indigenous, and Third World feminism as well as queer and postcolonial theory (Hankivsky, 2014), intersectionality stems from coalition-building and social justice–seeking movements. It "originally focused on transformative counter-hegemonic knowledge production and radical politics of social justice" (Bilge, 2013). The intersectional approach highlights social inequalities and inequities experienced by various marginalized populations (Collins & Bilge, 2016; Hankivsky, 2014). It rejects binary understandings of the world (e.g., woman/man, young/old, rich/poor, disabled/able-bodied) in favour of accepting the complexity that characterizes people with multiple intersecting identities or social locations, situated in systems of power structures such as sexism, racism, classism, patriarchy, ableism, and colonialism (Garry, 2011; Rice et al., 2019). Although several definitions of intersectionality exist, all are guided by the core concepts of social inequality, intersecting social categories, power structures and dynamics, social context, reflexivity, relationality between all concepts, and social justice, which is the ultimate goal of intersectionality (Collins & Bilge, 2016; Hankivsky, 2014).

We recognize that gender does not act alone and we are attentive to equity and social justice as essential objectives for decolonizing knowledge production and mobilization in global health (Abimbola & Pai, 2020)—adopting an intersectional lens is a key step toward decolonizing Canadian institutions for global health to become more equitable, diverse, and power-symmetric. To that end, we are informed by the work of Goodkind et al. (2021), who present four criteria for intersectional gender equity analyses: "(1) analyzes power, (2) interprets population and phenomena in context, (3) mutually constituted and interdependent category use, and (4) strategic and transparent social justice goals."

Drawing on Goodkind et al.'s criteria (2021), we have established points of investigation:

1. "Analyzes power"
   - Through looking at publicly available materials, we can assess if institutions "acknowledge, name, and analyze normative standards and power differentials" in their mandates, missions, objectives, and initiatives. If institutions do acknowledge, name, and analyze such norms and differences in power, *how* do they do this? What attention is given to these norms and power and in what way(s)? Is the motivation for these considerations

explicitly declared? How do institutions differ both in terms of how they talk about norms and power and their motivation, if at all?

2. "Interprets population and phenomena in context"
   - For institutions that consider different population groups and/or power differentials, are these standalone considerations or within a specific socio-politico-cultural context? If the latter is true, what broader equity considerations and gender-transformative measures (e.g., consequent gender budgeting) are afforded? Do patterns emerge, diverge, or present unexpected outcomes when comparing institutions' considerations across contexts? Do these emergent patterns reflect the work of these institutions and are there any opportunities to improve and/or further promote gender equity and intersectionality?
3. "Mutually constituted and interdependent category use"
   - Which women are represented within the organization's leadership and on boards of directors? For example, is attention paid to groups across race/ethnicity, age, and disability? This can be investigated through assessing the use of self-reported categorization of Black, Indigenous, and racialized people (BIR), age group, and those with differing levels of ability (i.e., both visible and invisible disabilities).
   - How do institutions represent this diversity or lack thereof? Are intersecting identities mentioned or discussed and if so, does this reflect authenticity in being inclusive of various perspectives or is it performative?
4. "Strategic and transparent social justice goals"
   - While this criterion does not yield lines of inquiry, we align our own investigation with their indicators:
     - "Background acknowledges past and present inequities as motivation and starting point for the research."
     - "Technical terms and analytic categories are clearly defined, including gender and other social categories."
     - "Report acknowledges social locations and backgrounds of the authors in relation to the groups studied and the authors' interpretation of findings."
     - "Report includes recommendations for equity-enhancing interventions."

FUTURE RESEARCH DIRECTIONS

With the focus of many global health efforts on the health of girls and women, given their particular disadvantage in many societies (World Health Organization, n.d.), it is crucial to ensure gender equity is not only sought for the populations targeted, but also *within* organizations that undertake this work. Representation of women in high-level positions in global health institutions has been lacking across the globe, including in Canada (Global Health 50/50, 2020). Institutions such as universities, research centres, non-governmental organizations, and many others need to be interrogated through a gender lens (e.g., gender composition, commitment to and follow through on gender equity initiatives). A better understanding of how we are performing as a nation will undoubtedly highlight gaps and opportunities for improvement. Canadians deserve to know who represents and governs these organizations and how women are represented and occupying positions where they are able to shape organizational decisions. Are these institutions committed to gender equity and intersecting identities, and if so, is this practised through resource allocation, explicit gender-affirming policies, and regular monitoring of their effects? Do these institutions reflect on power and privilege with the aim to overcome differences?

These and other questions require explicit attention in future research (Nielsen et al., 2018). Because gender inequities have downstream effects on the policies and programs that emanate from women's global health work, we believe this has the potential to have widespread and long-term influence. One key area of investigation is understanding gender equity and equality within academic institutions, specifically schools or departments of global health. Academic institutions are well positioned to lead by example and contribute to the elimination of harmful practices that perpetuate gender inequities. Universities educate and prepare the next generation of leaders for roles in global health research, policy, and practice. However, the vast field of global health encompasses a wide array of disciplines, expertise, and skillsets—ranging from community-based research to epidemiology, program evaluation, and policy development, among other aspects—making it difficult for one school or program to provide comprehensive training to sufficiently equip students for a plethora of potential career paths or to undertake projects in the field (Amri, 2017). Future research could also expand beyond academic organizations to investigate non-governmental organizations, faith-based organizations, the private sector, funding bodies, professional associations, and journals in the field of global health. Drawing on the World Health Organization's Gender-Responsive Assessment Scale (World Health Organization, 2011), we assert that assessing organizations based on "levels" but with additional considerations for intersectionality will help realize potential shortfalls and the need to move from "gender-unequal," "gender-blind," "gender-sensitive," and "gender-specific" towards "gender-transformative" (World Health Organization, 2011).

Ultimately, the aim is to cultivate equitable inclusion of cis women, as well as transgender, non-binary, and gender-nonconforming peoples in Canadian global health institutions, and those with intersecting identities, including intersections for those who are BIR. Such change requires bringing diverse perspectives together to: (1) understand the current state of representation; (2) articulate a collective vision for a more equitable future; (3) deliberate about the implications; and (4) identify policy and practice levers for transformative change.

CONCLUSION

This chapter argues for the generation of much-needed evidence on gender and intersectional equity in Canadian global health institutions. It invites the Canadian global health knowledge ecosystem to champion gender-transformative policies, programs, and practices. With glaring evidence of persistent gender inequities, our hope is that institutions will no longer accept the status quo. More precisely, we hope that our work will lead to, first, promoting a culture of increased transparency, self-reporting, and enhancing women's representation in positions of leadership. This in turn will positively enhance representation and improve gender equity and intersectionality in various areas, including broader academic publishing, and ultimately make global health practice more equitable and inspire future generations of women in global health. This is arguably the most important aim, albeit the most challenging.

Imagine a renewed global health enterprise where women are treated fairly and face reduced barriers to advance in their careers and extend their influence, and their voices and perspectives are thus better reflected and explicitly taken up in decision making and other global health work. Their perspectives then improve the design of global health programs and positively impact women and girls around the world who are benefiting from this inclusion and revitalized perspective. These girls and women may then be further inspired and assisted in challenging the levers of power in their communities as well as more broadly—accumulating justice-informed influence for generations to come.

CRITICAL THINKING QUESTIONS

1. How do you think global health institutions can both better demonstrate their commitment to gender equity and follow through with meaningful and concerted action?
2. In your opinion, what is one gender transformative approach that all Canadian global health organizations should adopt? How can we measure gender transformation?

KEY TERMS

global health
gender
leadership
equity

SUGGESTED FURTHER READINGS

1. Baobeid, A., Faghani-Hamadani, T., Sauer, S., Boum, Y., Hedt-Gauthier, B. L., Neufeld, N., Odhiambo, J., Volmink, J., Shuchman, M., Di Ruggiero, E., & Condo, J. U. (2022). Gender equity in health research publishing in Africa. *BMJ Global Health*, *7*(7), e008821. https://doi.org/10.1136/bmjgh-2022-008821
2. Carducci, B., Keats, E. C., Amri, M., Plamondon, K. M., Jeannie, S., Ako, O., Osler, F. G., Henry, C., Pai, N. P., & Di Ruggiero, E. (2022). Prioritizing gender equity and intersectionality in Canadian global health institutions and partnerships. *PLoS Global Public Health*, *2*(10), e0001105. https://journals.plos.org/globalpublichealth/article?id=10.1371/journal.pgph.0001105
3. Global Health 50/50. (2020). *The Global Health 50/50 report 2020: Power, privilege and priorities.* https://globalhealth5050.org/wp-content/uploads/2020/03/Power-Privilege-and-Priorities-2020-Global-Health-5050-Report.pdf
4. Nielsen, M. W., Bloch, C. W., & Schiebinger, L. (2018). Making gender diversity work for scientific discovery and innovation. *Nature Human Behaviour*, *2*(10), 726–734. https://doi.org/10.1038/s41562-018-0433-1
5. World Health Organization. (2011). WHO Gender Assessment Tool. In *Gender mainstreaming for health managers: A practical approach.* https://www.who.int/publications/i/item/9789241501057

NOTES

1. In public health, the term *inequalities* is widely understood as measured systematic, unfair, and unjust differences (i.e., inequities entail a moral commitment to social justice). See: Amri et al., 2021; Amri et al., 2020; Kawachi et al., 2002; Whitehead, 1990.
2. The caveat is that we assumed the authors' gender, as most journals do not require gender declarations upon submission.

CHAPTER 4

Stuck in a High Wire Act: Ways of Understanding Immigrant Women's Mental Health beyond Biomedicine

Nicola Gailits, Denise Gastaldo, Izumi Sakamoto, Celeste Bilbao-Joseph, Giselle Vazquez, and Lori E. Ross

LEARNING OBJECTIVES

1. Compare the difference between biomedical approaches to mental health and critical approaches that acknowledge ways of knowing outside of colonialism.
2. Understand how colonialism, capitalism, and patriarchy work collectively to create migratory distress.
3. Recognize the impact of validating the source of distress by changing mental health language.

> I don't know if it happened to you, but it happened to me that many times when I called [my family] to say "look how horrible [it is here], look how awful, look how sad everything is" ... I waited for [them to say] "come back, we are waiting for you, we are here for you" ... [*everyone in story circle nods*] ... and it never came ... they have an expectation in our countries that everything will be great and that we will be very successful and that we will never show a tear to them ... we will always show them the good side, the beautiful side ... "look how nice [it is here], look how successful [we are]." And it happens, but look what it costs us ... look how complex [this is], our anger with this process. It is partly because we have, we have a weight that we bring from there, that they put on us ... [*everyone nodding*] and we let them put it on us, when they say "you're going to Canada and you're going to be successful ... you can't come back here, you can't call me saying that, no, you didn't achieve [success], that you're a failure" ... [*everyone nodding*] ... then again the role of the strong woman, where you say, "I cannot tell my family that I am doing badly because they [would] kill me." They believe in me. They trust me. So how do I tell them that I'm not doing well? (Carolina)

This chapter explores the results of a community-based qualitative study, *Nos Escuchan?* [*Can You Hear Us?*]. This postcolonial narrative study was conducted in Spanish with 14 immigrant women from Latin America living in Canada, in partnership with the Centre for Spanish Speaking Peoples (CSSP) in Toronto. It used story circles, metaphorical drawings, and individual interviews as research methods, as well as a podcast as a knowledge translation tool. The research process was as important as its objectives: over five weeks together, participants collectively shared migration stories while building community. The study's goal was to examine the impact of migration on women's mental health, specifically exploring ways of understanding immigrant mental health outside of biomedical approaches.

Immigrant women who enter Canada as economic immigrants face highly stressful circumstances; as a result, they are often biomedicalized as having "mental disorders" post-migration. In fact, the majority of research on immigrant women's mental health has been focused on characterizing their mental health outcomes, and thus it is implicitly situated within a biomedical paradigm (Mills & Fernando, 2014). Within the biomedical model, illness is due to "individual biophysiological pathology" (Guruge & Khanlou, 2004, p. 38). Therefore, distress[1] that immigrants face is constructed as an individualized problem to be remedied by psychotherapeutic and pharmacological treatments (Summerfield, 2012). In this way, biomedical research locates mental health problems within the "disordered" immigrant body, removing the psychosocial distress from its socio-political context, including the impact of structural factors such as immigration policies, labour practices, and socioeconomic instability (Viruell-Fuentes et al., 2012).

Biomedical research on immigrant women's experiences frequently pathologizes migratory distress, erasing or depoliticizing distressing migratory experiences. This type of approach exemplifies an age of "psychiatric universalism," whereby only psychiatric knowledge is considered valid and, as such, risks reproducing colonial knowledge relations (Summerfield, 2012, p. 520). Furthermore, this repackaging of women's distress can be seen as epistemic violence, defined as practices that delegitimize or erase other forms of knowledge or worldviews (Fricker, 2007). As a result of epistemic injustice, poor mental health for immigrant women can go unrecognized in primary care. For example, when newcomers are interviewed outside of medical settings, "more patients report psychosocial stressors, which they sometimes are reluctant to reveal to physicians because they think such stressors are inappropriate topics for medical attention or they believe that their situation will not be understood" (Kirmayer et al., 2011, p. 963). This highlights the need for critical mental health approaches that validate other forms of knowledge and locate experiences within their socio-political context, often by focusing on the interactions among peoples and within communities instead of solely among individuals (Bhatia & Priya, 2021). In fact, some Latinx mothers associate "depression" with weakness, withdrawal, shame, and embarrassment and can be reluctant to verbalize their struggles with it (Vanderkruik & Dimidjian, 2019). However, if their experiences were listened to and not pathologized, perhaps they would have a different response.

This chapter examines four macro elements: the narrative of "Canada as a land of opportunity," structural instability, the loss of community, and the dominant narrative of needing to *perform strength*. Though the participants arrived in Canada as fiercely resourceful women, once these four elements combine, they are often too much for anyone to handle and the responses the women had were normal reactions to precarity, loss, and epistemic violence. Throughout the chapter, we explore ways of understanding immigrant women's mental health beyond biomedicine: this includes *holding on* [*aguantando*] as a reaction to structural instability, *migratory grief* as reaction to community loss, and *performing strength* as a reaction to gendered expectations.

STUDY OVERVIEW

Context of Immigration in Canada

There are four categories of immigrants in Canada: economic immigrants, family-class immigrants, humanitarian and compassionate applicants, and refugees; however, most are economic immigrants, selected for their capacity to contribute to the economy (IRCC, 2020). Immigrants arrive with either permanent residence (PR) or, for the majority, a temporary work or study permit (IRCC, 2020). In 2019, 70% of immigrants arrived on a work or study permit while only 30% arrived with PR in hand (IRCC, 2020). This creates extreme precarity, as very few of those with temporary permits are given PR each year; therefore, there is no guarantee they will be able to remain in Canada. In 2019, only 63,000 immigrants with work permits were given PR, but over 404,000 new work permits were issued (IRCC, 2020).

Immigrants with temporary permits must apply for PR and they are evaluated on whether they are deemed to be a "skilled immigrant" based on a points system. Points are assigned based on four main areas: English/French language ability, age, level of education, and Canadian work experience. To obtain PR, they need one year of work experience in Canada in "skilled" domains, including managerial, professional, or technical jobs (Government of Canada, 2021).

Participant Demographics and Context of Arrival

This doctoral study included 14 women who identified as Latin American, had documentation (visa/PR/citizenship), were aged 18 to 45 upon arrival, lived in the Greater Toronto Area, and arrived in Canada 3 to 10 years prior. While not all areas were reached, we prioritized inclusion of women within identity intersections often marginalized in research: those identifying as single mothers (n=1), sexual minorities (n=2 bisexual women), Black (n=1), or Indigenous (n=0). They had to identify as cisgender women, given that we had previously conducted research with trans Latina immigrants, and their migration experiences as trans women were very distinct (Gailits et al., 2021).

The participants arrived from Mexico, Colombia, Argentina, Honduras, Ecuador, Venezuela, and Dominican Republic. On average, they were 35 years old, had been in Canada for 5 years, and the majority arrived with temporary study or work permits. Only half the women were employed full time, and the women's median income was between $20,000 and $40,000. Most participants had a partner, and half of them had children. All participants were economic immigrants and therefore migration was ostensibly a choice: however, migration can also be understood as a response to socio-political instability in their country of origin, leaving them with little choice but to leave. Most participants left to find new opportunities for themselves and their children, as well as to escape unsafe and unstable living conditions (e.g., constant threats of robbery or sexual violence). Most participants explained that they sold off everything they owned and risked everything, emotionally and financially, to migrate.

Methodology

We used postcolonial narrative inquiry (PCNI), a methodology that was developed for this study (Gailits et al., forthcoming). PCNI can be used to counter damaging master narratives, decentre colonialist epistemologies, and challenge epistemic violence. It refocuses the research agenda toward deep listening while prioritizing the research process (including community building) as much as its outcomes. The primary researcher (NG), a non-Latinx Spanish speaker, had been collaborating with the CSSP for three years prior to the study. Two CSSP staff members co-facilitated the story circles (CBJ, GV), providing safety as they were mental health professionals as well as Latinx immigrants themselves. The story circles became a unique space for the participants, as many of them had not shared their migration stories before, even with close friends or family. This chapter is an incomplete account of the women's experiences of joy, victory, and triumph, and should be read alongside the PhD chapter "Migration as Transformation" (Gailits, 2023).

FOUR MACRO ELEMENTS AND THEIR IMPACT ON WELL-BEING

Here, along with challenging epistemic violence by describing distress outside of biomedical disorders, we examine four macro elements that impact women's well-being post-migration. The macro elements are grounded in colonialism, capitalism, and patriarchy.[2] Each macro element builds upon the previous one, highlighting how they intersect to aggravate distress. A final section describes experiences of crisis and pathologizing responses from mental health professionals. Lastly, the paper explores one way of imagining the women's cumulative experience: being "stuck in a high wire act." All participant quotes have been translated from Spanish, and all participant names are pseudonyms.

"Canada as Superior" Narrative: When Expectations Silence Reality

> Why don't we give ourselves permission to say, "yes, I came to Canada and it was awful" ... because there are many things that are different, there are many things that you lose ... there are many things that are not how you're told they will be. (Patricia)

Even before the women migrated, there were high expectations for their success, prosperity, and happiness in Canada. These expectations emanated from a dominant hegemonic narrative: "Canada as a land of opportunity." This master narrative stems from colonialism and the idea that Canada is "superior" to Latin America. The narrative's strength comes from both Global North and Global South, reinforced in Canada by calls for a prosperous, easy migration and in Latin America by the idealization of Canada. The women shared how their communities back home have ingested this narrative, with many believing that "here everything will be perfect" (Luz). They described how this narrative was sold to them back home, in advertisements and media: "Here [in Canada], it's a wonderland, that's how they sell it to you" (Veronica). The narrative was then further reinforced by well-meaning family members who pushed them to leave and then held high expectations of success for them. The narrative thus generated a fantasy idea, since there was a significant discrepancy between the expectation and reality of life in Canada: "This is something few immigrants talk about ... when we go to our country, it is all happiness, all joy, lots of money to spend ... but when we are here ... that is not our reality ... you practically save all year to go home" (Camila).

The discrepancy created a context where the women's emotions and experiences were silenced, producing distress. Participants described how they were unable to share difficult experiences with family members back home, both because it was hard to challenge the perfection of Canada and because family members did not want to hear that Canada was not a successful haven: "Everyone would have liked to be in my place at that time ... and how do I say, 'No, it's horrible' ... I didn't feel that was right ... I don't know why I thought it was not right to shatter that expectation" (Patricia). Additionally, some participants did know that migration would be challenging, but they felt equally silenced in speaking with their families because they had chosen to leave.

Many women began to hide their experiences and they then experienced fractures in their family relationships. Their family members did not want to hear about their distress, especially when the socio-political context at home was incredibly challenging. In response, some women began to *perform strength* (explored below) instead of sharing the reality of life in Canada: "I had to be a rock when I was talking to my dad. My dad wouldn't let me talk about anything that was negative. My dad always told me, 'the best thing you did was leave'" (Carolina).

The women described feelings of failure, disappointment, or shame because of not meeting the impossible expectations set for them. Some women described feeling alone in their failure, believing that all other immigrants were successful. The weight of this narrative also made the women feel stuck since it was impossible to return home, as they would have nothing to show their family. As one woman explained, "you question whether the decision you made [to come to Canada] was good because you're not meeting the expectations" (Gabriela).

In response, some women challenged the legitimacy of the narrative, speaking out about their reality. Some women shared how they fought back against the idea of the "grateful immigrant," instead offering a critical view: "Canada has grown so much because of the migrant workforce" (Gabriela). Most importantly, the story circles themselves created a form of resistance to the individualism embedded in the Canada narrative:

> I felt very defective, like what is wrong with me that I am not achieving all these dreams ... and the most beautiful thing about sharing [in the story circles] is like all of us, of course we have unique stories,

> but our processes are very similar, right? ... Those initial difficulties, those struggles of the spirit ... and also understanding that of course Canada invites us to come here because we are a qualified workforce ... so I think it's really beautiful to understand that we are not isolated people who are defective, but that we are very capable, and we are part of a very large social process. (Adriana)

Structural Instability: Holding On in Precarity

In contrast to the expectations of an easy, successful migration, the women described experiencing immense structural instability after arrival due to a lack of permanent documentation and financial instability. This instability is largely due to capitalist migration policies that create precarity by incentivizing arrival by work permit instead of PR (described in the introduction). Finding a job that qualifies for PR can take months to years, and therefore obtaining PR can often take three or more years. It is during this period that migratory distress can be highest. Even for participants who arrived with PR or citizenship, they described facing large challenges obtaining financial stability due to language barriers and invalidation of credentials.

Upon arrival, most women took any job to survive. Whether or not they were in the process of obtaining PR, the majority of women described needing to work non-stop for years, often attending school programs early in the morning and then working until late at night. Many worked precarious jobs in cleaning, hospitality, retail, transportation, and factories. For most of them, this was their first time working precarious jobs as they came from upper social classes and professional work: for example, one woman who was a journalist back home worked as a bathroom attendant. Only a few of the women had initial financial stability because they or their partners had gotten a job transfer to Canada.

After working precarious jobs, many women transitioned to jobs that could be used to qualify for PR. These jobs (e.g., call centre, customer survey company) were still precarious and very stressful, with high pressure and responsibility alongside low wages and a lack of job security. On top of that, the context produced additional distress because the women needed to push themselves to constantly excel at their job to achieve the one-year minimum for PR. Participants described "working like a machine" to obtain stability in Canada. At the same time, they were also feeling stuck because there was no guarantee they would be able to stay in Canada, regardless of how hard they worked. One woman pushed herself to the limit, producing triple the requested deliverables to obtain a managerial position to qualify for PR. Another woman described how her job and uncertain PR status led to insomnia and panic attacks:

> I already had all the pressure that I had to do a very good job and that I had to move up ... so with all that pressure I started to get panic attacks ... there was like [performance statistics] and if I didn't meet them then [I would be laid off] ... I saw how people were fired like that every day and so I was living so anxiously. (Luz)

In the face of structural instability, most women described *holding on* [*aguantando*]. Holding on was a response to remaining in an incredibly uncertain and unstable position, enduring extremely high stress levels. They described operating in survival mode for years, pushing themselves forward without stopping. Several women described blocking out thoughts and emotions to keep moving forward. The impact of this distress affected participants differently. Some experienced immediate effects; however, most women described how the distress accumulated over time and surfaced years later, once they were stable in Canada. One woman described how she started getting panic attacks only after she finished her college program: "I realized that this happened to me because during the first two years, my body was like a machine, fighting hard, hard, hard" (Carolina). The toll of constantly holding on through instability in the migration process is not validated or acknowledged in public health.

One woman shared how holding on led to severe illness. She arrived in Canada alone with two young children, while her husband had remained back home until they were financially stable. She experienced extreme stress for two years, barely sleeping while caring for her children, going to work, and attending school. She described moving without stopping or feeling: "Everything that was happening was so intense and so much responsibility that if I stopped to think, I was going to say ... 'I'm not going to be able to ... that adrenaline without stopping ... an adrenaline that allowed me to endure pain, emotional pain, plus stress and pressure" (Claudia). She explained the process of finding a job that would qualify her for PR: after applying to 120 jobs without success (due to lack of PR), she offered to work for free for several months, in desperation. She recounted the unimaginable stress: after two years, she felt pains in her body and was diagnosed with a severe illness, which she attributed to the structural instability of not having PR. She described her first moments following the diagnosis and how she only thought of her PR:

> The incredible thing is that I thought: "how am I going to make this work so that I don't miss work?" ... that was my first thought, instead of saying, "my children, me" ... because the stress was so

> much, my permanent residency had to work out and I had to stay in Canada because the sacrifice had been so great that that was my first thought ... I remember driving back from the doctor and I said, "How am I going to tell my boss I'm going to have to undergo treatment? How?" ... so I planned the whole surgery. I asked the doctor for [a surgery appointment] on a Friday so that I would only ask for one [work] day off ... imagine the degree of stress that I was under that my job was always the only thing that gave me the backing of being able to stay in Canada. (Claudia)

The capitalist structural instability found in Canada is the primary element creating the need to hold on. However, holding on can be better understood by examining its intersection with other elements (Figure 4.1). The distress of structural instability combines with the high expectations and pressure from the Canada narrative, and these two elements come together to silence and fracture family communication. Part of silenced communication and its resultant lack of social support is due to the need to perform strength (described below). When all the elements combine, the distress of holding on is exacerbated.

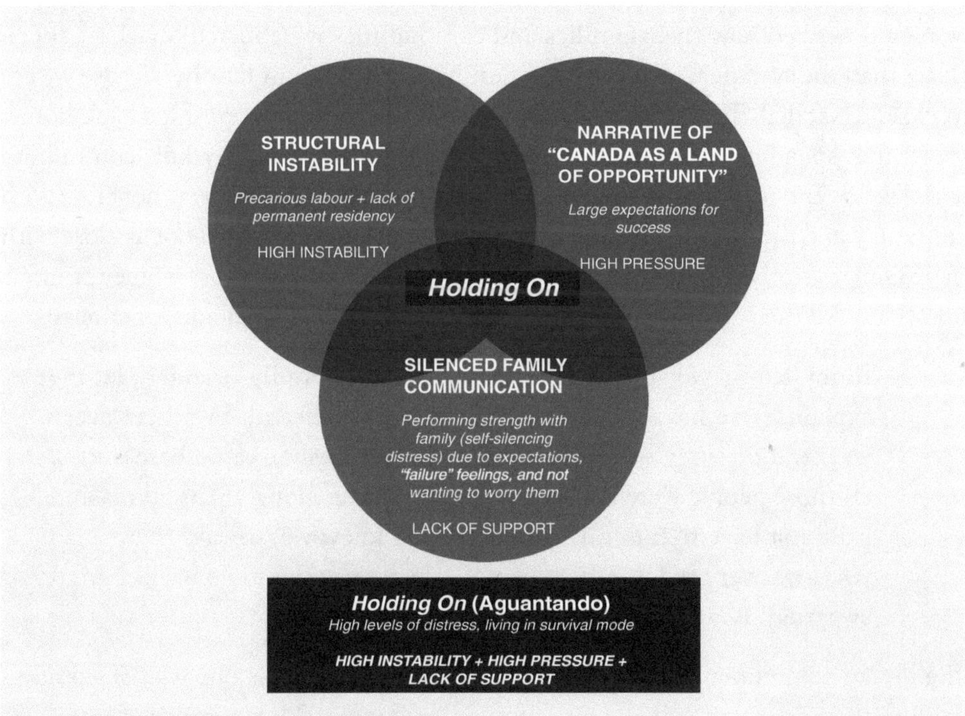

Figure 4.1. Holding On (*Aguantando*) as a Reaction to Intersecting Distress Elements

Even in the face of holding on, the women fought back against unfair labour practices and workplace harassment. One woman (who had Canadian citizenship), while working as a cleaner and restaurant server, faced manipulation and sexual assault from an abusive supervisor. She filed a formal complaint and started teaching new co-workers how to handle the supervisor. In the face of this difficulty, she shared: "I felt like superwoman because I did not stop for three years ... I needed to feel like 'I can do it all'" (Sofía). Another woman worked at clothing stores and described how the company specifically exploited immigrants by not paying their overtime work. When she was promoted to manager, she fought back: she taught newcomers their labour rights, helped women with their resumes, and battled management to follow labour laws. Despite holding on and fighting back, the women were also grieving the loss of their family at the same time, as seen in the next section.

Community Loss: Experiencing Migratory Grief

Migrating to Canada meant leaving behind parents, grandparents, extended families, and entire communities. The women not only lost the joy of being with their families and communities, but they also lost their support networks. Most of the women described how their families and communities were incredibly close, much closer than the average Canadian-born family: "we die for our family, because we are so close" (Natalia). They depicted strong extended family relationships back home, sometimes spending every weekend together, or having a tightly knit community with friends and neighbours close by. Only one of the participants was not close with her family and did not miss them; a couple other participants were not as close with their family as others but still felt very lonely in Canada. For most women, migration fractured their family connections and created intense grief and loneliness:

> In my family we are very Latino, we are very family-oriented, let me explain ... we have a "Thanksgiving" every weekend. We meet every weekend or every other weekend ... so obviously I came here and ... all those people were not there, I was walking along a path alone and I did not have that family support that I knew was always there ... so yes, I was very sad the first year ... I always wanted to go back. I cried every day. (Carolina)

The loss of community can be called *migratory grief*, which is one way of acknowledging this sorrow or sadness without medicalizing it. Migratory grief intersects with the colonial narrative of Canada and is exacerbated by capitalist migration policies that do not allow entire families to migrate together. Women described the grief as body weakness, feeling their soul hurting, a void or emptiness, or simply feeling incredibly sad and alone and not wanting to do anything or get out of bed. One woman shared: "I have gone through many moments of sadness, but of sadness crying, oh god, such awful pain in my chest from seeing myself alone" (Aziza). Other women described having depression or anxiety. They use biomedical words to recount their experiences, as there are no other words or language available. One woman reported developing anxiety from this loss and feeling it reflected in her body as muscle tension, joint pain, tiredness, sensitivity, and intense dizziness. Overall, the women described increased need to perform strength, only allowing themselves to cry when alone.

Since most participants were intimately connected with their families, many of them lost almost all their social and emotional support upon arrival. For participants who had children, they expressed no longer having the care and support they had back home. Furthermore, the pressure of structural instability prevented women from forming community, as they described needing to save every dollar and thus not having either the time or the money to socialize. The intensity of *migratory grief* prevented many women from being able to make new connections. They recounted closing themselves off in the face of distress. For one woman, she explained that she was unconsciously blocking out others. Another participant described slowly speaking less with her family, grieving the loss of in-person connections. She explained that she was "very depressed," and this closed her off from finding community: "I began to lose that connection with my family and with my friends, but I didn't find something here either. I couldn't find it because I think I was closed off. I didn't want to find it" (Patricia).

The women's experiences of migratory grief intersected with Canada's colonial narrative. They explained how in this narrative, migration to Canada is prized for its material assets—because of the capitalist mindset of prioritizing financial wealth above all else—while the emotional costs of migration are made invisible through the colonial narrative of migration that deliberately excludes the impact of the loss of community. In the words of one woman,

> When we say that it is hard, everyone talks about the physical or material things ... it is hard because it is really tough to earn money ... I think almost no one says that it is hard because you miss everyone, it's hard because you want to be with your family ... for me the hardest thing was the emotional part of everything that I had lost. (Patricia)

After three to five years, many women finally obtained structural stability. It was at this point that many described having the time and emotional capacity to open themselves up to finding community in Canada. Several women expressed how these moments of finding their "second family" changed everything. For example, one woman experienced years of migratory grief before meeting another Latina immigrant: "That was the day my life and my story started to change ... because all of a sudden I met someone who was in a similar situation to mine" (Patricia). For another participant, her greatest triumph in Canada was finding a drumming group for women: "when I was surrounded by a lot of women, I finally felt at home ... there were a lot of immigrant women too ... for me these women are my home, they are my family" (Natalia). Finding community helped some women break down the need to perform strength, which is explored in the next section.

Performing Strength: The Need to Hold Emotions Inside

One of the greatest sources of distress was a hegemonic narrative pushing the women to *perform strength*. In terms of mental health, this resulted in the women keeping emotions inside. In the context of high uncertainty and expectations, the need to perform strength intensified.

Performing strength can be seen as a reaction to patriarchal gender expectations and the expectation that women will put their family's well-being before their own. It is also a response to patriarchal narratives of how accepting help or showing vulnerability is seen as weak, for men and women alike. This is heightened in contexts of violence and insecurity: participants highlighted how their grandmothers took care of large families and often faced sexual violence but needed to stay strong, look beautiful, and persevere in highly distressing environments. One participant described her grandmother's world: "there are a lot of things that will continue to smack into your life, like the husband who beats you, money problems, not having enough to eat ... and you still have to get up the next day and push your family forward ... and look beautiful ... and keep being strong" (Natalia).

Women reported that while performing strength, they kept their emotions inside, feeling that they did not have the right to share. One woman explained, "we're pushing down everything that we are feeling and we're trying to be strong, but it is a very difficult process" (Adriana). In terms of performing strength for their family in Canada, one woman shared: "I had nowhere to put [my emotions] and I had to be there for my children, super strong ... [trying] to keep my children more emotionally stable" (Claudia). For their family at home, it meant not sharing distress:

> I didn't want to worry my parents, so I didn't want to tell them, "I'm sad, I feel lonely" ... because for them, the fact that I was here was security ... I had to put on a happy face [when I visited them] and say

> that everything was great ... but I wasn't okay. I wasn't happy and I was always trying to put a smile on for my son, so that he would be okay ... so that my husband would feel supported. (Patricia)

As detailed above, performing strength intersects with the Canada narrative of silencing emotions. With the added loss of community, there is no one in Canada to share with, and the need to keep emotions inside further increases. One participant who arrived alone recounted,

> I have always been very private with my emotions and with my family ... but [in Canada] it is even worse ... as soon as I arrived, bad things started to happen and I couldn't tell anyone because for everyone [at home], I was in the best country in the world.... On one occasion I tried and I felt that refusal to believe that [Canada] was not as good as it had been described, so I kind of gave up and I keep holding all [my feelings] in my [emotional] trunk that is already full ... I have always been quite reserved, but [in Canada] I was much worse. I had to become the real "strong woman." (Camila)

One facet of performing strength was performing success—which meant continually showing others they had a perfect and successful family. Even if they were feeling distressed, they had to pretend all was well and that they looked beautiful. This further exhausted the women: "I need to work really hard so that people do not realize how much I am suffering right now" (Veronica). With the high expectations for success, the need to embody a victorious migration increased distress. Only one participant did not perform strength at all: she fought back against her mother's pushes to dismiss emotions and shared openly with her loved ones. Over time, the women described slowly fighting back on the need to perform strength. They pushed themselves to be more vulnerable and care for themselves, searching out new friendships, finding support groups, or taking up hobbies. However, the continuous years of keeping emotions inside took an immense toll on their health, which is explored in the next section.

Migratory Distress over Time: Crisis and Epistemic Violence

Distress as a result of migration can be called *migratory distress*. Migratory distress impacted participants at different migration stages with varying intensities, the most severe being a health crisis or breakdown. This period of crisis occurred after the women had obtained structural stability (often after three to five years). They described experiencing an explosion of emotions or distress in their bodies following years of pushing through in survival mode, keeping emotions inside, and holding on: "for three years I was repressing, repressing, repressing, and when I reached the limit ... I exploded" (Patricia). Six women related experiencing "panic attacks" or "anxiety," two women described unintentionally exploding with verbal abuse at their children, one woman developed severe illness, and many reported "feeling depressed." One woman explained how and why this health breakdown occurred:

> It's the fact that you don't give yourself the time to feel, to breathe, so it's like a time bomb. You accumulate and accumulate and accumulate ... and you can't take it anymore, the bomb explodes. I think that it's something very common for many immigrants. You are so busy or so worried about everything that you have to do ... that you don't give yourself time to stop for a second and think about how all the change is affecting you ... and when you have that financial stability, that stability that the children are here and they belong, you have the chance to feel and see your emotions, and [that's when] your emotional stability breaks down ... when things calm down and you realize ... everything that happened ... how you felt ... everything falls apart and you get a super-intense slump ... I had depression, anxiety, with super-intense panic attacks. (Gabriela)

After experiencing a form of crisis, some participants sought support. However, in the process, participants faced epistemic violence from mental health professionals who pathologized or invalidated the migratory distress they had experienced. For one participant, she explained to a therapist that she was distressed because she had been unable to find fulfilling work in Canada due to her lack of documentation and the exorbitant cost of study programs for newcomers. When she shared this, the therapist individualized these systemic problems and negated the way she navigates the world as an immigrant: "She was like, 'No, but this depends on you' ... she spoke from her experience as a Canadian professional, as if she were speaking to anyone ... so I told her, 'No, my life in this country is different'" (Luz).

Another participant told of the way her family doctor brusquely prescribed her antidepressants without explanation. She was grieving the loss of family, and the interaction medicalized her loss. Pathologizing her experience as an individual problem led to her rejecting mental health support. Several years later, after she experienced a crisis, she saw a therapist who explained the distress in different terms: how it is normal for immigrants to experience distress after losing their immediate support circle. It was only after this validation of her experience as an immigrant that she could accept help.

To conclude, this chapter explores how the women's experiences are similar to being *stuck in a highwire act*, along with ways critical mental health research can combat epistemic violence.

DISCUSSION

Latin American immigrant women living in Canada often experience migratory distress, which is produced primarily by four macro-level elements grounded in capitalist, colonial, and patriarchal power. The colonial Canada narrative creates high expectations for life in the Global North, silencing the ability to share realities while generating feelings of "failure." Structural instability in Canada, grounded in capitalist migration policies, produces highly uncertain and stressful environments, creating a need to *hold on* despite increasing distress. Migration to Canada forces families to separate to obtain access to the idealized Global North (capitalism and colonialism), but this loss of community surfaces as *migratory grief.* Lastly, women *perform strength* as a response to patriarchal expectations.

When the four structural elements come together, the combined distress is even greater: the need to perform strength intensifies and the women describe self-silencing and keeping emotions inside, often to the point of crisis. One way of thinking about the distress experienced by immigrant women is being *stuck in a high wire act* (i.e., a tightrope, seen in Figure 4.2). There is only one way across, but there are thousands of ways to fall off, and it can happen at any time. To get to the other side, the women must survive a long period of hyper-demanding jobs but also must perform this act as if it is simple. They are stuck for many reasons: they cannot return home because their family's expectations for success are incredibly high and their countries of origin are too unstable, and they are forced to endure precarious work for years to obtain PR, with little social or emotional support.

Predominant research does not connect immigrant women's mental health to macro-level structures: it instead focuses on rates of depression and anxiety. As a result, biomedicine reduces women's experiences to biomedical disorders. This reductionism produces epistemic injustice: there is no collective language to describe or validate the women's experiences and identities, and thus their voices are dismissed. As women, Latin Americans, and immigrants, they bring together at least three distinct intersectional identities and are thus even more susceptible to having their experiences delegitimized.

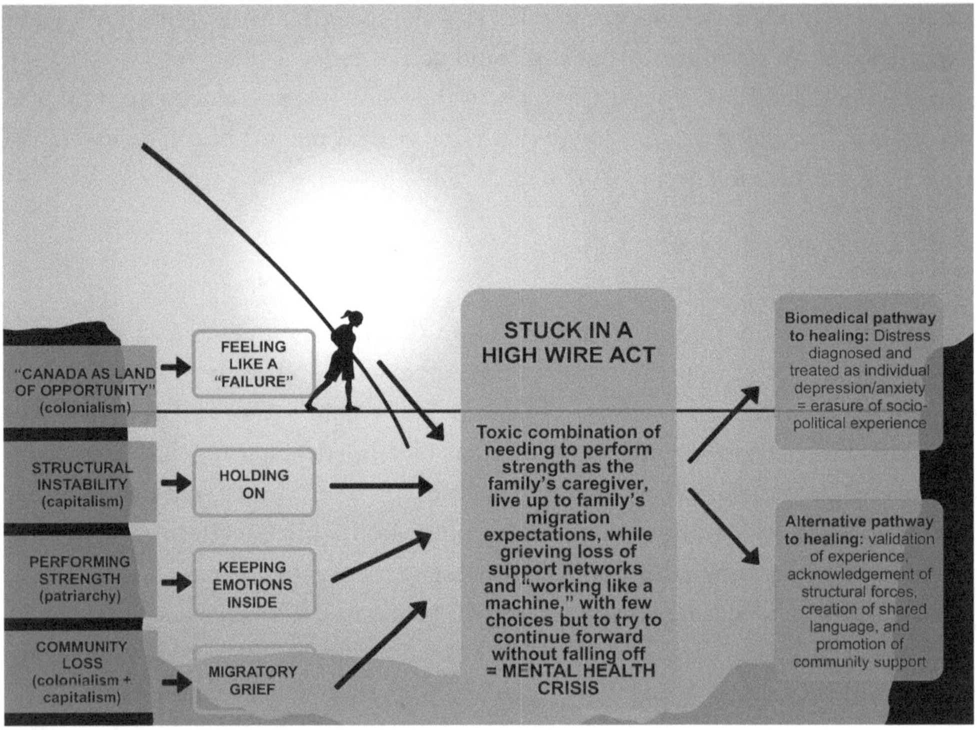

Figure 4.2. Stuck in a High Wire Act

Attributing their distress solely to biomedical disorders also hides the structural forces at play. Instead, the distress is seen as an individual problem that "resilient" women can handle. "Resilience" is often used to individualize the struggle to survive in a capitalist economy, creating "a constant internalisation of crisis and uncertainty as an opportunity to flourish" (Donoghue, 2022, p. 513). While immigrant women are incredibly fierce in their fight for stability in Canada, individualization of their distress feeds epistemic violence: capitalism, colonialism, and patriarchy work together, simultaneously creating distress while making their own role invisible by discharging it onto the individual.

A postcolonial feminist public health approach counters epistemic violence: it acknowledges the role of structural forces while affirming ways of knowing and being that are outside colonial biomedical approaches. Doing this has two important effects: it gives the distress a *scale* (structural, not individual) and it produces *new language* that validates a shared experience. This study argues for the use of non-biomedical language to describe immigrant women's experiences, including terms such as *migratory distress*, *holding on*, *performing strength*, and *migratory grief*. For example, migratory grief (described initially by Lakatos [1992]) can be seen as a normal reaction to the loss and fracturing of families and communities, but it is not currently socially recognized or accepted in our discourses. Replacing the term *depression* with *migratory grief* properly locates the source of distress within the migration process, not the person.

Immigrant women specifically have identified the need to *perform strength*: research with Black immigrant women in Canada describes their need to be a "strong Black woman" as a reaction to racism and gendered expectations. She is "physically strong, resists vulnerability, and suppresses emotion in order to survive" (Carter & Rossi, 2019, p. 291). Furthermore, *performing strength* to the point of crisis has also been described by Chinese immigrant women in Canada, who use "endurance" as a "coping strategy that prioritizes suffering through difficulties on one's own without showing distress." However, they used endurance until reaching a breaking point, attempting suicide as a way to escape their distress (Zaheer et al., 2016, p. 51). Zaheer et al. (2016) emphasize that "endurance" can be seen as a response to gendered expectations and oppression of women's agency. While racism did not emerge as a central feature of Zaheer's study or our own, the intersection with gender and the forms of gendered racism are important points of further research.

The need to self-silence is seen in women worldwide (Jack & Ali, 2010), but it is heightened in the context of migration. Colonial migration narratives individualize success and emphasize a need to embody gratefulness toward the host country, which leaves even less room to share experiences of distress. In our study, the pressure to self-silence to the point of crisis can be seen as a reaction to patriarchal gender roles, capitalist instability, and colonial expectations. In addition to validating new mental health language, we must bolster community sources of support: community-building spaces (including story circles) not only promote emotional and social support for newcomers, but they also combat harmful hegemonic narratives.

In conclusion, embracing experiences of distress as reactions to structural forces and hegemonic narratives means changing the way we understand mental health problems and what we decide is "the problem." In order to properly support individuals of multiple intersecting identities, we must listen to and legitimize their experiences, create new language, promote community building, and step outside of biomedicine to locate sources of distress in power structures instead of individuals.

CRITICAL THINKING QUESTIONS

1. Why does using a critical mental health approach matter (i.e., acknowledging the impact of patriarchy, capitalism, and colonialism)?
2. What difference does it make to use the term *migratory grief* instead of *depression*?
3. Are the experiences of *performing strength* and *holding on* unique to migration?
4. Why is there such a large gap between the women's expectations for Canada and the reality they found upon arrival?
5. How would experiences of racism, xenophobia, homophobia, transphobia, or ableism further exacerbate migratory distress?

KEY TERMS

critical mental health
immigrant health
women's health
epistemic violence

SUGGESTED FURTHER READINGS

1. Mills, C. (2015). The psychiatrization of poverty: Rethinking the mental health–poverty nexus. *Social and Personality Psychology Compass*, *9*(5), 213–222.
2. Morrow, M., & Malcoe, L. H. (2017). *Critical inquiries for social justice in mental health.* University of Toronto Press.
3. Ndlovu-Gatsheni, S. J. (2018). *Epistemic freedom in Africa: Deprovincialization and decolonization.* Routledge.

NOTES

1. We use the term *distress* as a way of acknowledging adversity without pathologizing it.
2. Racism and xenophobia are equally important macro-level elements, but they were not a central feature mentioned by the women. However, this does not mean they were not present in their lives.

CHAPTER 5

Spurring the Witch Hunt: Abortion, Colonialism, Stigma, and Indigenous Knowledges in Canada

Arie Ross

LEARNING OBJECTIVES

1. Gain an understanding of the history of abortion access in Canada and stigma surrounding abortion.
2. Explore traditional knowledges around reproductive health among Indigenous communities in Canada.
3. Recognize the influence of religion and colonialism on stigmatizing views of abortion and reproductive autonomy among Indigenous communities in Canada.

INTRODUCTION

Public health feminism provides a framework for increasing justice and equity. It requires us to dismantle systemic inequities and structures of oppression found in public health models to create a safer and healthier future for all. This chapter reflects on the goals of reproductive justice (RJ) to explore the history of abortion access in Canada, abortion stigma, the influence of religion on abortion stigma and abortion in Indigenous communities, and it highlights current work to improve abortion access and reduce abortion stigma. A public health feminist lens acknowledges that traditional reproductive knowledges and practices surrounding bodily autonomy and self-determination exist(ed) in Indigenous communities on Turtle Island pre-contact. This chapter aims to acknowledge and honour these knowledges and practices to reduce abortion stigma in Canada today.

It is important to note that abortion is not exclusively a gendered health service. Though most of the literature on abortion is explicitly gendered, not all who have abortions identify as female, as abortion impacts trans, non-binary, two-spirit, and other gender-diverse individuals (Moseson et al., 2021). Any gendered language in this chapter is due to direct quotes from the existing literature. However, we must move beyond the gender binary in discussions of abortion and sexual and reproductive health and rights overall. This may help to improve health outcomes and to realize public health feminism and RJ.

SELF-LOCATION

I was raised on the territories of the Tsawwassen First Nation and spent most of my adult life on the traditional territory of the Tsleil-Waututh, Musqueam, and Squamish peoples in "Vancouver." I am now a grateful, uninvited guest on the traditional territories of the Lekwungen, Songhees, W̱SÁNEĆ, and Esquimalt peoples in "Victoria." I consider myself a steward of these lands and spent most of my twenties defending them from extractive resource projects like the Kinder Morgan and Enbridge pipelines as a community organizer.

I am a fourth-generation settler of mixed Central and Eastern European Jewish descent, and Scandinavian, Central, and Western European descent. I hold unearned privilege and power due to my identities as a cisgender, heterosexual white woman with an invisible disability. I have experienced sexual violence and was able to access resources relatively easily due to my privileged identities, but I know this is not the case for many.

Public health feminism requires us to identify and consider the intersecting lived experiences that shape our identities and realities. Self-sufficiency in Jewish communities was necessary due to historic oppression. There is a history of forced sterilization among Jewish people at the hands of Nazi scientists surrounding the Holocaust. My lineage has endured genocide and assaults to our reproductive rights. Though experiences are unique and not interchangeable, Jewish and Indigenous Peoples have historically endured systematic attacks on our very existence, and there is now an urgency to reproduce to rebuild our populations. As Kim Anderson states, "it's simple: when a people are under siege, it becomes imperative to reproduce" (Anderson, 2003, p. 175).

Rabbi Lori Koffman notes that in Judaism, protecting the life of the pregnant parent is paramount and a fetus does not have independent rights (Koffman, n.d.). This means abortion is not only permitted but may be required if pregnancy threatens the well-being of the parent (Koffman, n.d.). This is often in contrast with prevalent anti-abortion sentiments of many other mainstream religions (Abortion Rights Coalition of Canada, 2017; Koffman, n.d.). I am called to this work to help realize equitable access to reproductive health services in Canada and to build a just future that honours experiences, traditional knowledges, and respects self-determination.

DEFINING REPRODUCTIVE JUSTICE

The term *reproductive justice* (RJ) was coined at the Black women's caucus in Chicago in 1994 (Cattapan et al., 2021; Kirby, 2017; SisterSong, n.d.). RJ emerged from Black women's experiences and subjugated knowledge excluded by the mainstream pro-choice movement based on the perceived "lower" social location of Black women (Ross, 2017; UN Women, 2020). RJ embodies a broad vision of reproductive rights, including the ability to access abortion and effective birth control methods, the rights to have or not have children, to control birthing options, to parent the children one has, and to raise them in safe and healthy communities (Cattapan et al., 2021; Kirby, 2017; SisterSong, n.d.). Public health feminism acknowledges that RJ is requisite for equitable health outcomes.

WHY WE NEED REPRODUCTIVE JUSTICE

Barriers to accessing reproductive health services disproportionately impact racialized communities (El-Mowafi et al., 2021; Kirby, 2017; Monchalin, 2021). Yet abortion has commonly been described as a white woman's issue, focusing on reproductive rights rather than RJ, pointing to needs that privileged white women often take for granted (Burnett, 2018; Kirby, 2017; Ross, 2017; SisterSong, n.d.), such as the rights to have and raise children and to access basic health services. In contrast, inequitable access to reproductive health services for racialized communities is commonly ignored (Burnett, 2018; El-Mowafi et al., 2021; Garcia & Sharif, 2015; Kirby, 2017; SisterSong, n.d.). The inaccessibility of basic healthcare may be seen in mandatory birth evacuations from remote and northern Indigenous communities (Cattapan et al., 2021; Kirby, 2017; Lawford & Giles, 2012) and in the widespread forced sterilization of Indigenous Peoples across Canada (Agecoutay, 2022; Burnett, 2018; Rasmussen, 2019). We need RJ to reduce systemic barriers to accessing abortion services for Indigenous Peoples in Canada.

ABORTION ACCESS IN CANADA

Abortion was criminalized in Canada until 1969, when the Criminal Code was amended to only decriminalize it in certain circumstances (Ackerman & Stettner, 2019; Kirby, 2017; Sethna & Doull, 2013; Shaw & Norman, 2020). Providing abortion was only allowed if the pregnant person's life was threatened by the pregnancy, the abortion was performed by a physician in hospital, and it was approved by a "therapeutic abortion committee" (Shaw & Norman, 2020, p. 51). These requirements kept safe abortions inaccessible for many communities (Kirby, 2017; Shaw & Norman, 2020). In response to this injustice, a caravan of protestors stormed the Canadian Parliament in 1970 and chained themselves inside, calling for decriminalization and safe abortion access (Shaw & Norman, 2020).

The Supreme Court of Canada struck down the restrictive abortion law through the historic *Morgentaler* decision in 1988 (Kirby, 2017; Shaw & Norman, 2020). The *Morgentaler* decision made abortions induced by a medical doctor safer and more accessible and affordable for some (Kirby, 2017). Henry Morgentaler, Holocaust survivor, physician, and abortion rights advocate, stated,

> The fact that I am a survivor of the Holocaust played a tremendous part in my decision to break the [anti-abortion] law ... because while I was in a concentration camp, I was there lawfully ... laws should be rational, in the interest of people. A law which is unfair and cruel like the abortion law, which condemns women to die horrible deaths and to seek illegal abortion and to abort themselves, is not a law which I can respect. (Musée de l'Holocauste Montréal, 2019, 0:05)

Morgentaler rightly argues that just because something is the law, does not make it right (Musée de l'Holocauste Montréal, 2019). Canada is now one of only four countries globally to have no restriction against abortion in law (Ackerman & Stettner, 2019; Kirby, 2017; Monchalin, 2021; Myran & Bardsley, 2018; Shaw & Norman, 2020).

Unfortunately, legal abortion does not equal safe and accessible abortion for all (Monchalin, 2021). Lack of knowledge about abortions and how to access them, and geographic and financial barriers, blocks safe access to essential abortion services for many (Kirby, 2017; Monchalin, 2021; Myran & Bardsley, 2018; Shaw & Norman, 2020). Abortion services in Canada are generally only available in major cities (Mehta, 2019; Shaw, 2013); five provinces and territories in Canada have no rural access to abortion services (Action Canada for Sexual Health and Rights, n.d.). In Prince Edward Island, Yukon, and Northwest Territories, there is one provider for each of these jurisdictions (Action Canada for Sexual Health and Rights, n.d.; Loreto, 2020). Abortion options include a surgical procedure up to 25 weeks gestation and the medical abortion, which involves taking two medications, Mifepristone and Misoprostol, sold together under the brand name Mifegymiso, and is approved for use up to 9 weeks gestation (BC Women's Hospital and Health Centre, n.d.). Abortion access is restricted after 12 weeks and 6 days in

Prince Edward Island (Government of Prince Edward Island, 2021), and after 15 to 16 weeks in Newfoundland and Labrador (Planned Parenthood, 2020), Yukon (Opal Clinic, 2022), Nova Scotia (Halifax Sexual Health Centre, n.d.), and New Brunswick (Horizon Health Network, 2022).

Importantly, barriers to accessing health services are disproportionately experienced by racialized communities with intersecting identities, such as Indigenous women and two-spirit people, who also experience severe disparities in social determinants of health and their outcomes (Allan & Smylie, 2015; Monchalin, 2021; Reading & Wien, 2009; Shaw, 2013). For example, Indigenous Peoples experience homelessness, unemployment, and violence at a rate higher than non-Indigenous peoples in Canada (Allan & Smylie, 2015; Monchalin, 2021; Reading & Wien, 2009). Indigenous women also face sexual violence at a rate three times higher than non-Indigenous women, indicating a potentially greater need for abortion access (Cohen, 2020; Monchalin, 2021; National Inquiry into Missing and Murdered Indigenous Women and Girls, 2019).

ABORTION STIGMA: A SNAPSHOT

Abortion stigma is a social process that devalues and discriminates against people who are associated with abortions (Belfrage et al., 2020; Cockrill et al., 2013; Erdman, 2016; Ipas, 2018; Kumar et al., 2009), and several studies have shown that many abortion seekers face such stigma (Astbury-Ward et al., 2012; Belfrage et al., 2020; Cockrill et al., 2013; Hanschmidt et al., 2016; Shellenberg & Tsui, 2012).

Abortion stigma has been defined in various ways in the literature (Cockrill et al., 2013; Hanschmidt et al., 2016; Ipas, 2018; Kumar et al., 2009). For the purposes of this chapter, abortion stigma includes internalized or self-, anticipated, perceived, felt, and enacted or experienced stigmas (Cockrill et al., 2013; Hanschmidt et al., 2016; Ipas, 2018). As a result of abortion stigma, people who have abortions may face social and self-judgment and a desire to keep abortions private (Belfrage et al., 2020; Hanschmidt et al., 2016; Kumar et al., 2009). This may perpetuate secrecy and reinforce the myth that abortion is abnormal, uncommon, and shameful.

Abortion may be seen as socially deviant, going against "traditional" gender roles and social norms (Belfrage et al., 2020; Erdman, 2016; Kumar et al., 2009). As Joanna Erdman (2016) writes,

> Abortion, the decision and act to terminate a pregnancy, has long been linked to undesirable moral qualities in the individual—sins of lust and gluttony, the sins of desire.... A woman who wishes to or does terminate a pregnancy challenges gender and moral codes, and

> so unsettles, if not threatens, communal norms. She is, for this reason, a "public enemy." The criminalization of abortion in the nineteenth century traded on this idea, reflecting general anxieties of modernity and its effects on the moral fabric of society. (Erdman, 2016, para. 5)

Abortion stigma contributes to secrecy around abortion experiences (Belfrage et al., 2020; Cockrill et al., 2013; Hanschmidt et al., 2016), which is problematic as abortion cannot be normalized if no one talks about it (International Planned Parenthood Federation, 2016). Shellenberg and Tsui (2012) explored the prevalence of perceived stigma among abortion patients in the United States and found that 66% expected to be looked down on by at least some people due to their abortion. Quantitative studies reveal that secrecy is used to manage stigma, but evidence has demonstrated the consequences, including social isolation (Astbury-Ward et al., 2012; Belfrage et al., 2020; Cockrill et al., 2013; Ipas, 2018), poor mental health (Belfrage et al., 2020; Hanschmidt et al., 2016; Major & Gramzow, 1999) and diminished social support resources accessed (Belfrage et al., 2020; Cockrill et al., 2013; Hanschmidt et al., 2016; Ipas, 2018; Shellenberg & Tsui, 2012).

The consequences of abortion stigma are far reaching. Internalized, self-directed shame may impact emotional, mental, and social well-being, and the ability to cope (Ipas, 2018; Shellenberg et al., 2011). Secrecy and shame may also reduce the accessibility of abortion services, which may lead to healthcare avoidance and seeking unsafe abortions (Ipas, 2018; Monchalin, 2021). It has been noted that people "who want an abortion will put their lives on the line to get one" (Gilmore, 2020, para. 8) and this may mean resorting to unsafe methods to terminate their pregnancies. Abortion stigma among providers may also contribute to further barriers for people seeking safe and prompt abortion services (Freedman et al., 2010; LaRoche et al., 2020). However, this stigma has not been thoroughly examined in the Canadian context.

Abortion stigma is inextricably linked with forms of power and oppression, including sexism, racism, classism, and wealth (Belfrage et al., 2020; Kumar et al., 2009; LeTourneau, 2016). Shout Your Abortion is an online space to talk about abortion experiences, aiming to normalize and destigmatize abortion (Shout Your Abortion, n.d.). A contributor shared that "getting an abortion did not traumatize me. Abortion stigma traumatized me" (Shout Your Abortion, n.d.). This demonstrates the harmful impacts of abortion stigma on a person's well-being. Addressing abortion stigma can reduce associated harms, like loneliness, depression, and trauma (Action Canada for Sexual Health and Rights, 2019; Ipas, 2018; Stangl et al., 2019).

THE INFLUENCE OF RELIGION AND COLONIALISM ON ABORTION STIGMA

Stigmatizing views on abortion are socially constructed and may be influenced by religious values within community (Belfrage et al., 2020; Hanschmidt et al., 2016; Kumar et al., 2009). Catholicism is the predominant religion in Canada and currently advocates against abortion to prevent taking a life that has received "its soul" (Abortion Rights Coalition of Canada, 2017, para. 2), though it should be noted that many Catholics believe in a pregnant person's right to choose.

Colonial religious ideologies and beliefs are prominent in Indigenous communities in Canada due to the ongoing effects of colonialism, residential schools, and the Sixties Scoop (Anderson, 2003; Burnett, 2018; Monchalin, 2021; Redvers, 2019). Kim Anderson (2003) states that "the church was undoubtedly the greatest obstacle to the practice of traditional birth control" (p. 181). Colonial influence degraded traditional Indigenous knowledges, deeming them unscientific, inferior, and "witchcraft" (Anderson, 2003, 2011; Redvers, 2019). As Nicole Redvers writes, "Traditional medicine and Indigenous spirituality were deemed by the church as being devil's work, and to this day those feelings still linger in the hearts of many who experienced those judgements" (2019, p. 215). This stigmatization spurred a "witch hunt" against traditional Indigenous knowledges and Peoples. This set the stage for colonial violence against ways of being and doing that challenged predominant colonial norms.

Populations influenced by Catholic and other Christian ideals may be more likely to hold negative views about abortion (Anderson, 2003; Belfrage et al., 2020; Hanschmidt et al., 2016; Shellenberg & Tsui, 2012). For example, Christian women were significantly more likely to perceive abortion stigma than non-religious people in two quantitative studies (Cockrill et al., 2013; Shellenberg & Tsui, 2012). Religious contexts may contribute to fears of being judged and feelings of guilt and shame among people with abortion experience (Belfrage et al., 2020; Hanschmidt et al., 2016; LeTourneau, 2016; Shellenberg et al., 2011). This sentiment may be influenced by interpretations of the Bible that claim it prohibits abortion and that an unborn child is a "sacred human life" (Abortion Rights Coalition of Canada, 2017). Further, Christian religious organizations have historically stated that abortions are sinful and that people who have them are bad (Abortion Rights Coalition of Canada, 2017; Belfrage et al., 2020). It is important to explore how religious influences have perpetuated stigma against traditional knowledges and abortion among some Indigenous Peoples in Canada.

COLONIALISM, TRADITIONAL KNOWLEDGES, AND ABORTION STIGMA AMONG INDIGENOUS PEOPLES IN CANADA

Public health feminism acknowledges that traditional reproductive knowledges and practices existed before settler contact and continue to this day (Monchalin, 2021). A public health feminist lens reveals how the intersection of colonialism, racism, and gender impacts Indigenous Peoples' lived experience (Burnett, 2018; Monchalin, 2021). It also highlights that traditional medicines were effective and used to prevent and/or end pregnancies in Indigenous communities pre- and early contact (Anderson, 2003, 2011; Burnett, 2018; Monchalin, 2021; Redvers, 2019), but colonial stigma prevented their continued use. For example, Elder Maria Campbell describes how Catholic morality prevented her mother from taking life-saving traditional medicine to control dangerous pregnancies (Anderson, 2003).

A toolkit created by the Native Youth Sexual Health Network quotes Elder Joanne describing how Indigenous medicines and knowledges existed to control birthing options (Monchalin et al., 2015). Elder Joanne describes that judgment and stigma around contraceptives was not a traditional Indigenous practice:

> In our traditional way, we knew how to stop pregnancies. There were medicines. So, we knew, when women found out they were pregnant, they would know how to get un-pregnant. It is not our traditional way to pass judgment on that, the Creator always gives us choice. (As quoted in Monchalin et al., 2015, p. 18)

These practices were made illegal by early settlers and knowledges were suppressed and systematically undermined, forcing communities to bring the knowledges "underground" (Anderson, 2003, 2011; Burnett, 2018; Monchalin, 2021; Redvers, 2019). Indigenous reproductive health knowledges were "replaced by Christian morals and a Western medical paradigm that gave birth, pregnancy and female sexual and reproductive health matters over to male doctors" (Anderson, 2003, p. 181). In present contexts, this colonial and state-sanctioned violence against Indigenous Peoples' RJ shows up as systemic racism in the health system, with attempts to control Indigenous Peoples' birthing through forced sterilization, child apprehension, and coerced abortion (Anderson, 2003, 2011; Burnett, 2018; Cattapan et al., 2021; Dyck & Lux, 2016; Monchalin, 2021; Rasmussen, 2019).

These compounding barriers to abortion access for Indigenous Peoples in Canada have resulted in lost and fractured intergenerational knowledge systems, cultural discontinuity, and feelings of shame around abortion (Anderson, 2003,

2011; Burnett, 2018; Cattapan et al., 2021; Kirby, 2017; Lawford & Giles, 2012; Rasmussen, 2019; Redvers, 2019). Abortion stigma often persists in communities where abortion is not seen as "traditional" (Anderson, 2003, 2011; Monchalin, 2021). Colonial Christian ideas that stigmatize reproductive autonomy may now be seen as "traditional" in some Indigenous communities (Anderson, 2003). Métis scholar Kim Anderson quotes Métis Elder Maria Campbell and writes,

> Maria asks the question about what we mean when we say "traditional," suggesting that a lot of what is considered traditional is steeped in Christian thought, morality and ethics. (Anderson, 2003, p. 177)

Many Indigenous communities' perspectives were not always against abortion. Rather, stigmatizing views of abortion were introduced through colonization and reinforced through colonial violence (Anderson, 2003, 2011; Burnett, 2018; Redvers, 2019). Before settler arrival, traditional contraceptives and abortifacients were used in Indigenous communities, often given by grandmothers and aunties (Anderson, 2003). This knowledge was passed down intergenerationally (Anderson, 2003, 2011). Now, with racism in health services, pressure to reproduce due to genocide, and early feminist notions that abortion is a "white woman's issue," access to abortion for Indigenous Peoples has been ignored (Anderson, 2003; Burnett, 2018; Kirby, 2017; Monchalin, 2021). However, even as the settler-colonial state systematically condemned and denigrated Indigenous reproductive knowledges, settler women sought out Indigenous knowledges for reproductive and sexual health in early contact as Christian, particularly Catholic, morality forbade birth control and restricted reproductive autonomy (Anderson, 2003; Burnett, 2010, 2018; Monchalin, 2021; Rasmussen, 2019).

Colonization, racism, social exclusion, and a lack of self-determination play a key role in the disparities between Indigenous and non-Indigenous people's health (Allan & Smylie, 2015; Coen-Sanchez et al., 2022). To improve access to abortion services, there is a need to reduce stigma, bridge Indigenous and Western medical knowledges, and honour Indigenous ways of knowing and doing around controlling birthing options and reproductive autonomy (Monchalin, 2021; Redvers, 2019).

INITIATIVES TO IMPROVE ABORTION ACCESS AND REDUCE STIGMA

There is a light at the end of the abortion stigma tunnel. Despite the obstacles presented above, many communities and organizations are taking action. For example, Abortion Support Services Atlantic is a grassroots, volunteer-run group providing non-medical, trauma-informed support to anyone seeking abortion care in the Atlantic provinces, including emotional or peer support, travel, and/or accommodation (Abortion Support Services Atlantic, n.d.). The ekw'í7tl Indigenous doula collective is a network of Vancouver-based Indigenous doulas providing full-circle support to families during pregnancy, labour, birth, postpartum care, abortion, and beyond (ekw'í7tl, n.d.). They provide abortion companionship and non-judgmental post-abortion care for Indigenous parents considering and/or electing to have an abortion (ekw'í7tl, n.d.). The Northern Reproductive Justice Network is a collective that holds politicians and the healthcare system accountable, works to destigmatize abortion, provides information and resources surrounding abortion, and creates a safe environment to seek peer support and share abortion stories (Northern Reproductive Justice Network, n.d.). Northern Manitoba Abortion Support is a grassroots organization offering compassionate and non-judgmental support for people having abortions in northern Manitoba (Northern Manitoba Abortion Support, n.d.). They offer Abortion Aftercare Support Kits to people in Northern Manitoba who have an abortion (Northern Manitoba Abortion Support, n.d.). Action Canada for Sexual Health and Rights and the Abortion Rights Coalition of Canada are also breaking down barriers by providing accurate and accessible abortion information, including where to find abortion services nearby (Abortion Rights Coalition of Canada, n.d.; Action Canada for Sexual Health and Rights, n.d.). Shout Your Abortion, as mentioned, provides a safe space to share experiences, build community, and destigmatize abortion. They are a network of individuals who are creating resources, campaigns, and media intended to eliminate abortion stigma (Shout Your Abortion, n.d.). Grassroots, community-based organizations are leading the way in improving access to abortion services while reducing surrounding stigmas.

CONCLUSION

Despite abortion being legal, stigma against it persists. The legacy of colonial policy in Canada contributes to the ongoing stigmatization of Indigenous knowledges, abortion, and reproductive autonomy. Indigenous communities honoured individual choice until contact with religious settlers, who often condemned and outlawed traditional Indigenous reproductive practices. However, effective Indigenous reproductive knowledges have continued to be shared. Abortion stigma exacerbates access barriers among Indigenous Peoples in Canada, contributing to poor health outcomes. To improve abortion access, there is a need to reduce stigma and honour Indigenous ways of knowing and doing that honour reproductive autonomy.

CRITICAL THINKING QUESTIONS

1. Explore your own history and lineage. What do you find around "traditional" reproductive knowledge and abortion/reproductive autonomy?
2. How, and in what ways, have religious ideologies influenced your personal and/or community beliefs about abortion? What harms and benefits might this cause?
3. What are the dangers and harms of abortion stigma? How do they manifest in your life and/or your community? What can you do to combat those harms?
4. What are the ways in which your identity privileges or undermines your ability to access health services safely? How can you contribute to greater equity in health services in Canada?

KEY TERMS

abortion
stigma
Indigenous knowledges
reproductive justice

SUGGESTED FURTHER READINGS

1. Anderson, K. (2003). Vital signs: Reading colonialism in contemporary adolescent family planning. In K. Anderson and B. Lawrence (Eds.), *Strong women stories: Native vision and community survival* (pp. 174–191). Sumach Press.
2. Burnett, K. (2018). Different histories: Reproduction, colonialism, and Treaty 7 communities in Southern Alberta, 1880–1940. In S. Stettner, K. Burnett, and T. Hay (Eds.), *Abortion: History, politics and reproductive justice after Morgentaler* (pp. 35–54). UBC Press.
3. Cattapan, A., Moore, S., & Lawford, K. (2021, March 1). *Reproductive justice and Indigenous women in Saskatchewan: Overview and recommendations.* Johnson Shoyama. https://www.schoolofpublicpolicy.sk.ca/documents/research/policy-briefs/jsgs-policybriefs-reproductive-justice-and-indigenous-women-in-sk.pdf
4. Monchalin, R. (2021). Novel Coronavirus, access to abortion services, and bridging western and Indigenous knowledges in a postpandemic world. *Women's Health Issues*, *31*(1), 5–8. https://doi.org/10.1016/j.whi.2020.10.004

CHAPTER 6

Deconstructing Ableism in Healthcare

Maren B. Akyürek and Natalie Frandsen

LEARNING OBJECTIVES

1. Describe the impacts of ableism on students in healthcare education.
2. Describe how public health feminism can be used to critique the institution of healthcare education.
3. Describe how structural violence leads to inequities for persons with (dis)abilities.

A NOTE ON TERMINOLOGY

Throughout the chapter, the term *(dis)ability* will be used rather than *disability*, *disabled*, or *dis/ability*. The brackets around *dis* bring awareness to what disability is: not just an identity but a social category that has been constructed and shaped throughout history by dominant culture. In Schalk's work, she describes her use of *(dis)ability* as it "gestures toward the mutually dependent nature of disability and ability" (2017, para. 3). The brackets also bring a form of disjointedness to the word, causing the reader to question what (dis)ability is each and every time it is read: is it permanent or is it fluid? As Schalk asserts, "The parenthetical curve helps highlight how the boundaries between disability and ability are uneven, contestable, and context dependent" (2017, para. 3). However, *disability* will appear in its original form in quotes or in the names of theories (e.g., social model of disability).

INTRODUCTION

Ableism pervades our culture and higher education in varied and insidious ways. Ability is defined by the status quo, and thus so is (dis)ability, which subsequently impacts access to healthcare education. Definitions based on and influenced by ableism and stigma create barriers. There has recently been a push for more diversity (e.g., racialized people, people with (dis)abilities, and those who identify as 2SLGBTQIA+) among healthcare professionals; however, until we critically evaluate healthcare professional programs, deconstructing the structural violence caused by ableist rhetoric embedded into their fabric, a more diverse healthcare system is unattainable. Through the use of public health feminism to deconstruct and disrupt ableist structures in healthcare education, this chapter will unpack how ableism in healthcare education leads to structural violence for all people with (dis)abilities.

Healthcare students with (dis)abilities often face discrimination and ableism (discrimination based on (dis)ability) in the academic setting. This results in structural violence: avoidable injury or disparity caused by a system or institution (Galtung & Fischer, 2013). Diverse healthcare teams are stronger and lead to better patient outcomes (Cohen, Gabriel, & Terrell, 2002). When patients encounter healthcare practitioners with the same background, studies show they are more likely to consistently access care and follow-up, leading to better health outcomes (Allan et al., 2020; Saddler, Adams, Robinson, & Okafor, 2021).

CONCEPTUALIZATIONS OF DISABILITY

The ways in which (dis)ability is defined or conceptualized influence the creation of accessibility-related laws, policies, programs, and services, which in turn have a direct impact on who is included in and excluded from educational opportunities. Therefore, one must be aware of the diverse conceptualizations of (dis)ability to examine (dis)ability-related issues in post-secondary education. The concept of *disability* has been described and understood in a variety of ways over time, including medical and social orientations. Wolforth (2016) wrote that

> [p]rior to the 1980s, disability was seen very much from the perspective of a medical or rehabilitation model, and people with disabilities were treated as having inherent defects and limitations that could not be fixed, as though they were lacking some measure of "normal" humanity. (p. 139)

Thus, the medical model or rehabilitation approach views (dis)ability as an issue inherent in the individual. Consequently, the focus is on curing, eliminating, managing, or minimizing the illness or (dis)ability (Goering, 2015). Scholar Beth Pickard (2020) notes one of the common critiques of this model is that it positions "disability as deficit in the disabled individual as opposed to misinformed assumptions in the non-disabled 'viewer'" (p. 395). For example, many people who have been blind from birth view their blindness as a neutral way of being rather than being a problem (Goering, 2015); however, others may assume their blindness is a deficit. Even as recently as 2019, the World Health Organization's (WHO) definition of disability was medically oriented. It described disability as

> an umbrella term, covering impairments, activity limitations, and participation restrictions. An impairment is a problem in body function or structure; an activity limitation is a difficulty encountered by an individual in executing a task or action; while a participation restriction is a problem experienced by an individual in involvement in life situations.

The main critique of the medical model of disability is the misplaced focus on an individual's "impairments" (Crow, 2010). Problems or limitations resulting from a (dis)ability are seen as intrinsic to the individual (Wolforth, 2016) as opposed to resulting from structural or societal barriers imposed on the individual. Bioethics scholar Cristina Richie (2019) critiques the medicalization of (dis)ability and contends that, "for disability advocates, the medicalization of disability marginalizes individuals and denigrates the unique diversity of humankind" (p. 383). This model fails to consider the social, cultural, and environmental contexts in which individuals with (dis)abilities live, work, and play. Sara Goering (2015) argues that the medical model causes harm. "One result of the common medical understanding of disability is that people with disabilities often report feeling excluded, undervalued, pressured to fit a questionable norm, and/or treated as if they were globally incapacitated" (p. 134). She goes on to suggest that in the medical model of disability, the focus of attention is misplaced:

> For many people with disabilities, the ***main*** disadvantage they experience does not stem directly from their bodies, but rather from their unwelcome reception in the world, in terms of how physical structures, institutional norms, and social attitudes exclude and/or denigrate them. (p. 134)

For example, people born with limb differences may learn to function as well with one arm as someone born with two. However, because of discrimination and social attitudes, they may wear a prosthetic limb to "pass" as able-bodied (Wright, 2019).[1] In this case, wearing the prosthetic is not to enhance function or to limit any presupposed "disability," but rather to fit in and avoid judgment or to make other people comfortable. Educational systems subscribing to medical conceptualizations of (dis)ability focus on the limitations or deficits that students have and consequently focus on altering learning design elements (e.g., assessments) through remedial accommodations rather than building more broadly accessible learning environments (Dolmage, 2017; Richie, 2019).[2] Inclusive post-secondary institutions cannot be created when policies are driven exclusively by the medical model and accommodations are understood to be the sole approach to achieving accessibility.

Critical disability studies emerged in response to the medicalization of (dis)ability, and the social model became a recognizable critical perspective that challenged the medical model of (dis)ability (Goodley, 2014). The field of (dis)ability studies is interdisciplinary, takes a critical approach to (dis)ability, prioritizes the experiences and perspectives of people with (dis)abilities, and is grounded in (dis)ability rights (Dolmage, 2017). "Critical disability studies view (dis)ability as both a lived reality in which the experiences of people with disabilities are central to interpreting their place in the world, and as a social and political definition based on societal power relations" (Reaume, 2014, p. 1248). Feminist disability studies is allied with the broader field of critical (dis)ability studies and shares a similar orientation. (Dis)abilities scholar Rosemarie Garland-Thomson (2005) writes about the complexity of the field of feminist (dis)ability studies and highlights key features that align with the earlier description of critical (dis)ability studies, such as dismantling existing stereotypes, situating the experience of (dis)ability within the context of rights and exclusions, defining (dis)ability from a socio-cultural viewpoint versus a medical one, and attending to the effect of power relations.

In the early 1980s, Mike Oliver, the first professor of (dis)ability studies and a world-renowned (dis)ability researcher-activist, developed the "social model of disability" (Oliver, 2013). Following the lead of the social determinants of health orientation, which focuses on socioeconomic and structural influences on health as opposed to individual health-related behaviours, the social model of disability differs from the medical model by centralizing the impact of societal structures on people with (dis)abilities. That is, it posits that people are marginalized, disadvantaged, and (dis)abled *by society* (McSpadden, 2022). (Dis)ability is conceptualized as a manifestation of barriers within the environments in which the person lives, works, and studies (Wolforth, 2016); it is considered in the context of external factors, including social oppression, cultural processes, discrimination, exclusion, and social and environmental barriers (Crow, 2010; Goering, 2015; Mulvany, 2000; Shakespeare, 2018). That is, in the social model of disability, (dis)ability relates to the impacts of inaccessible socially constructed environments on a person with an impairment,[3] rather than being something inherent *in* people with (dis)abilities (Oliver et al., 2006). In this way, (dis)ability is conceptualized as a social, not a medical, problem (McSpadden, 2022). Over 10 years ago, disabled feminist scholar Liz Crow[4] talked candidly about the personal impact of the social model of disability in *Including All of Our Lives: Renewing the Social Model of Disability* (2010), where she says,

> For years now the social model of disability has enabled me to confront, survive and even surmount countless situations of exclusion and discrimination. It has been my mainstay, as it has been for the wider disabled people's movement. It has enabled a vision of ourselves free from the constraints of disability (oppression) and provided a direction for our commitment to social change. (p. 124)

Like Goodley (2014), Crow contends that the adoption of this model has saved and continues to save lives. As she goes on to say, "The contribution of the social model of disability, now and in the future, to achieving equal rights for disabled people is incalculable" (p. 125).

Almost 20 years ago, the United Nations (UN) Convention on the Rights of Persons with Disability (UN, 2006) adopted the social model, signifying a global shift in paradigm away from the medical model.[5] This shift was concurrent with the movement in the field of public and population health away from the medical model and toward the model of population health and health promotion. Both the social model of disability and the model for population health and health promotion advocate for attention to be paid to the structural, societal, and environmental factors that influence people's health and experience with (dis)ability. This global shift continues, and evidence of more recent adoption comes from the World Health Organization (WHO). That organization now centres social barriers instead of personal limitations and defines (dis)ability as

> the interaction between individuals with a health condition (e.g., cerebral palsy, Down Syndrome and depression) and personal and environmental factors (e.g., negative attitudes, inaccessible transportation and public buildings, and limited social supports). (WHO, 2022)

Critics argue that the social model is too rigid and simplistic. Under this model, when (dis)ability and impairment are depicted as two distinct entities, there is a failure to recognize the relationship between impairment and (dis)ability (Owens, 2015; Shakespeare & Watson, 2010). Thus, the social model has the potential to ignore the impairments that are experienced by people with (dis)abilities. Shakespeare and Watson (2010) posit that, "while environments and services can and should be adapted wherever possible, there remains disadvantage associated with having many impairments which no amount of environmental change could entirely eliminate" (p. 63). Crow (2010) and Goering (2015) suggest that some nuance is required when considering how (dis)ability is conceptualized. They acknowledge the need to consider the disabling effects of the impairment (e.g., inability to work due to episodic pain or depression) *and* the disabling effects of discrimination and inaccessibility. While the social model has been critiqued for ignoring the medical needs of people with (dis)ability, proponents of it do not deny the importance of having access to care and advice from medical professionals. Rather, the focus moves from medical needs and impairments to the way in which care and advice are provided. "What is different is the overall approach to treatment: it responds to the expectations of the patient, not those of the institution" (UN Human Rights, 2014, p. 10).

Public health feminism situates ableism within greater systems of oppression and power, illuminating the interconnected (Aguayo-Romero, 2021) and intersectional effects: decreased levels of education (Statistics Canada, 2015), poorer health outcomes (Rios, Magasi, Novak, & Harniss, 2016), and higher levels of poverty and financial insecurity (Government of Canada, 2021). Although persons with (dis)abilities make up 15% to 20% of the population, one American study showed that less than 5% of medical students had a disclosed (dis)ability (Meeks et al., 2020). Within the healthcare education context, public health feminism examines ableist policies and practices in healthcare education that lead to structural violence in education and society.

(DIS)ABILITY IN CANADA

Almost everyone will experience either a permanent or temporary (dis)ability in their lifetime and 15% of the global population has at least one (dis)ability (WHO, 2022). In Canada, that number is higher: just over one in five Canadians over the age of 15 live with one or more (dis)abilities (Morris, Fawcett, Laurent, & Hughes, 2018). (Dis)ability disproportionately affects women and marginalized populations. For First Nations and Métis[6] living off reserve, the number is nearly as high as one in three (Hahmann, Badets, & Hughes, 2019). Women report higher rates of (dis)ability than men: 24% versus 20% (Statistics Canada, 2022). Although there are limited statistics, there is a push in Canada for more statistics on the people from racialized and 2SLGBTQIA+ communities who have disabilities (Kimpson, 2021). In Canadian universities, Indigenous students and students of colour are more likely to report a (dis)ability. Also in academic settings, students with (dis)abilities graduate with more debt (NEADS, 2018).

The cascade of inequities, from lower levels of education to increased poverty, is apparent. People with (dis)abilities are less likely to hold a university certificate, diploma, or degree at the bachelor's level: 14% versus 27% (Arim, 2015). Only 59% of those with (dis)abilities are employed versus 80% for those without (dis)abilities. Of persons with severe (dis)abilities, 28% live in poverty, whereas only 10% of those without (dis)abilities live in poverty (Morris et al., 2018). However, these statistics likely underrepresent the prevalence and thus the impacts of (dis)ability because (1) a dearth of primary care providers leads to a lack of continuity of care to document health challenges to *prove* their (dis)ability (Crooks, Agarwal, & Harrison, 2012); (2) the application to become a *person with a (dis)ability* (for income assistance or tax purposes) is complex and difficult; and (3) definitions of (dis)ability are rigid (Rios et al., 2016).

The Canadian Charter of Rights and Freedoms (1982) and the Canadian Human Rights Act (1985) are the primary pieces of legislation that protect people with (dis)abilities from discrimination and promote inclusion within Canadian society (Government of Canada, 2018). Canada has demonstrated commitment to protecting the rights of people with (dis)abilities. In 2010, Canada ratified the United Nations Convention on the Rights of Persons with Disabilities, which requires government to promote, protect, and ensure the full and equal enjoyment of all human rights by persons with (dis)abilities (Government of Canada, 2017). In 2019, the Accessible Canada Act was passed; its purpose is to make Canada "barrier free" by 2040 (Employment and Social Development Canada, 2020).

(DIS)ABILITY AND POST-SECONDARY EDUCATION IN CANADA

Everyone in Canada has an equal right to an education that meets their needs (Canadian Human Rights Commission [CHRC], 2017), and post-secondary institutions have a legal responsibility to ensure that students with (dis)abilities have access to their programs and services (British Columbia Human Rights Code, 1996, s. 8). The educational environment includes, but is not limited to, service providers (instructors and other staff), institutional policies (admissions, attendance, course load, or graduation requirements), campus facilities (classrooms, laboratories), and equipment (such as computers). Under the British Columbia Human Rights Code (1996), organizations have a "duty to accommodate," up to the point of undue hardship,[7] to ensure that people with (dis)abilities can fully participate in all aspects of their lives (including education, employment, and leisure). In the post-secondary context, the duty to accommodate is often operationalized as academic accommodations, the purpose of which is to reduce or eliminate barriers to participation so that students with (dis)abilities have equal access to learning and services in the educational environment (Alberta Human Rights Commission, 2010; Queen's University, 2016; Simon Fraser University, n.d.). Accommodations are based on negotiated agreements with students, typically through university (dis)ability support units (DSUs).[8] In most situations, this means providing some accommodation (e.g., extra time for exam writing, extensions for assignments, provision of note takers, and physically accessible classrooms and laboratories).

(DIS)ABILITY WITHIN HEALTHCARE EDUCATION PROGRAMS

In Canada, each province regulates healthcare professionals through legislation. Each profession has their own regulatory body, and there are more than 30 regulated healthcare professions across Canada (Aldridge, 2008), including nurses, doctors, midwives, pharmacists, social workers, dental hygienists, and respiratory therapists. Programs range from 2 years (dental hygienist) (Vancouver Community College, 2022) to over 10 years (medical doctor) (Carleton University, 2022). To become a healthcare professional, a student must graduate from an accredited program and pass their respective association's exam. The majority of programs only offer full-time enrolment, and most have applied learning in the field (e.g., in hospitals or other healthcare facilities). Although there are a few online programs, the majority require in-person learning. Modified programs (such as decreased course load) are rare.

There are no specific statistics on students with (dis)abilities in healthcare education; however, a Canadian study shows that 8.8% of students with self-disclosed (dis)abilities are in a health program or related area of study (Furrie, 2017). In American medical schools, 4.3% of students have a self-disclosed (dis)ability (Meeks et al., 2020), which is less than a third of the proportion of persons with (dis)abilities in the general population. To understand why there is a smaller proportion of students with (dis)abilities enrolled in healthcare education compared to the persons with (dis)abilities in the general population, the barriers that they face need to be identified and addressed.

ABLEISM TAKES HOLD

Rather than focusing on the definition of (dis)ability, here we wish to analyze ableism. Schalk and Kim (2020), feminists of colour, challenge the idea that (dis)ability is an identity to be negotiated; rather, they contend that (dis)ability arises from a relationship of power derived from ableism, white supremacy, race, gender, class, and citizenship status. Ableism positively values able-bodiedness (Dolmage, 2017) and describes the negative attitudes and oppression based on stereotypes, discrimination, and prejudices towards people with (dis)abilities and the devaluation of (dis)ability (Dunn, 2019). It is insidious, systemic, and "has to be seen as a series of entrenched structures—not just the action of an individual or of individuals" (Dolmage, 2017, p. 58). An intersectional approach can be used to understand how influences such as white supremacy, patriarchy, heterosexism, transphobia, colonialism, and poverty are inextricably tied to ableism (Schalk & Kim, 2020). This approach encourages an examination of "dynamic and contradictory power dynamics" (Goethals, DeSchauwer & Van Hove, 2015, p. 78).

The *intersectionality approach* has been used to analyze how determinants of health interact to influence health outcomes. Kimberlé Crenshaw coined this term in 1989, naming "the structural convergence among intersecting systems of power that created blind spots in antiracist and feminist activism" (Collins, 2019, p. 26). Intersectionality is a recognized form of critical inquiry and praxis that may guide practitioners and policymakers in their efforts to address structural forms of inequality (Collins, 2019; National Collaborating Center on Healthy Public Policy, 2015). Consequently, this approach is relevant to work done in the health *and* education sectors; more specifically, it is relevant when exploring issues related to (dis)ability, accessibility, and inclusion.

Gender and (Dis)ability

To demonstrate how embedded ableism is into culture, let us compare two social constructs: gender and (dis)ability (Garland-Thomson, 2005). Just over a hundred years ago in Canada, women could not vote, had limited access to education and the job market, and were cast as second-class citizens (Canadian Encyclopedia, 2022). This was based on the social construct of gender which purported that a woman was *less than* [a man]. The constructs of (dis)ability and gender have similar barriers: access to equal education, access to public space, and increased odds of living in poverty. Women did not struggle because they were incapable, but rather due to sexist policies. Similarly, rigid mandates and the lack of inclusive policies hinder persons with (dis)abilities.

Through repeated exposure to constant ableist attitudes, ableist microaggressions, and stigma towards people with (dis)abilities, students with (dis)abilities may develop internalized ableism, also known as self-stigma or internalized stigma (Kattari, Olzman, & Hanna, 2018; Lett et al., 2020). It is the negative attitudes a person has toward themselves and is the result of internalizing negative public attitudes (Ahmedani, 2011; Corrigan & Rao, 2012), in this case, with regards to (dis)ability. Additionally, internalized ableism may also affect the collective identity of persons with (dis)abilities by isolating people with (dis)ability from one another (Kumari Campbell, 2006). This affects students with (dis)abilities because they are unable to support each other. Students are not always cognizant of internalized ableism and often minimize their own conditions by comparing themselves to peers with (dis)abilities (Kattari et al., 2018).

Garland-Thomson (2002) describes two parts to the (dis)ability identity: (1) the public—the way one is viewed—and (2) the private—the way one views themselves. Within different spheres, these two identities are constantly challenged and negotiated, influenced by the oppression from ableism (Garland-Thomson, 2005; Schalk & Kim, 2020). This is pertinent for students with invisible (dis)abilities because their (dis)ability is *hidden*. Invisible (dis)abilities refer to ones that are not always, or ever, apparent to others (Kattari et al., 2018; Mullins & Preyde, 2013). People with invisible (dis)abilities find that their bodies are policed (Kattari et al., 2018), and the onus is on them to *prove* their illness or (dis)ability (because people with (dis)abilities have adapted to not look ill). However, the invisibility also allows them to *hide* their (dis)ability and pass as able-bodied, "escap[ing] the negative consequences of stereotyping and discrimination" (Nario-Redmond et al., 2019, p. 737).

ACADEMIA: NAVIGATING POWER STRUCTURES

Public health feminism aims to deconstruct power structures and build upon existing feminism, (dis)ability studies, and public health approaches. Colonialism is often absent from (dis)ability studies, although Grech (2015) introduces the concept of *colonial normativity*, which continues today: The *ideal* body (able-bodied) is based in colonial notions of fitness and the body's ability to contribute to the economy. Public health feminism, through its combining of both (1) a feminist lens to disentangle the structural oppression towards students with (dis)abilities and (2) public health outcomes for students with (dis)abilities, can help to identify the structures and systems that perpetuate colonial normativity and the notion of an ideal body. With these two lenses it can further uncover and make sense of the entrenched inequities built into the fabric of institutions (Garland-Thomson, 2002).

Although there are power dynamics between educators and healthcare students, institutional rules around accommodation deepen the dynamic. Educational systems subscribing to medical conceptualizations of (dis)ability focus on the limitations or deficits that students have and consequently focus on altering learning design elements (e.g., assessments) through remedial accommodations rather than building more broadly accessible learning environments (Dolmage, 2017; Richie, 2019). Overreliance on academic accommodations fosters an Othering environment (e.g., for those with executive functioning challenges, neurodivergence, learning (dis)abilities, and hearing impairment) rather than an inclusive one. Inclusive post-secondary institutions cannot be created when policies are driven exclusively by the medical model and accommodations are understood to be the sole approach to achieving accessibility.

Healthcare students with (dis)abilities face institutionally created barriers and inaccessible spaces (e.g., a lack of ramps and accessible washrooms), limited adoption of universal design for learning, inflexible course design, and requirements to maintain full course loads (Bailey & Mobley, 2018). Universal Design for Learning (UDL) is an effective philosophy, framework, and set of principles for creating and delivering course materials to diverse students, and there is evident demonstrating that it improves the learning process for all students (Al-Azawei, Serenelli, & Lundqvist, 2016; Capp, 2017; Hall, Meyer, & Rose, 2012).

Within ableist healthcare education institutions that rely on academic accommodations as the main tool for accessibility, students are required to disclose details of their (dis)ability to multiple people (e.g., (dis)ability support staff and instructors). Results from a large systematic review (n = 36 studies and 5,174 participants) (Lindsay et al., 2018) focused on the barriers to and facilitators of disclosure and accommodations in post-secondary institutions. The most common barriers were stigma and discrimination, which negatively influence a student's choice to seek support. Processes inherent in the accommodation model give space for stigma and discrimination. For example, instructors and (dis)ability support staff have gatekeeper functions, determining if accommodations will be approved and implemented. Accommodation-related decisions by instructors and DSU staff are based on knowledge of (dis)ability-related impairments and influenced by socially constructed attitudes and bias (NEADS, 2018). The act of disclosing a (dis)ability for healthcare students with (dis)abilities requires effort, adds an emotional burden (Bulk et al., 2020) and decreases their perceived power as they navigate negative attitudes (e.g., paternalism, pity, stigma, and invalidation [Nario-Redmond et al., 2019]). These negative attitudes can be magnified for healthcare students with (dis)abilities who belong to other marginalized communities (Bailey & Mobley, 2018).

Canadian research by Epstein et al. (2021) focused on the experiences of clinical nursing instructors and nursing students who self-identified as having a (dis)ability. Results from their scoping review, based on the findings of 27 papers published between 1999 and 2018, indicated that nursing students with (dis)abilities felt labelled, excluded, and judged by instructors because of their (dis)ability. The most startling and disheartening finding was related to the magnitude of stigma and discrimination experienced by the students: "Students experienced more problems with health care professional attitude than with managing their disabilities" (p. 113). Consequently, students with invisible (dis)abilities respond by masking their (dis)abilities and choosing not to access their accommodations (Kattari et al., 2018). Rather than being supported, students may be accused of "faking it, queue jumping, or asking for an advantage" (Dolmage, 2017, p. 10) and further, they may be required to educate others about their conditions and needs (Kattari et al., 2018). Their fear of discrimination limited or completely inhibited their ability to seek support. Although this scoping review is focused on the experiences of students during clinical nursing placements, the findings have broader relevance. Most Canadian post-secondary institutions offer professional certificates and degrees that include required field work/cooperative learning/clinical placements.

Under federal law in Canada, service-providing organizations, including post-secondary institutions, have a duty to accommodate students with (dis)abilities. However, almost 30% of post-secondary institutions in Canada failed to provide students with a process for accommodation (NEADS, 2018). This leaves students without an avenue to seek the support they deserve with their studies, demonstrating that students with (dis)abilities are not always being considered in institutional policies. Up to 14% of students with (dis)abilities leave post-secondary institutions before obtaining their desired level of attainment due to barriers such as insufficient institutional support (CHRC, 2017), long and complex academic accommodation processes, negative attitudes and stereotypes, ineffective accommodation dispute-resolution mechanisms, and lack of individualized support (Ontario Human Rights Commission, n.d.).

TOWARDS A MODEL OF INCLUSION

The current biomedical model of *accommodation* in post-secondary education focuses squarely on the student and on the *needs* that they have. This medical conception of inclusion fails to consider larger—ableist—structural issues and in doing so, it erects barriers to education, underutilizes universal design, and perpetuates ableism (Dolmage, 2017). It meets the needs of a segment of the population of students with (dis)abilities. Students are entitled to receive academic accommodations if they can provide evidence to the university DSU that their (dis)ability results in functional impairments that prevent or limit their ability to participate fully in their academic programs (Condra et al., 2015). This registration process requires students to navigate medical systems *and* post-secondary bureaucratic processes, which requires time, financial and human resources, and access to medical professionals. Obtaining required medical documentation may not be feasible due to insufficient availability of healthcare services and/or limited personal resources (Canadian Mental Health Association, 2017; Condra et al., 2015; Moroz, Moroz, & D'Angelo, 2020; Xiao et al., 2017). The use of personal resources to access accommodations—which could be used towards completing schoolwork—detracts from disabled healthcare students' education.

Accessible learning in the context of post-secondary education has been defined as "the process of designing courses and developing an approach to teaching that leads to meeting essential requirements and that maximizes the learning outcomes to meet the needs of individuals from a variety of backgrounds, abilities, and learning styles" (Canadian Standards Association, 2020, p. 12).[9] Accessible education celebrates diversity among learners, does not compromise academic rigour, is proactive and inclusive, reduces the need for specialized adaptations and utilizes principles of UDL (Ontario Universities Accessible Campus, 2017). Accessible and inclusive educational environments are created and fostered, in part, by the instructors who teach infinitely diverse groups of students. To make post-secondary institutions safer places for students with (dis)abilities, we must decrease stigma and normalize (dis)abilities, include students with (dis)abilities within healthcare education, and consult with peoples of varying abilities (Dolmage, 2017). Additionally, providing opportunities for current healthcare providers and educators to be open about their (dis)abilities may help to promote inclusive learning environments.

STRUCTURAL VIOLENCE: A PRODUCT OF ABLEISM

Structural violence was a term coined by Galtung, a peace researcher, in 1969 (Galtung & Fischer, 2013). Given that "violence is any avoidable insult to basic human needs ... [it] lowers the real level of needs satisfaction below what is potentially possible ... and hurts and harms body, mind and spirit," structural violence is a "structure at work, churning out harm, causing basic human needs deficits ... un-intended [or] indirect" (Galtung & Fischer, 2013, p. 35). According to Galtung, structural violence impacts four areas: survival, wellness, freedom, and identity (Galtung & Fischer, 2013). Further, it is so entrenched in dominant systems that its use and presence feel normal, not wrong, and part of the status quo. Just as structural violence underpins domestic violence (Hyman et al., 2016), it also underpins academic violence towards students with (dis)abilities. Within academia, this violence manifests as the gross inequities faced by oppressed populations (specifically, students with (dis)abilities) due to institutional policies.

Structural violence is highlighted in analyses of reported (dis)abilities in higher education in the United Kingdom. There is an inverse trend between the percentage of disclosed (dis)abilities and education level: With an increase in education level, there is a decrease in the percentage of students who disclose (dis)abilities (Brown, 2021). However, the report does not speak to the etiology of this trend. Furthermore, the structural violence is apparent whether the disclosure of (dis)ability threatens academic careers or if there is decreased accessibility in higher education for students with (dis)abilities, causing an exodus of students with (dis)abilities from higher education. If there are fewer healthcare students with (dis)abilities at the master's level, the careers and economic disposition of persons with (dis)abilities is affected. This trend is consistent with data from Canada in that persons with (dis)abilities are less educated (Arim, 2018). The structural violence enacted within education has far-reaching effects on other spheres. Successful completion of post-secondary education leads to better job opportunities, higher wages, and, because of improved socioeconomic status, better health, and more opportunities and privileges within society (PHAC, 2019). Having a diverse workforce that is reflective of the population can lead to increased productivity, cultural awareness, and organizational efficiency (Inegbedion et al., 2020; Mickahail & Andrews, 2017).

A DIVERSE WORKFORCE LEADS TO BETTER HEALTH OUTCOMES

Public health feminism enables us to link the oppression of healthcare students with (dis)abilities with the barriers faced in the longer-term health outcomes of persons with (dis)abilities. Healthcare education institutions are built on colonial values that perpetuate ableism. As healthcare education environments are not supportive of healthcare students with (dis)abilities, there are proportionately fewer persons with (dis)abilities within healthcare education programs than in the general population. This leads to a decrease in the representation among healthcare providers of persons with (dis)abilities. Persons from marginalized communities who access healthcare providers from their community are more likely to have better health outcomes.

Public health feminism can bring together (dis)ability studies, feminist studies, and public health approaches to highlight these decreased health outcomes for persons with (dis)abilities. The ableist, structural inequities in healthcare education—a system of accommodation, fewer students with (dis)abilities, and ableist policies—that stem from oppression (e.g., colonialism, racism, sexism, homophobia, white supremacy) lead to less representation among healthcare professionals. By helping us to understand how the structural violence that begins in healthcare education impacts persons with (dis)abilities as a whole, public health feminism can work towards identifying, naming, and decreasing barriers rooted in ableism and oppression, improving the representation of and health outcomes for disabled persons through the education and training of more healthcare providers with (dis)abilities.

CRITICAL THINKING QUESTIONS

1. How does ableism in the academic setting contribute to structural violence?
2. How can public health feminism be used to identify inequities for students with (dis)abilities in healthcare education?
3. What are the benefits of a diverse healthcare system?

KEY TERMS

ableism
healthcare education
structural violence
(dis)ability
academia

SUGGESTED FURTHER READINGS

1. Dolmage, J. (2017). *Academic ableism: Disability and higher education.* University of Michigan Press.
2. Hamraie, A. (2017). *Building access: Universal design and the politics of disability.* University of Minnesota Press.
3. Price, M. (2011). *Mad at school: Rhetorics of mental disability and academic life.* University of Michigan Press.
4. Schalk, S. (2022). *Black disability politics.* Duke University Press.

NOTES

1. *Disability passing* refers to the ways people conceal social markers of impairment to avoid stigma and to pass as "normal" or the ways they exaggerate a condition to receive benefit. It also includes the ways others impose (dis)ability or non-(dis)ability identity on others. According to Brune and Wilson (2013), "The topic of disability passing reveals the dynamic nature of disability and identity and provides insight into what is at stake when it comes to disability and nondisability identification" (p. 1).
2. Dolmage (2017) notes the significant challenge of this orientation, suggesting that when "accommodations are intended to simply temporarily even the playing field ... in a single class or activity, it is clear that these retrofits are not designed for people to live and thrive with a disability, but rather to temporarily make the disability go away" (p. 70).
3. In the social model, impairment is viewed as the physical, cognitive, mental, or sensory deficit or limitation (e.g., paralysis, blindness, diminished executive function, memory loss, hypersensitivity to noise), and (dis)ability is the social oppression and exclusion (Shakespeare, 2018). "Impairment relates to an embodied difference in terms of the functioning of the body or brain" (Goodley, 2014, p. 7).
4. Disabled feminist scholar is how Liz Crow identifies.
5. Canada signed the Convention in March 2007 (UN Treaty Collection, 2011).
6. This is the language used in the report.
7. Under subsection 15(2) of the Canadian Human Rights Act, undue hardship can be claimed when "the duty to accommodate would cost too much or create risks to health or safety" (CHRC, 2010).
8. In Canadian post-secondary institutions, these units were established in the mid-1980s (Cox & Klas, 1996).
9. The existence of innate "learning styles" has been contested and described as a pervasive myth or misconception about cognition. The learning style myth asserts that individuals learn better when they receive instruction that is tailored to the person's visual, auditory, or kinesthetic learning style (Nancekivell et al., 2020, p. 221). With evidence lacking to support assessing for and teaching to learning styles, the focus ought to be on building on pre-existing knowledge using diverse teaching methods for all learners (Pashler et al., 2009). The term *learning styles* is used here when taking direct quotes from the literature.

CHAPTER 7

Queer and Trans Perspectives on Obstetric and Gynecological Violence: Centring Those at the Margins to Capture the Intersectional Effects of the Phenomenon

Mylène Shankland and Ivy Lynn Bourgeault

LEARNING OBJECTIVES

1. Appreciate the multilayered nature of the power dynamics intertwined in obstetric and gynecological violence (OGV).
2. Understand the importance of capturing intersectional experiences of OGV to eliminate discrimination in obstetric and gynecological care and services.
3. Delve into existing queer and trans literature to include all birthing and bodies with uteruses' experiences of OGV.
4. Develop critical thinking around the systemic dimension of OGV and its implication for queer and trans people.

INTRODUCTION

Obstetric and gynecological violence (OGV) denotes acts, behaviours, and practices in the provision of reproductive healthcare that are not consensual and as such are considered disrespectful and abusive by those who experience them. Some increasingly point to the systemic nature of this abuse embedded into the patriarchal nature of the healthcare system (Sadler et al., 2016). To date, OGV has been documented and discussed predominantly from heterosexual cisgender women's perspectives, excluding queer and trans people whose reproductive healthcare and services can also be described and experienced as discriminatory, disrespectful, and in some cases abusive.

By *queer*, we refer to individuals with sexual orientation differing from heterosexuality. By *trans*, we refer to individuals whose gender differs from the one assign at birth. Both queer and trans people challenge the normative rules of sexuality and gender (Love, 2014). Because of their shared criticism of sexual and gender normativity, we used the term *genderqueer* to suggest "the intimacy between trans and queer" (Love, 2014, p. 173). We choose to discuss broadly the intersection of sexualities, genders, and OGV to open the discussion about LGBTQ+ realities and challenges.

In this chapter, we analyze the literature on discriminatory practices in maternity care towards queer and trans people to centre their marginalized experiences. We choose to name the violence from the perspectives of those who have faced it, notably to increase their empowerment and centre the experiences of the victims (Lévesque & Ferron-Parayre, 2021).

OGV was first described in 2010 in the Venezuelan Law on the Right to Women to a Life Free of Violence as *obstetric violence*:

> the appropriation of the body and reproductive processes of women by health personnel, which is expressed as dehumanized treatment, an abuse of medication, and to convert the natural processes into pathological ones, bringing with it loss of autonomy and the ability to decide freely about their bodies and sexuality, negatively impacting the quality of life of women. (Pérez D'Gregorio, 2010, p. 201)

Shortly thereafter, in 2014, the World Health Organization (WHO) declared the phenomenon a worldwide public health issue (WHO, 2015). Community-based groups had already begun to organize, notably in Quebec, Canada (Regroupement-Naissances-Respectées, 2019), in Brazil (Sadler et al., 2016), and in Argentina (Quattrocchi, 2019) to denounce OGV as a violation of reproductive rights. This growing international recognition has been strengthened by the United Nations Special Rapporteur on violence against women and girls, who affirmed OGV as a violation of human rights (Garcia, 2020).

TERMINOLOGY MATTERS

Using OGV instead of "disrespect and abuse" or "mistreatment" allows us to make visible the systemic dimensions of the phenomenon and extend our analysis beyond the dichotomous relationship between individual healthcare providers and individual patients (Sadler et al., 2016). Moreover, examining OGV from the perspective of genderqueer people allows us to broaden our focus beyond the traditional conception of motherhood to parenthood and include as a problematic concern regarding all reproductive healthcare and services. This enables the inclusion of existing queer and trans literature that denounces the stratified reproduction embedded in social comprehension of motherhood. We build on arguments that there are limits to exclusively conceptualizing OGV around motherhood (Hill, 2019), since this does not allow us to capture all manifestations of this kind of violence, including stigma and discrimination, toward all birthing bodies. Taking an explicit genderqueer perspective, we build our case around the appropriation and control of bodies with uteruses, thus reflecting the gender inequality and power relations into the healthcare facilities (Katz et al. 2020; Savage & Castro, 2017) and society more generally.

CONCEPTUALIZATIONS AND LIMITS OF OGV

A body of evidence on OGV is growing. Bohren and colleagues (2015) conducted a systematic review of 65 studies in 34 countries regarding the mistreatment of women during childbirth. Their results identified seven domains of this mistreatment: "1) physical abuse, 2) sexual abuse, 3) verbal abuse, 4) stigma and discrimination, 5) failure to meet professional standards of care, 6) poor rapport between women and providers and 7) health system conditions and constraints" (Bohren et al., 2015, p. 5). A complementary conceptualization is offered by Claire Michel and Claire Squires (2018), who described OGV according to two specific characteristics: not consensual and not justified.

Similarly, Birth Monopoly, a scientific organization that advocates for women's reproductive rights by focusing on obstetric violence manifestations, birth trauma experiences, and the dysfunction of the American model of maternity care, developed a pyramid of the gradation of OGV (Figure 7.1). This pyramid lists a variety of behaviours and practices considered to be OGV by those who experience them. People can rate the experience of no pain to the more serious forced Caesarean without medical reasons (Birth Monopoly, 2022). This model highlights aspects of the established feminist studies literature on gradations of violence and the insidious nature of the phenomenon.

The literature likewise reports numerous negative outcomes from these experiences: post-traumatic stress; negative impacts on the relationships with partner/s, sexual life, and the relationship with the newborn; and feelings of distress, anxiety, stress, suffering, insecurity and abandonment (Bowser & Hill, 2010; Hodnett, 2002; Olde et al., 2006; Schroll et al., 2013). Bohren et al. (2015) state that the experiences of mistreatment in maternity wards lead women to mistrust the healthcare system and choose to give birth outside of institutions and instead surrounded by supportive carers.

A key limitation of this growing literature on OGV is that it currently tends to focus on the experiences of childbirth and motherhood, neglecting other forms of sexual and reproductive health services as well as parenthood without heterosexual

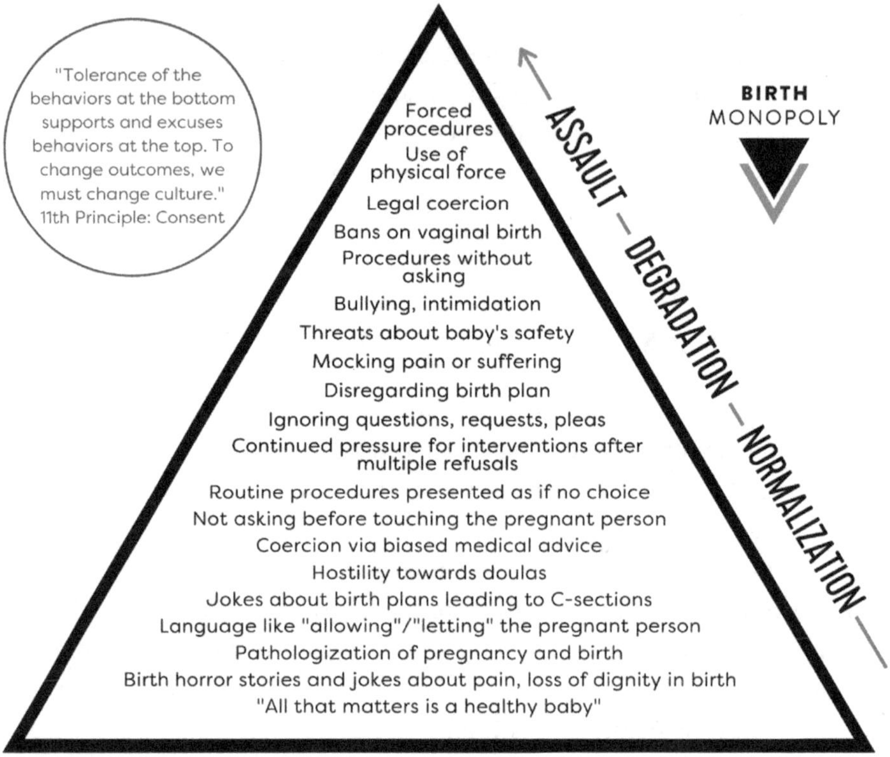

Figure 7.1. Pyramid of OGV

Image courtesy of Birth Monopoly (2022), https://birthmonopoly.com/obstetric-violence/

and cisgender female identity. This assumed connection with childbearing can serve to reinforce the intrinsic link between the social role and the natural function of bodies with uteruses. It is important to highlight how the roots of OGV may lie in this representation of social roles of women (Shabot, 2016). Feminist advocates and scholars encourage us to deconstruct these assumptions about the "nature" of women.

The existing literature on OGV also has yet to focus on the experiences of pregnancy and reproductive care beyond childbirth. We argue that an intersectional lens allows us to capture the more fulsome scope of the phenomenon. In addition, we assert that the discrimination and stigma associated with OGV also manifest in broader gynecological care and so OGV concerns more than obstetrical care services.

Assumed societal rules about parenting—as binary, heterosexual, cisgender, Euro/colonial, and supported by the medicolegal system—align femininity and maternity. Scholars such as Sara Cohen Shabot (2016, 2021) and Shabot and Keshet Korem (2018) argue that dominant conceptualizations of birthing bodies are restricted to heterosexuality and femininity. Even if we agree with these observations, we can raise how these arguments are cisnormative and fail to capture the reproductive constraints and barriers that prevent genderqueer people from becoming parents in their own ways. Western culture has traditionally presented pregnancy and childbirth as "strictly and exclusively female experiences and desires" (MacDonald et al., 2021, p. 18). Michelle Walks (2017) argues that there is an obsession with the traditional model of parenthood, specifically on the obligation to identify and meet female gender expression norms. Trevor Kirczenow MacDonald and colleagues (2021) point out that gender binarism restricts the desire to experience pregnancy exclusively in accordance with the female gender. In this order, using the neutral expression "birthing people" is insufficient to address the cisnormative nature of OGV conceptualization.

Consequently, the empirical literature on OGV has only focused on cisgender experiences of pregnancy and birthing and has not looked more fully into the literature on queer and trans experiences to uncover the larger scope of OGV from a genderqueer perspective. Heidi Moseson and colleagues (2020), for example, note that reproductive health research has always focused on cisgender women relative to this specific topic and thus has yet to generate relevant data for queer and trans people. This provides additional justification to open the discussion on OGV with reference to the literature on queer and trans experiences that expands OGV conceptualizations.

THE INTERSECTIONAL NATURE OF OGV

To support the need to intersect sexism with heteronormativity and cisnormativity, there is a need to expand the conversation beyond the actual comprehension of OGV with an intersectional approach. Intersectionality is used by feminist scholars to explain the variety of lived experiences of a singular phenomenon across different social identities, based on Kimberlé Crenshaw's (1991) theorizing of intersectionality as the interweaving of oppressive systems that amplifies lived discriminations. An intersectional lens allows us to look specifically at the sexist, heterosexist, and cissexist nature of OGV.[1] Although intersectionality recognizes the fluidity of various identities, Jasbir K. Puar (2007) enriches this conceptualization with *assemblage theory*, which was first developed by Deleuze and Guattari. Leah Warner and colleagues (2020) explain that this theory

> considers identity not as an attribute of individuals, but rather as an event or action, whereby a multitude of factors such as historical context, geographic location, and social context contribute to the experience of "identity." Thus, rather than orienting around identities,

> scholars orient around assemblages: patterns of affective, discursive, embodied, and material relations built around these events and actions. (p. 266)

In this sense, we believe that assemblage theory allows for a more global (historical, cultural, and political) context that supersedes individual social identities and thus allows a light to be shone on the systemic elements and effects of OGV.

Many have become interested in OGV from an intersectional lens, particularly concerning race, migration status, and class (Sadler et al., 2016; Vedam et al., 2017, 2019). Vedam and colleagues (2019) have demonstrated that in the United States,

> Indigenous women were the most likely to report experiencing at least one form of mistreatment by healthcare providers (32.8%), followed by Hispanic (25.0%) and Black women (22.5%). Women who identified as White were least likely to report that they experienced any of the mistreatment indicators (14.1%). (p. 8)

Some have focused on other intersections, such as Rachel Chadwick (2020), who explored the experiences of young mothers who are often infantilized and their capacity to mother minimized. Others point to the infantilization reported by parents living with disabilities; child protection services are often alerted by healthcare personnel because the parents are seen like children themselves (Rice et al., 2020). Little research has been undertaken on a genderqueer intersection despite some authors calling for us to broaden our perspectives to include sexual and gender identities in our research (Vedam et al., 2019).

OGV studies have yet to focus on the unique experiences of genderqueer people. Empirical analyses have shown the heterosexist and cissexist nature of the interaction with healthcare personnel, healthcare facilities, and social institutions more broadly (Burrow et al., 2018; Hoffkling et al., 2017; Light et al., 2017; Shankland & Abergel, 2022). Mari Greenfield and Zoe Darwin (2021) have conducted a scoping review showing that there is no research directly addressing traumatic birth and its related factors with genderqueer populations. This is a remarkable absence in the scientific literature given the high rates of postpartum depression in this population (Light et al., 2017), which may be attributed to OGV and the demonstrated connection between inappropriate behaviours and childbirth trauma (Rodríguez-Almagro et al., 2019).

THE MULTILAYERED NATURE OF OGV

We build on Diana Bowser and Kathleen Hill (2010), who argue that disrespect and abuse is a multilevel phenomenon, notably individual but also rooted in the structural and political dimension. Analyses of OGV have been slowly integrated into the literature, particularly in the social sciences, to make visible the systemic dimension of the phenomenon. The systems operate in function of dominant culture, influencing the perceptions and social norms conveyed by healthcare providers on the patients who need obstetric and gynecological care (Savage & Castro, 2017). In this regard, we first review the existing literature about cisnormative and heteronormative beliefs, discrimination, and stigma by healthcare personnel and the environment in which they are operating. Then, we point to the structural and political levels that twist the meaning of consent and the barriers associated with it.

THE EXPERIENCE OF OGV AT THE INDIVIDUAL LEVEL—THE ROLE OF HEALTHCARE PERSONNEL

Many studies report on negative healthcare experiences from queer and trans people's perspectives, notably in sexual and reproductive health (Dean et al., 2016; Light et al., 2017; Pyne, 2012; Shankland & Abergel, 2022; Wingo et al., 2018). The vulnerability of genderqueer people is reinforced by the heteronormative and cisnormative context (Burrow et al., 2018; Dean et al., 2016; Dutton et al., 2008; Wingo et al., 2018) and by the healthcare personnel not having specific skills with this population (Hoffkling et al., 2017) or not appropriately applying the skills they have (Wingo et al., 2018). In this regard, Alexis Hoffkling and colleagues (2017, p. 12) identify six components in this lack of competencies:

1. addressing the patient with the wrong title or pronoun
2. calling the patient by their legal name rather than the name they use
3. presuming to know the shape of a patient's genitals by their name or face
4. ignoring intake forms that ask patients' gender
5. presuming that a patient has, or should have, a given relationship with their body
6. discussing gender identity as though it is sexual orientation

Misgendering[2] is an explicit manifestation of stigmatization toward trans peoples, which can be part of the experience of OGV in Bohren and colleagues' (2015) categories of mistreatment during childbirth. The conceptualization of sex and gender as mutually exclusive by healthcare personnel reinforce the cisnormative assumptions of gender and of the role of a mother who is a cisgender woman, heterosexual, and feminine. This type of behaviour illustrates intolerance toward familial models outside of traditional norms and reinforces the global social system—and consequently the health system—as binary and normative (Shankland & Abergel, 2022).

Besides misgendering, some people are confronted by medical barriers to becoming parents. Many studies raise that queer and trans people would like to or judge important to be informed about the impacts of gender-affirmation therapies on their future reproductive options (Hoffkling et al., 2017; Light et al., 2017; Pyne, 2012; Shankland & Abergel, 2022). To make free and informed decisions, there is a need to have complete information, including what science knows and does not know (Hoffkling et al., 2017). One could argue that failing to inform patients about their reproductive options can be included as a form of OGV in that it *de facto* controls reproduction, circumscribing who can become a parent.

Some practices are insensitive to genderqueer realities and can cause unnecessary discomfort. For example, intrusive exams necessitate prolonged exposure of genital parts. In Hoffkling and colleagues (2017), the situation was described as having no medical basis, equating it to a form of medical voyeurism. The lack of sensitivity about gender for trans people and the pathologization and stigmatization attached to their identity can lead healthcare personnel to doubt trans people's ability to be parents, notably because of the association between femininity and mothering. Thus, humanizing obstetric and gynecological care needs to extend beyond a patient-centred approach and personalization of care to fully meet the needs of genderqueer people (Richardson et al., 2018).

Some question the objectivity of the terminology of OGV, how it is conceptualized in the literature, and how it inherently levels blame towards healthcare personnel (Swartz & Lappeman, 2021). Others recognize that healthcare personnel have difficulty seeing themselves as the perpetrators of these forms of violence because of the inherently risky nature of obstetric and gynecological practices (Jardim & Modena, 2018). Regardless of intent, it is necessary to analyze the systemic nature of individual acts that can be described as violent by those who experience them.

In sum, providing safe, competent, and appropriate medical care adapted to the realities of queer and trans people points to a need to use individualized and respectful language that recognizes genderqueer identities (Greenfield & Darwin, 2021). On the contrary, not adapting practices is a symptom of the cisnormative specificity of OGV.

OGV AT THE STRUCTURAL LEVEL: THE ROLE OF HEALTHCARE FACILITIES

Healthcare facilities are not exempt from gender discrimination ideology since they are structurally embedded within patriarchal and cisnormative social systems (Burrow et al., 2018; MacDonald et al. 2021). It is assumed that a person who needs obstetric and gynecological care is necessarily a woman. The forms in these units are not adapted to genderqueer people because from a heteronormative and cisnormative view, it is assumed that sex and gender are aligned, as discussed previously. Even when some clinics portend to integrate inclusive practices, healthcare personnel do not always apply these practices (Hoffkling et al., 2017), and sometimes they do not apply them correctly (Wingo et al., 2018). Similarly, hospital electronic systems are formatted in a way that categorizes services into those for "women" or "men" (Hoffkling et al., 2017; MacDonald et al., 2021). For example, MacDonald and colleagues (2021) reported that someone faced refusal to receive pain relief because the computer did not allow an order of anesthesia for a man.

Thus, healthcare facilities structure their expectations on heteronormative and cisnormative protocols and other procedures, and in doing so, genderqueer people are made to fit into dominant sexual norms (Burrow et al., 2018; MacDonald et al., 2021; Wingo et al., 2018). In this regard, birthing rooms can be recognized as historical and political places constructed on heteronormativity and cisnormativity (Burrow et al., 2018; Dutton et al., 2008; MacDonald et al., 2021; Walks, 2005, 2014), and consequently they devalue the experiences of genderqueer people because the latter do not conform to femininity standards. For example, the birth planning unit environment is largely cisgender and reflects the expectations of femininity toward birthing people, with posters exclusively about women and the right way to parent, as well as a lack of all-gender bathrooms (Pyne, 2012). These places create discomfort, because little documentation is adapted to genderqueer people (Pyne, 2012) and consequently fails to be inclusive (Burrow et al., 2018), exacerbating their feelings of disrespect and isolation (Greenfield & Darwin, 2021). Being in such unsafe places can increase traumatic experiences because of a structural lack of recognition (Greenfield & Darwin, 2021; Pyne 2012).

Confronted with these numerous stereotypes, the literature on OGV reports that birthing people activate defence mechanisms to confront trauma by withdrawing themselves from the birthing process to protect themselves and their newborn (Briceño Morales et al., 2018). Some prefer to silence themselves as a queer or trans person to get through it, while others affirm their identities (Dean et al., 2016; Light et al., 2017; Walks, 2005). Being permanently out increases their vulnerability, and the possibility of being assigned into femininity by healthcare personnel can be seen as a form of OGV based on discrimination and stigmatization. Also, it has been documented that some trans individuals choose a homebirth or an elective Caesarean to control the circumstances of their birth (Greenfield & Darwin, 2021). This situation shows that the options are limited and that the chosen one is not necessarily by full and free consent.

The individual and structural levels can also be deconstructed to reveal the broader social organization of women's roles, already well defined in the literature.

Intersecting the notions of consent and control in OGV literature with the role of authoritative institutions allows us to question the meaning of consent in a social context that prohibits some people from existing authentically.

OGV AT A POLITICAL LEVEL: THE ROLE OF AUTHORITATIVE INSTITUTIONS

Examining OGV at the political level enables us to locate the roots of the phenomenon from queer and trans perspectives. Walks (2014) argues that many Canadian and provincial policies have historically discriminated against genderqueer people by stratifying those who can and cannot have children. The state demonstrates control of who can be a mother and what they should look like: heterosexual, cisgender, and most of all feminine. Walks (2014, p. 77) mobilizes Colen's (1986, 1995) analysis to support that there are "expectations and respect related to *biological* reproduction, but also to the physical, emotional, and mental labour of raising or enculturing children." Historically, all provinces and territories obligated trans people to undergo gender reassignment surgery to change their legal gender identified by the state. While these barbaric practices are no longer in place, the Quebec Caquist government (2018–present) tried to reinstate this obligation with Bill 2, An Act respecting family law reform about filiation, and amending the Civil Code in relation to personality rights and civil status by awkwardly distinguishing sex and gender.[3] This type of policy toward queer and trans people is rooted in OGV since it is a means to control their reproductive capacities to obtain legal recognition of their gender. The government addressed the criticisms by revising Bill 2 to further respect the reproductive autonomy and rights of queer and trans people.

Damien W. Riggs and Clare Bartholomaeus (2020) introduce the concept of trans reproductive justice to explain how obstetric and gynecological care controls who should have children:

> to ensure that reproductive justice narratives are inclusive of transgender and non-binary people, Nixon (2013) suggests that such narratives must go beyond abortion, and instead also focus on the intersectional aspects of reproduction that can stop transgender and non-binary people from being able to: (1) have children when they want to and (2) parent their children. (p. 316)

Thus, acts of imposed sterilization can be conceived as reproductive violence, lacking regard for bodily autonomy by the state and as a manifestation of cisnormativity. Indeed, we assert that the literature and analysis of OGV should more directly address trans reproductive justice, moving beyond feminine representations to address the systemic level and its effects beyond a cisgender lens.

These overarching reproductive social norms constrain what should be free and informed consent. Indeed, the fact that discrimination and stigmatization create barriers for some people in their reproductive options is another political manifestation of OGV. Being forced to choose certain reproductive options to avoid cissexist violence does not allow for free decision making. In this sense, we argue that the notion of consent is not applicable in such a binary and exclusive cultural context because not all options are truly available.

OGV can be seen as an instrument for reinforcing normativity that perpetuates the inferiority of bodies with uteruses and discourages genderqueer people from obtaining and exercising bodily autonomy. The exclusion of their realities and experiences is a sign of intolerance and stigmatization. Understanding the scope and meaning of OGV from a queer and trans perspective highlights the impacts of heterosexism and cissexism on sexual and reproductive health inequalities and power relations.

CONCLUSION

The recognition of the multilayered nature of OGV requires changes at interpersonal, structural, and political levels to enable a more inclusive and fulsome conceptualization of gender-based violence (Katz et al., 2020; Savage & Castro, 2017). OGV is normalized because of the natural appearance of patriarchal and cisgender norms and their internalization by healthcare personnel and by every birthing body.

Cultural images of women and motherhood impose a specific reproduction status allowing control of bodily autonomy as well as abuse and coercive norms on bodies and sexualities (Briceño-Morales et al., 2018; Jardim & Modena, 2018; Sadler, 2016; Shabot, 2016). Sexual and reproductive health research has mainly focused on cisgender women who were mostly heterosexual, and as such it has generated little relevant data for queer, trans, and non-binary individuals (Moseson et al., 2020). From explicitly queer and trans perspectives, we unpack the ways in which homophobia and transphobia amplify and broaden experiences of OGV.

We argue for extending categorization of the phenomenon outside of motherhood and to consider a bigger picture as part of the solution. A perspective more inclusive of queer and trans experiences allows us to capture the phenomenon even before the possibility to become pregnant to conceptualize it as also encompassing reproductive care. The conceptualization of OGV should include the appropriation and the control of the bodily autonomy of people with uteruses at any stage of life and any types of sexual and reproductive healthcare and services. This chapter contributes to a larger understanding of OGV by taking into consideration genderqueer experiences of sexual and reproductive healthcare and services.

QUESTIONS FOR CRITICAL THOUGHT

1. Which OGV characteristics highlight the heteronormative and cisnormative nature of motherhood?
2. Is empowerment possible in obstetric and gynecological care and services for queer and trans people in a heteronormative and cisnormative healthcare system?
3. How does intersectionality allow us to capture the discriminatory roots of OGV?
4. Is it possible to change obstetric and gynecological service structures without generating social change in the comprehension of parenthood?

KEY TERMS

obstetric and gynecological violence (OGV)
maternity care
sexual and reproductive healthcare and services
queer and trans experiences
genderqueer

SUGGESTED FURTHER READINGS

1. Burrow, S., Goldberg, L., Searle, J., & Aston, M. (2018). Vulnerability, harm, and compromised ethics revealed by the experiences of queer birthing women in rural healthcare. *Journal of Bioethical Inquiry*, *15*(4), 511–524. https://doi.org/10.1007/s11673-018-9882-5
2. Greenfield, M., & Darwin, Z. (2021). Trans and non-binary pregnancy, traumatic birth, and perinatal mental health: A scoping review. *International Journal of Transgender Health*, *22*(1–2), 203–216. https://doi.org/10.1080/26895269.2020.1841057
3. Sadler, M., Santos, M. J., Ruiz-Berdún, D., Rojas, G. L., Skoko, E., Gillen, P., & Clausen, J. A. (2016). Moving beyond disrespect and abuse: Addressing the structural dimensions of obstetric violence. *Reproductive Health Matters*, *24*(47), 47–55. https://doi.org/10.1016/j.rhm.2016.04.002
4. Walks, M. (2014). Stratified reproduction: Making the case for butch lesbian's, transmen's and genderqueer individual's experiences in British Columbia. In S. Paterson, F. Scale, & M. K. Sokolon (Eds.), *Fertile ground: Exploring reproduction in Canada* (74–93). McGill-Queen's University Press.

NOTES

1. The phenomenon of intersectionality was first developed by Combahee River Collective (Ross, 2017) before academia appropriated it. This advocate group of Black American women pointed to the universalization of sexist and misogynist experiences around privileged white women. In doing so, the simultaneous effects of sexism, racism, and class were excluded from feminist fights.
2. Misgendering is the violent practice of addressing someone with the wrong pronoun, and it refuses to recognize a person's gender identity and strengthens the association between sex and gender. It may cause distress or gender dysphoria to trans, non-binary, and genderqueer individuals.
3. It should also be noted that the minister of justice, Simon Jolin-Barrette, who is responsible for the reform of family law, is also responsible for the fight against homophobia and transphobia.

CHAPTER 8

Black Feminism in Critical Public Health Research, Policy, and Programming: Theory and Practice for Promoting the Health and Well-being of Black Women

Tola Mbulaheni, Fiqir Worku, Falan Bennett, Nakia Lee-Foon, and Kimberly Robinson

LEARNING OBJECTIVES

1. Describe the historical and social contexts that shape the realities of Black communities and contribute to Black women's health disparities in Canada.
2. Employ a Black feminist approach to (re)orient understandings of social and health inequities faced by Black women.
3. Prompt critical reflection of current policy environments and considerations for effective policy responses to redress Black women's health inequities.

INTRODUCTION

Central to a public health feminist approach to program and policy responses is thinking critically of women's relationships to power when examining their health inequalities. Yet racialized forms of gendered power that sustain these inequalities for Black women remain peripheral in feminist discourses across the health sciences. Poorer health outcomes are further disconnected from Black women's experiences of intersectional marginalization and their knowledge towards redressing it. In this chapter, we begin by situating anti-Black racism as a legacy of slavery and colonization and make strong connections to Black women's present-day social realities. We present core principles of a Black feminist framework to support reconceptualizing Black women's health in Canada. We apply these principles to case studies focused on reproductive health, personal support work and the COVID-19 pandemic, and HIV/AIDS to critically consider how they can help us reframe health inequities and inform policy considerations and recommendations.

In presenting this critical examination, it is important to note that the social realities of Black women are often under/mis/unrepresented in scientific literature due to multiple barriers that impede the production of knowledge, particularly within a Canadian context. We hold that the structural discrimination shaping the disparate health outcomes of Black women also shape research institutions and processes that sustain barriers to meaningful research. While we actively and intentionally cite Black (feminist) and Canadian scholarship, remaining knowledge gaps reflect a paucity of literature rather than a lack of citational and scientific rigour.

PART 1: A BRIEF HISTORY OF BLACK PEOPLE IN CANADA

Black Migrations/Displacements into Canada

Black populations have been migrating into Canada from around the world since the 17th century and have actively contributed to Canadian society since their arrival. The first known person of Black-African descent to set foot in Canada was Mathieu de Coste (Winks, 1997). Arriving in 1608, de Coste was an interpreter of the Mi'kmaq language for the governor of Acadia—a region that encompassed parts of the current-day Maritime provinces (Winks, 1997). After the American Revolutionary War, thousands of Black people who sided with the British Crown were granted emancipation from enslavement and safe passage into Canada (Walker, 1992). Many of these now-emancipated people settled in Acadia while others, who remained enslaved, came to Canada with their Loyalist enslavers. From 1783 to 1785, over 3,000 free Black people settled in Nova Scotia, the Prairie provinces, and other parts of Canada, where they built vibrant communities despite encountering hostility, racial segregation, poor working conditions, and social inequality (Hill, 1992; Vernon, 2020).

Transatlantic Slavery: A Canadian Institution

Although Canada is often framed as having been a safe haven for Black peoples escaping enslavement in the United States, the country has its own violent history of slavery, which was practised in Canada for over two hundred years. In the early period of colonization, enslaved Black people were a legalized source of exploited labour towards expanding Canada's economic growth (Winks, 1997). Black women were specifically valued for their ability to reproduce Black children as property (Elgersman, 2013). A commonly perpetuated myth is that people enslaved in Canada were treated better than their American and Caribbean counterparts. However, many were subjected to physical, sexual, and psychological violence at the hands of their enslavers. Yet they resisted in various ways. Some briefly left their enslaver's property without permission, feigned illness to get out of forced labour, or ran away in pursuit of freedom (Cooper, 2007). Slavery was later abolished across the British Empire (which included present-day Canada) in 1834 (Winks, 1997).

Flows of Black Migration

Migrations of Black people into Canada from the United States continued until the early 20th century. In 1910, migration was thwarted when the Canadian government implemented the Immigration Act, which limited the entry of Black and other racialized populations as they were deemed "undesirable races" (Kelley & Trebilcock, 2000). Black migration increased slightly with the introduction of the West Indian Domestic Scheme (Lawson, 2013). This program allowed single women from Caribbean countries to be employed as domestic workers as a pathway to citizenship (Henry, 1968). It was not until 1967 that the Canadian government eliminated race-based immigration laws, which prompted a significant increase in immigration from African and diaspora countries (Kelley & Trebilcock, 2000). The points-based immigration system prompted greater economic migration by skilled workers who were highly ranked based on education, age, and knowledge of Canada's official languages. Over 40% of Black newcomers came to Canada through this economic program between 2011 and 2016 (Statistics Canada, 2019).

Transatlantic slavery and colonization have fundamentally shaped Black people's presence in Canada and laid the groundwork for its current political, social, and economic infrastructure. These institutions undergird anti-Black racism, which informs how Black people are perceived and treated within immigration, employment, healthcare, and other social institutions shaping their life opportunities and health outcomes (Maynard, 2017).

PART 2: SOCIAL REALITIES OF BLACK WOMEN IN CANADA

Social Realities of Black Women in Canada: The Research Gaps

The social realities of Black women are fundamentally influenced by histories of anti-Black racism in their gendered forms. However, research that speaks to racial inequalities often takes a generalized approach, inadvertently erasing the unique impact of such disparities on Black women (Collins, 2002). It is important to note that there is even less data on Black women who navigate queerphobia, transphobia, disability, and other systems of oppression. However, the research available strongly supports that Black women face extensive barriers navigating immigration, education, and employment. Consequently, they experience disproportionate levels of poverty and poorer health outcomes (Statistics Canada, 2020a).

Immigration

In 2016, immigrants comprised 21.9% of the Canadian population and in the same year, 13.4% of recent immigrants were born in Africa, a percentage four times higher than reported in the 1971 census (3.2%) (Statistics Canada, 2017). Thus, describing immigration and settlement in Canada and how it shapes the lives of immigrant and Canadian-born Black women is essential to characterizing their social realities.

Black women who come to Canada as economic immigrants are often deskilled via the non-recognition of foreign credentials, their lack of "Canadian experience," and discrimination due to their accents. They are subsequently, streamlined into employment that doesn't reflect their training, skills, or experiences (Creese & Wiebe, 2012). Considering these factors, Black women are more likely to navigate employment precarity and difficult economic environments that create multiple barriers to achieving a higher socioeconomic standing.

Many Black women also come to Canada as refugees and refugee claimants. Immigration policies and settlement practices can foster structural barriers to the equitable integration of Black immigrant women into Canadian society (Mooten, 2021).

Education

Narrated experiences of Black women and girls make clear that intersectional discrimination plays a fundamental role in their engagement with Canada's education system (Neeganagwedgin, 2013). They identify differential treatment, lack of Afrocentric curriculum, and the absence of Black teachers as prominent issues. Further, they are more likely to be streamed into general and basic-level academic programs despite demonstrated ability and achievement (Human Rights Council, 2017). This systemic discrimination at the primary and secondary education level creates barriers to attaining post-secondary education and ultimately affects employment opportunities and income-earning potential. However, data show that both immigrant and Canadian-born Black women are achieving post-secondary education at increasingly higher rates (Statistics Canada, 2020b).

Employment

Despite high levels of post-secondary education and representation in the labour market, Black women faced a 10% unemployment rate in 2016, compared to 6% for women in the rest of the population (Statistics Canada, 2020b). When employed, there is often a high rate of overqualification, as 25% of Black women with a university degree in Toronto worked in a position only requiring a secondary diploma (Stapleton, 2019). Moreover, employment is often precariously characterized by low pay, with few prospects of upward mobility (Block, Galabuzi & Tranjan 2019). The pay gap was exceptionally wide, as Black women were paid 59 cents for every dollar non-racialized men were paid (Katshunga & Massaquoi, 2019). Data suggests that they do not fare better intergenerationally. Black women exhibited the highest rates of becoming the working poor in subsequent generations. Between 2006 and 2016, the rate of working poverty among Black women rose from 9.7% to 12.2% (Statistics Canada, 2020b).

Health Inequalities

Research increasingly demonstrates that the effects of racism and other forms of systemic discrimination over the life course adversely impact the health and well-being of Black women in Canada (Human Rights Council, 2017). The available data show that they are disproportionately represented in the national rates for diabetes, cardiovascular disease, and hypertension (Chiu et al., 2015; Veenstra & Patterson, 2015) and that racial discrimination plays a critical factor in sustaining these disparities (Siddiqi et al., 2017). The differential impacts of the ongoing HIV/AIDS and COVID-19 pandemics have also been documented (Massaquoi et al., 2021). Overall, the multiple and intersecting forms of discrimination that Black women navigate sustain poorer health outcomes and access to quality care.

PART 3: (RE)CONCEPTUALIZING BLACK WOMEN'S HEALTH INEQUITIES: A BLACK FEMINIST FRAMEWORK

A Black (Canadian) Feminist Framework

Black feminist thought is a political and intellectual intervention that aims to paradigmatically shift how Black women are constructed and treated in society. It emerged from a genealogy of thought and activism rooted in the experiences, oppressions, and resistances of Black women (Collins, 2008). Black Canadian feminist thought specifically illustrates the structural contexts of Canada and the ways it uniquely shapes the experiences of Black Canadian women (Massaquoi & Wane, 2007). For example, immigrants comprised about half of the Black population in 2016 (Statistics Canada, 2019). Thus, the ways Canada's immigration policies and practices sustain discrimination and social exclusion for Black Canadian women is integral to redressing their social and health inequities.

Principles of a Black Feminist Framework

We articulate the following core principles in defining our use of a Black feminist framework (BFF) in this chapter.

1. Standpoint Epistemology

Standpoint epistemology holds that social groups who experience marginalization are best positioned to make claims about its meanings and impacts (Richie, 2012). This principle asserts that Black women occupy a social location that affords them the expertise to describe the discrimination they experience and the impact it has on their health and lives (Collins, 2007). Therefore, centring Black women and their experiential knowledge offers a more accurate analysis of the issues, better informing changes to institutional policy and practice (Richie, 2012). Standpoint epistemology also challenges conventional understandings of who is positioned as "the expert." It further requires locating this authority with experiential knowledge holders which is typically conferred on researchers, policymakers, and others who do not have embodied access to this standpoint (Collins, 2007). This principle highlights the importance of centring Black feminist epistemologies in the development and implementation of public health responses and Black women playing a leadership role in these endeavours.

To employ standpoint epistemology, we, the authors (Black women, graduate and postdoctoral scholars, and Black feminist thinkers), intentionally ground the contents of this chapter within Black (feminist) scholarship. We draw from both traditional sources of data (e.g., epidemiological data), as well as qualitatively informed evidence including the narrated experiences, perspectives, and histories of Black women.

2. Intersectional Thinking

Intersectionality, a term coined by Kimberlé Crenshaw (1989), emerged from the standpoint epistemology of Black women's historical and ongoing experiences of discrimination and activism, traditionally excluded from white feminist and anti-racist movements (Combahee River Collective, 1983). Intersectionality acknowledges how multiple, interlocking, social identities (race, gender, sexuality, immigration status, etc.) shape the distinct experiences, marginalizations, and privileges of diverse groups of people. Conceptualizing Black women's health intersectionally also requires examining their structural environments, which comprise interconnected systems of oppression (e.g., racism, sexism, queerphobia, immigration systems). A BFF holds that an intersectional approach is vital to understanding the diverse and differential impacts of social and health inequities on Black women's lives.

This chapter aims to elucidate how these systems and institutions not only converge to sustain discrimination, but also differentially impact Black women's social realities, configure health risks, and inform their related decision making.

3. Social Construction of Black Womanhood

"Controlling images" are stereotypes that are used to misrepresent a group of people based on discriminatory ideas of them (Collins, 2002). Dominant ideas of Black women are tacitly held to be genetic or biologically inherited traits rather than socially constructed beliefs rooted in histories of slavery and colonization. These stereotypes have been mainstreamed and influence how they are perceived and treated across institutions in Canadian society (education, healthcare, criminal justice, immigration, etc.). By critically situating social and health inequities within larger structural and social frameworks and calling attention to the ways controlling images are operationalized, this chapter asserts that Black women's health outcomes are a product of systemic discrimination rather than inherent "deficiencies."

It is imperative to discuss how medicine (and the health sciences more broadly) have played an integral role in not only animating these ideas of Black women in research and practice, but also rationalizing them through a "scientific" logic (Gilman, 1985). This long history of medical racism perpetuates negative stereotypes of Black women as hypersexual, socially immoral, clinically non-compliant, and pain tolerant. Examining social constructs of Black womanhood also exposes the ways stereotypes are deeply entrenched within healthcare systems, shaping the care they receive and their subsequent health outcomes.

We highlight how these long-standing notions of Black women continue to shape how they are constructed in Canadian society and inform the social structures that marginalize them.

4. Social Justice/Action-Oriented Approach

A social justice orientation affirms that activism is an integral part of knowledge generation rather than antithetical to it (Ritche, 2014). This orientation provides an interpretive framework for approaching the production of knowledge as a tool for political and social change. The purpose of social justice as a Black feminist praxis in public health is to produce action to ultimately dismantle the oppressive systems that keep Black women and all disenfranchised communities marginalized. We assert policy recommendations grounded within a BFF towards supporting a social-justice, action-oriented approach to knowledge discussed in this chapter.

PART 4: CASE STUDIES: APPLICATIONS OF A BLACK FEMINIST FRAMEWORK

Introduction

We apply a BFF to three case studies that discuss specific health issues and their impacts on Black women. The case studies aim to demonstrate how a BFF can support a conceptual shift in how we think about and respond to Black women's health inequities. We implicate policy in structurally shaping poorer health outcomes for Black women and provide policy recommendations towards redressing them.

Case Study 1: (Re)conceptualizing Black Women's Reproductive Health: A Reproductive Justice Model

In this case study, we discuss why shifting from a reproductive rights to a reproductive justice (RJ) model is necessary for informing policy that rectifies Black women's reproductive health inequities (Richie, 2012; Ross & Solinger, 2017). The lack of scientific data on the state of reproductive health for Black women in Canada is striking and also serves as a structural barrier to developing effective policy. Yet we know that 8.9% of Black babies born in this country were preterm in 2016, compared to 5.9% for their white counterparts (McKinnon et al., 2016). Although the rates in the United States are markedly higher (12.7% and 8.0%, respectively) (McKinnon et al., 2016), it is clear that the racial *disparity* of preterm births in Canada is comparable. However, we assert that Black women's reproductive health extends far beyond concerns of conception, fertility, and the perinatal period and encompasses social and health issues related to parent- and childhood. This case study applies a reproductive justice approach towards conceptually shifting what constitutes reproductive health and how we critically engage related issues pertinent to Black women. We specifically speak to the ways their reproductive health is shaped by intersectional systems of oppression (racism, sexism, classism, etc.) and how they inhibit their capacity to freely and safely parent their children across the life course.

Histories Informing the Reproductive Health of Black Women

It is important to emphasize that reproductive health disparities are a legacy of slavery as Black women have historically lacked personal bodily autonomy and parental decision-making power (Hogarth, 2017). During enslavement, their sexuality and reproductive capacities were controlled and exploited; their agency to choose sexual partners, to become or stay pregnant, and to parent the children they gave birth to was denied (Ross & Solinger, 2017). Further, Black women's bodies have been sites of violent medical experimentations that were foundational to developing the fields of obstetrics and gynecology (Owens & Fett, 2019).

Reproductive Rights and Reproductive Justice

A reproductive rights framework is conceptually premised on the legal rights of the individual. Policy discourses in Canada have limited their purview to the individual's right to access contraceptives and safe abortions. However, this framework presumes individual agency free of systemic barriers that inform access. While one's right to an abortion is protected under the Canadian Charter of Rights and Freedoms, it is implied that one is therefore *able* to freely access this procedure

Anarcha, Lucy, and Betsey ... and Nine Others

Between 1845 and 1849, 12 enslaved Black women—Anarcha, Lucy, Betsey, and nine others—survived and supported one another through experimentations without anesthesia. Conducted by Dr. James Marion Sims (1813–1883), these atrocities led to the development of procedures and tools that established modern gynecology (Dudley, 2016). Such experimentations were accepted at the time due to common beliefs that Black people held a "subhuman" status (Hogarth, 2017). While medical racism is implicated in Black women's poorer reproductive health outcomes, this particular history of modern medicine is often not considered in discourses of reproductive rights.

(Stettner, Burnett & Hay, 2017). Critically reflecting on the historical and social contexts that not only structurally impede Black women's access to such reproductive health services but also influence their ability to birth and parent altogether, it becomes evident that operationalizing a reproductive rights framework cannot provide equitable access to the rights Black women need and have been historically denied. It further negates the multiple barriers they face across the life course as parents.

Examining Black women's reproductive health instead compels us to engage reproductive justice (RJ). RJ is a social justice framework used to interrogate the web of structural and systemic conditions in which reproductive health is embedded (Richie, 2012; Ross & Solinger, 2017). Defined and conceptualized by Black feminists in 1994, RJ holds that anti-Black racism, patriarchy, and other forms of oppression intersect and manifest through systems that structure our political, economic, and social lives. The three primary tenets of RJ are the right to not have a child, the right to have a child, and the right to parent children in safe and healthy environments. To achieve these rights, RJ asserts the need to examine the totality of reproductive experiences beyond abortion and contraceptives (Ross & Solinger, 2017). Therefore, Black women's lifelong experiences of parenthood (and the experiences of their children) are integral to a RJ framework. When we then expand the scope of reproductive rights to include the right to parent within a larger social context, institutions across Canadian society become strongly implicated. We assert that the child welfare system, for example, becomes a legitimate and necessary site of both critical interrogation and intervention if reproductive justice for Black women is to be recognized.

Impeding the Right to Safely and Freely Parent: The Child Welfare System

It is important to state that controlling images strongly factor into conceptions of Black motherhood. These social constructs often portray Black women as unfit, lone parents of an inherently dysfunctional household (Collins, 2007). Black women are thus often thought of and treated as bad mothers by society and by the state in particular. Grounded in these ideas of respectability and morality is a long history of the state surveilling Black families in Canada, often resulting in the systematic removal of children/youth from the home (Maynard, 2018).

One of the major barriers to realizing RJ's third tenet for Black women is exemplified through the similarly disproportionate representation of Black children in Canada's child welfare system. Black youth are reported to continuously be overrepresented in child protective services in Western countries, naming racial discrimination at the intersection of gender and socioeconomic status as a significant factor (Cénat et al., 2021). This disparity often denies them a supportive family environment. While there continues to be a dearth of data, we know that in Toronto in 2016, 40.8% of children in state care were Black although they comprised only 8.5% of the city's population (Turner, 2016). Black families were more likely than their white counterparts to be investigated by child welfare services (King et al., 2017) and to be retained in care (Turner, 2016). Further, Black children were at higher risk of experiencing abuse, neglect, and violence in alternative care (United Nations Committee on the Rights of the Child [UNCRC], 2022). These data support narratives from diverse Black communities detailing their extensive experiences of discrimination when in contact with the child welfare system (Ontario Human Rights Commission, 2018).

Anti-Black racism, sexism, and poverty have created a web of structural marginalizations that converge on Black mothers and their families through state surveillance and discrimination by child welfare workers. RJ holds that a critical examination of the child welfare system, along with other systems that are complicit in criminalizing Black families (Perrit, 2020), is fundamental to understanding Black women being unable to parent in safe and healthy environments. Furthermore, RJ emphasizes the continuity of criminalization targeting Black families. Carceral overrepresentation occurs beyond the child welfare system and extends to imprisonment in adulthood. Data from Public Safety Canada (2022) reports that between 2019 and 2020, Black people were 8.1% of incarcerated individuals despite comprising only 3.5% of Canada's population (Statistics Canada, 2019).

Policy Recommendations/Considerations

Policy recommendations/considerations include but are not limited to

- Funding and implementing Black Family and Child Services agencies that handle child welfare cases involving Black youth from a community-centred, pro-Black feminist, and intersectional lens (Turner, 2016)
- Requiring child welfare agencies to engage Black Child and Family Services agencies in cases involving Black families (Turner, 2016)
- As a preventative measure, provide/refer Black families to support services, including counselling and community-based programs/resources (UNCRC, 2022)

Case Study 2: The Continued Exploitation of Black Women in Care Work

In this case study, we discuss how immigration pathways have and continue to streamline Black women into care work, an industry that precariously employs and exploits their labour. We underscore how precursory immigration programs draw Black women into Canada's care economy, specifically as personal support workers (PSWs). A BFF implicates this long history of precarious work and immigration status, converging on the care industry, in creating conditions for Black women's health risks during the COVID-19 pandemic. This case study facilitates critical thinking about COVID-19 vulnerabilities beyond individual/interpersonal risk/behaviours and identifies immigration policy and workers' rights as integral to addressing the disparate effects of the pandemic on Black women's lives.

Streamlining Black Women into the Precarity of Care Work

The current state of the care economy, at the intersection of immigration, reflects long-standing policies and practices that exploit Black and racialized labour and maintain barriers to acquiring permanent immigration status in Canada. Care work can be defined as activities undertaken to maintain the health and well-being of others in private or public settings and can incorporate paid or unpaid work (Canadian Women's Foundation [CWF] et al., 2020). Legacies of slavery and domestic servitude have informed the care work infrastructure in Canada, systemically gendering and racializing care work through its immigration pathways. Racialized women continue to make up the backbone of the country's care sector, an industry that is sustained by employment and immigration precarity, low wages, and limited access to and enforcement of workers' rights. The current infrastructure of Canada's care economy is a major contributor to the social realities of poverty for Black women and their subsequent health and well-being (CWF et al., 2020).

Black Women and the West Indian Domestic Scheme in Canada

In 1955, the Department of Citizenship and Immigration initiated the West Indian Domestic Scheme (WIDS) as a pathway to citizenship. This program targeted Black women from the Caribbean to migrate for work as domestic workers in the homes of Canadians (Henry, 1968). Women were eligible if they were single, aged between 18 and 35, childless, in possession of at least an 8th grade education, and considered to be of a "high moral character" (Lawson, 2013). While WIDS supported the migration of Black women and their families, they also faced challenging and exploitative working conditions, including enduring racial discrimination and being overworked and underpaid (Parks Canada, 2022). Although the WIDS formally ended in 1967, the program's criteria remained in place well into the 1970s and continued to recruit Caribbean women for domestic labour (Lawson, 2013). The program was eventually replaced by a points-based system that granted temporary work permits. For years thereafter, Black women continued to migrate to Canada for domestic work through this system. It is notable that this immigration policy has since evolved and continues to channel Black and other racialized women into the precarity of Canada's care economy (Foster, 2021). Extending beyond domestic workers, this sector now includes PSWs and live-in caregivers (CWF et al., 2020) and continues to sustain conditions that foster employment and immigration status insecurity.

The Impacts of Precarious Employment and COVID-19 on Black PSWs

The COVID-19 pandemic has exemplified not only the necessity but also the precarity of care work in Canada and its adverse impacts on workers' health and well-being. Racialized women distinctly make up a significant portion of the PSW workforce in Canada (Lum, Ying & Sladek, 2015). One study reported that 35.7% of healthcare workers who tested positive for COVID-19 were women (compared to men, who comprised 9.2%) and of these women, 44.9% were immigrants or refugees (Guttman et al., 2020).

"Save the Seven"

In a landmark case, seven Jamaican women who entered Canada in the mid-1970s under terms similar to the WIDS's were to be deported on the charge that they had not disclosed their family status as mothers. Elaine Peart, one of the seven, stated that "we were brought here to clean rich folks' homes and now we're not cleaning rich folks' homes so you want to throw us out" (Leah & Morgan, 1979). Their case garnered a great deal of public attention under the slogan "Save the Seven" and symbolized the exploitative nature of immigration policy and the expendability of Black women's labour. This case has also highlighted the controlling images informing the WIDS that dually perceive Black women as natural caregivers and inevitable single mothers (and thus future burdens on Canada's resources) in need of moral management by the state (Lawson, 2013).

Several recent studies have highlighted the ways that the health and well-being of Black PSWs in particular have been negatively impacted by the pandemic (Ahmed et al., 2021; Hapsari et al., 2022; Pinto et al., 2022). In these studies, Black PSWs comprised the majority of the sample and most were women and immigrants (often without citizenship). A substantive segment were precariously employed. A disproportionate number of Black PSWs were employed in long-term care facilities, a site of increased prevalence and mortality rates (Ahmed et al., 2021; Pinto et al., 2022). They subsequently were at higher risk of contracting COVID-19, and no access to paid sick days or extended health benefits compelled many to continue working despite testing positive (Pinto et al., 2022). A lack of a financial safety net further impacted their ability to stay home and fully recover. Many PSWs experienced extreme fatigue due to understaffing and increased workloads as well as inadequate wage increases and delays in compensation (Hapsari et al., 2022). PSWs also navigated limited access to personal protective equipment (Hapsari et al., 2022) and infrequent COVID testing (Sathiyamoorthy, 2020).

The cumulative dangers of this role puts Black women PSWs at greater risk of exposure to COVID-19 (Mianda, 2020). These effects are compounded at the intersection of economic and immigration insecurity that characterizes so many PSWs' lives. Although care work has been critically important to the maintenance of Canada's healthcare system, particularly throughout the pandemic, it meets few of the decent work indicators set by the International Labour Organization (2022) and puts the health of Black women at greater risk. The similar working environments currently imposed on PSWs to those of Black women domestic workers recruited through the WIDS program demonstrate the ways care work is continually undervalued along with those who undertake it.

Policy Recommendations/Considerations

Policy recommendations/considerations include but are not limited to

- Permanently increasing wages to rates comparable to other healthcare workers (Workers Action Centre [WAC], 2020)
- Providing paid sick leave and health benefits for PSWs and other low-wage care work (WAC, 2020)
- Establishing provincial regulatory bodies for PSWs to develop legislated healthcare practices, standardize training and educational programs, and provide oversight for workers' rights violations (the Government of Ontario recently introduced the Health and Supportive Care Providers Oversight Authority Act, 2021)

Case Study 3: Erasure of Black Women's Risk in HIV Prevention Discourses

Structural barriers greatly contribute to Black women's suboptimal access to biomedical HIV prevention interventions (e.g., HIV testing, pre-exposure prophylaxis, antiretroviral therapy). In this case study, the Canadian guideline for pre-exposure prophylaxis and the national HIV surveillance system will be examined to exemplify Black women's erasure from prevention discourses and interventions. Policy recommendations centre the prevention needs and gaps for Black women.

The Disproportionate Impact of HIV on Black Women

In its fourth decade, the current public health response to the HIV epidemic in Canada includes extensive epidemiological research and the delivery of innovative biomedical HIV prevention interventions (e.g., HIV testing). However, HIV continues to disproportionately impact Black communities, particularly Black women. In 2019, Black people made up 25.5% of all reported HIV cases in Canada (Haddad et al., 2021) while comprising only 4.3% of the country's population (Statistics Canada, 2022). In the same year, Black women accounted for 42.1% of all reported HIV cases among women (Haddad et al., 2021).

Social Realities Shaping HIV Risk and Prevention

Black women's aforementioned social realities in Canada fundamentally shape their HIV risk environments (Tharao & Massaquoi, 2001). These social and economic conditions can, for example, increase their financial dependence on male partners and limit their ability to autonomously negotiate safer sex practices, thereby increasing HIV risk (Williams et al., 2009). Their realities also sustain access barriers to HIV prevention services, despite higher prevalence rates (Logie et al., 2018). However, what is often not considered are the discursive practices that precede service delivery and how they erase Black women in HIV prevention research and policymaking. These discourses inform how services are designed and, ultimately, for whom they are designed. The subsequent marginalization of Black women in service provision can profoundly affect their HIV risk and overall health outcomes.

Erasure of Black Women's Risk from PrEP Discourses

Biomedical HIV prevention technologies are medical interventions that aim to reduce the risk of HIV transmission. One such intervention is pre-exposure prophylaxis (PrEP), which is the use of antiretroviral treatment as a prevention method (CATIE, 2016). It can significantly reduce infection rates via sexual intercourse by 85% to 92% when taken on a regular basis or during periods of heightened risk (Baeten et al., 2012). Approved by Health Canada, PrEP (in combination with safer sex practices) can be part of an effective HIV prevention strategy for Black women. Yet many are still unaware of it. While cost remains a barrier to PrEP use, a critical consideration is needed of the ways that Black women are erased from PrEP discourses and ensuing interventions.

Negating Black Women's Risk in the Canadian PrEP Guidelines

In Canada, individuals must be assessed by a physician and deemed to be at significant risk of HIV infection to be prescribed PrEP. This assessment is informed by the Canadian Guideline on HIV Pre-Exposure Prophylaxis and Nonoccupational Postexposure Prophylaxis (Tan et al., 2017). Although the guideline is touted as a way to help healthcare providers determine appropriate candidates for PrEP, it excludes the social and structural factors that forge risk environments and, thus, cannot accurately capture how these factors contribute to Black women's HIV risk (Nelson et al., 2019). For instance, the guideline constructs "heterosexual exposure" within the context of serodiscordant couples (an intimate partner relationship where one person is HIV positive and the other is HIV negative) as an indication for PrEP. This is the only available category that Black women can be classified within in order to be considered for PrEP. However, among a sub-sample of cisgender, heterosexual Black women living with HIV, 96% stated that pre-diagnosis, they did not know their sexual partners were HIV-positive (Tharao et al., 2018). Black women were therefore at significant risk but unaware of their increased vulnerability. By reducing focus to heterosexual serodiscordant couples as the only vulnerable group that Black women can be categorized within, the current guidelines dually presume their heterosexuality and awareness of the serodiscordant status of their relationship. The guideline's narrow framing of risk both erases the diverse ways Black women can be vulnerable to HIV transmission and eliminates their eligibility as PrEP candidates (Nelson et al., 2019).

Queer Black Women's Erasure in the HIV Surveillance System

The Public Health Agency of Canada monitors the epidemic through the HIV/AIDS Surveillance System. This system passively collates non-nominal data voluntarily submitted by each province and territory (Haddad et al., 2021). To capture a national epidemiological profile of HIV, it classifies reported positive cases within exposure categories premised on social groups at greatest risk (men who have sex with men, injection drug users, etc.). Yet, the surveillance system conceptually reduces Black women to a heterosexual identity, as the only categories for women include "heterosexual contact," "injection drug use" or "other." Black queer women are not afforded visibility, as the majority of Black women are classified within the "heterosexual contact" category due to the way they acquired HIV. At the intersections of race, gender, and sexuality, many Black queer women in Canada enter into consensual and non-consensual sexual relationships with men for diverse reasons, including queerphobia (or protection from its effects) and socioeconomic security (Logie & Gibson, 2013). They then face multiple and unique forms of marginalization, exclusion, and violence that increase their HIV risk—yet they are largely excluded from HIV prevention discourses due to their social invisibility and erasure from HIV surveillance frameworks. Data retrieved from Canada's surveillance system is utilized to inform the development of evidence-based programs and services. Prevention services informed by surveillance data subsequently promote compulsory heterosexism where it is assumed that all Black women are (or should be) heterosexual (Logie, 2015). Services positioning them as heterosexual then overlook their specific HIV prevention needs as queer Black women living with or at greater risk of acquiring HIV.

As a result of their erasure, Black queer women continue to be impacted by the HIV epidemic while confronting a complexity of structural barriers to accessing HIV services. This invisibility can result in the delay or loss of HIV care and perpetuate Black queer women's experiences of exclusion and discrimination within prevention responses (Logie et al., 2011).

Policy Recommendations/Considerations

Policy recommendations/considerations include but are not limited to

- Developing a provincial/national HIV prevention strategy for Black women designed to address their culturally and gender-specific service needs
- Revising HIV prevention guidelines to reflect an intersectional lens and supporting healthcare providers to exercise clinical discretion that considers socio-structural contexts when performing risk assessments (Nelson et al., 2019)
- Reconceptualizing the HIV surveillance exposure categories to reflect the intersectional identities and systems that shape HIV risk environments

CONCLUSION

This chapter aimed to reconceptualize how we think about the health disparities Black women face and to reposition how they are constructed in public health discourses. We hold that a BFF is vital as it requires a recovery of Canada's histories of enslavement and colonization and the structural continuities that make Black women more vulnerable to poverty as a social determinant of health. Critically and intersectionally taking up these issues through a Black feminist lens can inform effective research, policy, and programmatic responses that work towards actualizing health equity and social justice for Black women and for all.

CRITICAL THINKING QUESTIONS

1. How does a Black feminist approach expand and challenge dominant, biomedical ways of thinking about marginalized communities and their health risk?
2. What additional policy considerations are needed to ensure that the health inequities faced by Black women navigating intersections of homophobia, transphobia, ableism, Islamophobia, or other forms of systemic oppression are meaningfully redressed?
3. Applying the Black feminist framework outlined and applied in this chapter, what do you think is Black women's role in developing policies that meet the social and health needs of Black women and communities?

KEY TERMS

Black populations
Black feminism
anti-Black racism
reproductive health
COVID-19
HIV/AIDS
precarious work
immigration

SUGGESTED FURTHER READINGS

1. Abdillahi, I. (2022) *Black women under state: Surveillance, poverty & the violence of social assistance*. ARP Books.

2. Cole, D. (2020). *The skin we're in: A year of Black resistance and power.* Doubleday Canada.
3. Maynard, R. (2017). *Policing Black lives: State violence in Canada from slavery to the present.* Fernwood Publishing.
4. Walcott, R., & Abdillahi, I. (2019). *BlackLife: Post-BLM and the struggle for freedom.* ARP Books.
5. Wane, N. N., & Massaquoi, N. (2007). *Theorizing empowerment: Canadian perspectives on Black feminist thought.* Inanna Publications and Education Inc.

CHAPTER 9

Taking a Reproductive Justice Lens in Public Health Policy: A Case Study on Family Law for 2SLGBTQIA+ Parents and Families

Michelle W. Y. Tam and Lori E. Ross

LEARNING OBJECTIVES

1. Introduce the foundational principles of a reproductive justice framework, an interdisciplinary framework to address reproductive rights through a social justice lens.
2. Define reproductive justice in relation to reproductive public health and public health policy.
3. Demonstrate the role of legal systems and public health policy in 2SLGBTQIA+ family expansion, parenting, and reproductive capacity.
4. Apply a reproductive justice lens through a case study on family laws for 2SLGBTQIA+ people in Canada.

INTRODUCTION

In this chapter, we examine how a reproductive justice (RJ) lens can help us understand the possibilities to transform public health policy in relation to 2SLGBTQIA+ family expansion. RJ offers public health feminism and public health policy a lens to interrogate the latter and the impact it can have on the intersectional lived experiences of diverse communities. Aligned with the tenets of public health feminism, RJ argues that reproductive oppression is inextricably linked to—and a result of—structural oppressions, including heteropatriarchy, sexism, and racism. Reproductive oppression refers to the controlling of communities through the regulation of bodies, sexuality, labour, and reproduction (Ross & Solinger, 2017).

This chapter aims to describe RJ and apply it to public health policy through a case study of 2SLGBTQIA+ family expansion. In this introduction, we establish why reproduction and family expansion are public health issues in Canada. We then briefly cover the impact of government policies on 2SLGBTQIA+ family expansion, defining a RJ framework and how it is helpful in examining why and how family expansion is regulated. In the following section, we describe ways in which 2SLGBTQIA+ people in Canada encounter formal legal barriers to family expansion and we subsequently present a case study of family law for 2SLGBTQIA+ people in Canada by applying RJ to help us understand current practices and how they can be changed. Lastly, we will provide some key takeaways on applying a RJ approach to public health policy.

Why Are Reproduction and Family Expansion Public Health Issues?

The Canadian government acknowledges that reproductive and sexual health disparities are issues pertinent to human rights and gender equality in Canada and around the world. In the last decade, Canada has increased its funding support for sexual and reproductive health and rights globally (Global Affairs Canada, 2017). However, nationally, there are reports that reproductive and sexual health information and services in Canada are nonetheless underfunded (Action Canada, 2021). Although reproductive and sexual health are recognized as human rights, a lack of funding, programming, and policies means that not everyone is able to access these rights in the same way. Addressing the full range of reproductive and sexual health and needs of all people is essential to ensure equitable access and promote the health of all Canadians.

Public health in Canada is concerned with population health through "programs, services, and policies that protect and promote the health of all Canadians." This definition includes reproductive health as part of primary healthcare, providing services for contraception, abortions, maternal and child health, and sterility. Put another way, reproduction as a public health issue, or reproductive public health, is concerned with family planning or management of fertility. Reproductive public health, historically and presently, acts as a strategy of population control through services, programs, and policies of fertility regulation. Reproductive access in Canada changes according to policy and service access shifts and differs across time and space (provincially and territorially), illustrating that reproduction—and hence population control—is regulated by the government and not only determined by individual choice; who is able to have a child and when is determined by policies and changes in government that may result in reversals between policies that promote or limit access.

REPRODUCTIVE JUSTICE

RJ is helpful for examining why and how reproduction and family expansion are regulated, as well as what needs to be done to address reproductive health access. RJ is an interdisciplinary framework rooted in Black feminist thought, critical race theory, and critical feminist theory (Combahee River Collective, 1997; Crenshaw, 1989; Davis, 1982). RJ combines reproductive rights and social justice to draw attention to the social conditions in which individuals live and make decisions (Ross & Solinger, 2017). It is a movement and praxis that recognizes reproductive oppression as inherently interconnected with multiple intersections of other oppressions, including sexism, homophobia, racism, classism, health status, and access to healthcare (Asian Communities for RJ [ACRJ], 2005; Ross & Solinger, 2017). RJ focuses on power and abuses of power—specifically, intersectional forces of power that shape decision making around parenting and reproductive capacity (Ross, 2017; Ross & Solinger, 2017). Beyond an analytical framework, the RJ movement aims to challenge the structural conditions that control communities through regulation of sexuality, reproduction, and parenting (Ross & Solinger, 2017).

The concept of RJ was "birthed" in 1994 by 12 Black feminists working on reproductive health and rights while attending a pro-choice conference in Chicago (Ross, 2017). RJ is situated outside of the pro-choice/pro-life binary; rather, it reframes the problem (Ross, 2006): as a consumer and market-based ideology, "choice" does not capture the complexities that constitute reproductive lives (Ross, 2006; SisterSong, n.d.). In this reframing, RJ is concerned with the lived conditions that constitute a person's reproductive decisions, including access to resources and healthcare, familial elements, cultural values, educational opportunities, and other familial and community needs (Ross & Solinger, 2017). After its conception, SisterSong Women of Color RJ Collective (1997) was the first organization to actively promote and propel the movement. The RJ movement continues to reposition public debates, awareness, and practice through activism, academia, research, and advocacy. It has since been taken up as a framework for policy development in international contexts (Macleod et al., 2017; Chiweshe et al., 2017), with sexual and reproductive health activists in Canada calling for an adoption of a RJ framework into policymaking (Kirby, 2017; Women's Earth Alliance & Native Youth Sexual Health Network, 2016).

RJ is concerned with the integrative, rather than additive, impacts of racism, sexism, misogyny, transphobia, homophobia, and classism in reproduction and parenthood (Ross, 2006). As Loretta Ross and Rickie Solinger (2017) write, "these oppressive forces do not emerge or act independently of each other; they depend on each other, they feed on each other, and they gain strength from each other: they are integrative" (p. 75). It is not just about diverse identities but the confluence of them. These integrative forces interact to shape how one experiences the social world, institutions, and policy systems. RJ teaches us to understand a person as a whole, within the multiple and integrative structural conditions that constitute their lived experiences.

The foundational framing of RJ is that although we all have the same human rights, not everyone is able to access these rights in the same way, and "not everyone is oppressed the same way, or at the same time, or by the same forces" (Ross & Solinger, 2017, p. 72). There are three core tenets of RJ: (1) the right to have a child and birth a child under conditions of one's choosing; (2) the right not to have a child; and (3) the right to parent children in safe and healthy environments (Ross & Solinger, 2017). These three core tenets are situated within the understanding that each individual's reproductive and parenting capacities are experienced through intersecting social locations, including their race, class, gender, sexuality, family structure, and access to healthcare (Ross, 2017).

REPRODUCTIVE JUSTICE AND REPRODUCTIVE PUBLIC HEALTH

Although public health is concerned with programs, services, and policies that protect and promote the health of "all Canadians," not everyone is able to access the programs, services, and policies in the same way. Furthermore, in reproductive public health policy, not only is access an issue, but programs, services, and policies have been actively harmful for some people. Historically and presently, Canada controls and regulates fertility through legislated and non-legislated coerced sterilizations as a form of mass birth control for Black, Indigenous, and racialized people, as well as 2SLGBTQIA+ people in Canada (Murphy, 2012). In 2017, a class action lawsuit was launched by Indigenous women who reported experiences of coerced and forced sterilization (*M.R.L.P. and S.A.T. v. The Attorney General of Canada et al., 2017*). In 2019, Canada's Standing Senate Committee on Human Rights studied evidence on continued forced and coerced sterilization of persons in Canada, including intersex people, trans people, women and girls with disabilities, Indigenous women, and Black women (Senate of Canada, 2019). Pointedly, the Canadian government has always been interested in controlling who is allowed to and who cannot have children. It is a patriarchal and colonial form of control disguised as protecting and promoting the health of all Canadians, when the government can very squarely decide who and who does not get to have a child based on its services, programs, and policies. Therefore, the control and regulation of fertility and reproduction are reproductive public health issues and RJ is an approach that we need to understand reproductive public health.

This chapter focuses on two major tenets of reproductive justice: the right to have a child and the right to parent children in safe and healthy environments. Historically and presently, the government regulates who is legally allowed to become a parent and whose legal status is protected as a parent. Family law defines who "counts" as a parent, whether on the basis of biology, birthing, or relationship to the birthing person. As of 2023 in Canada, all provinces and territories, except Ontario and Manitoba, default in defining the birthing person as the mother of the child. The Vital Statistics Acts, defined by each province, register births and in turn parentage, and they regulate who can be named as a parent and how. Additionally, there are regulations through laws and policies related to adoption, custody, child welfare, and access to and funding for assisted reproductive technologies. When we apply RJ, we can see that the recognition of parenthood, as implicitly defined through laws and policies that define who can become and/or be legally protected as a parent, is constructed around heteronormative ideals of race, gender, class, sexuality, sexual behaviour, and family structure. The standard for fit is often predicated, legally and socially, on the basis of a middle-class white nuclear family structure, and those located outside of this structure are stigmatized and can face challenges in their rights to have a child and parent their children. What and who is defined as "bad" parents, "bad" mothers, "bad" fathers reside outside of the confines of a middle-class white nuclear family structure, in conditions that are deemed standard, normal, and safe (Ross & Solinger, 2017). For example, Black women, Indigenous women, women of colour, immigrants, and 2SLGBTQIA+ people are often portrayed as hyperfertile and in need of regulation (Murphy, 2012; Ross & Solinger, 2017). Racist and xenophobic stereotypes of Black, Indigenous, and racialized people and immigrant parents, as well as homophobic representations of queer parents, are found in Canadian public discourse (media, news) and public opinion (Alaazi et al., 2021; Hunter, 2015; Morrison et al., 2008). Parenting outside the confines of a middle-class white nuclear family structure is pathologized and framed as inferior (Alaazi et al., 2021; Bjork-James, 2020). The pathology of these populations is present in legal and policy systems that regulate reproduction and govern who can be a legal parent. These biased constructions of "fitness" have led to the removal of children from their parents' custody, as well as legislated and non-legislated coerced sterilizations (Senate of Canada, 2019). The right to have a child is regulated by the state through multiple mechanisms, such as biological reproductive capacity and the ability to have legal parent status. As such, 2SLGBTQIA+ people, who also have intersectional identities of race, sex, and disability, have been subject to ongoing regulation by the state with respect to parentage. In the next section, we will present a case study applying a RJ framework to explore Canadian legal regulation of the right to parent for 2SLGBTQIA+ people. We will make the argument that the right to have a child is connected to the right to parent children in safe and healthy environments, including the social supports that ensure safety, health, and dignity for children and their parents. We will close with key takeaways for family law with a RJ lens that support 2SLGBTQIA+ family expansion.

HOW ARE 2SLGBTQIA+ PEOPLE AFFECTED BY GOVERNMENT POLICIES RELATED TO FAMILY EXPANSION?

2SLGBTQIA+ people have always formed and expanded their families even as legal systems have created barriers in rights and recognition. From a legal perspective, it appears that in the last two decades 2SLGBTQIA+ people are increasingly able to form legally recognized families. The passing of anti-discrimination laws, reproductive rights, and legalization of same-sex marriage in Canada appear to have given more access to family recognition for 2SLGBTQIA+ people. Although 2SLGBTQIA+ procreation is not explicitly legally regulated, in practice, family law that defines legal parentage, and related processes such as legal birth registration, have presented barriers to full and equal inclusion of 2SLGBTQIA+ people in family building processes. Discrimination on the basis of sexual orientation is still widespread (Kite & Bryant-Lees, 2016) particularly when it comes to the right of sexual minority people to form families (Patterson, 2013). Discrimination on the basis of gender identity (e.g., transphobia) is even more widespread (Norton & Herek, 2013). When it comes to family expansion, 2SLGBTQIA+ people can face discrimination on multiple levels, including interpersonal discrimination based on individual interactions and institutional discrimination based on structural mechanisms such as policies or practices that do not allow 2SLGBTQIA+ people to adopt children or have legally recognized parentage.

2SLGBTQIA+ people become parents in myriad ways, including domestic adoption, international adoption, adoption by a second or third parent, pregnancy, surrogacy, conceiving through in vitro fertilization, sexual intercourse, artificial insemination, and sperm and egg donations. In 2000, same-sex couples obtained the right to legally adopt a child in Canada. However, despite legislation providing institutional support for 2SLGBTQIA+ people to apply for adoption, the accessibility of adoption services is not consistent (Fantus & Newman, 2019; Ross et al., 2009). As reproductive technologies have advanced, more people have been able to have biological children. In the case of assisted reproduction, as services have increased, the legislation has not followed suit to provide legislative support for 2SLGBTQIA+ parents. As a policy application of PHF with an RJ lens, we will present a case study on family law for 2SLGBTQIA+ people in Manitoba.

Heteronormativity is relevant to understanding the social and legal conditions of family expansion. Heteronormativity is commonly defined as a system of regulation and normalization that ascribes power, privilege, and normative status to heterosexual sexuality and relationships. In applying a RJ framework to family law, we draw on Cathy Cohen's extended conceptualization of heteronormativity. Cohen is a long-time activist, distinguished scholar, and Black feminist. Cohen (1997, 2019) argues for a conceptualization of heteronormativity and queer politics that is rooted within "ways in which heteronormativity works to support and reinforce institutional racism, patriarchy, and class exploitation" as integral to "how we problematize current constructions of heterosexuality" (Cohen, 1997, p. 455). For Cohen, an understanding of heteronormativity pays attention to power, normativity, and the structures—including race, gender, and class—that uphold heterosexuality as dominant in society. Heteronormativity emphasizes an understanding of sexuality that goes beyond a queer/heterosexual binary to include sexuality and sexual deviance from a socially constructed norm. Put another way, not all heterosexual people experience heterosexual privilege or heteronormativity in the same way. Cohen offers a powerful example of the stigma and demonization of single moms, primarily poor women of colour, because they are often perceived to have non-normative sexual behaviour and family structures. This example illustrates the usage of sexuality and sexual deviance to uphold heteronormativity even for those who identify as heterosexual. Thus, non-normative sexuality and sexual behaviour are punished, but how and who is punished is also informed by race, gender, and class. Cohen's definition of heteronormativity centres the white supremacist roots of heteronormativity that regulate sexuality through legal systems to deem what a family looks like, who is "fit" to be a parent, or who can access the right to be a parent. RJ and heteronormativity help us to understand the socially constructed norms around the right to have a child and right to parent children in safe and healthy environments.

CASE EXAMPLE: FAMILY LAW AND 2SLGBTQIA+ PARENTING

In Canada, family law governs and legislates relationships between spouses and between parents and their children. *Legal parentage* is a term used in family law that refers to the process of establishing the legal parents of a child. Birth registration is the process of officially documenting a birth, including the baby's parents. In Canada, legal parentage and birth registration are governed by provincial and territorial legislation—and therefore, such legislation is inconsistent across the country. As each jurisdiction has its own laws, there are vast differences in how progressive and how recently revised the policies are toward legal parentage (Snow, 2016).

With the advancement of assisted reproductive technologies (ART) and more parents, including 2SLGBTQIA+ parents, using ART to expand their families, parentage policy has become a legal barrier for many intended parents in various jurisdictions. It is estimated that up to 25% of fertility clinic users in urban areas of Canada identify as 2SLGBTQIA+ (Green et al., 2012). Same-sex male couples and single men make up approximately 32% of intended parents using ART in Canada (Dixon et al., 2019). Yet, parents who form families using assisted reproduction face barriers and discrimination when trying to be legally recognized and affirm their rights under law. To keep up with the reality of ARTs and expansive family structures, legal parentage across Canada has undergone policy changes in some jurisdictions and continues to need policy change in others. Reform of provincial legislation around legal parentage has largely arisen through legal changes brought forward by 2SLGBTQIA+ parents and families.

Section 15 of the Canadian Charter of Rights and Freedoms has been used to challenge policies and affirm 2SLGBTQIA+ rights (Snow, 2017). Section 15(1) states,

> Every individual is equal before and under the law and has the right to the equal protection and equal benefit of the law without discrimination and, in particular, without discrimination based on race, national or ethnic origin, colour, religion, sex, age or mental or physical disability.

In 1995, sexual orientation was also declared to be recognized as an equivalent ground on which claims of discrimination can be made. This addition to section 15 of the charter has been important in securing legal rights for 2SLGBTQIA+ people at the federal and provincial levels. Thus, section 15 has been used to challenge provincial parentage policies that are discriminatory towards 2SLGBTQIA+ parents. In the next section, we will discuss a case study of parentage policy change in Manitoba, Canada.

THE FAMILY MAINTENANCE ACT AND THE RIGHT TO HAVE A CHILD

The Family Maintenance Act (FMA) determines legal parentage in Manitoba. Under the FMA, legal parentage outlines obligations and rights around custody and access. The legal status of parents is important for the upbringing of children, including having legal rights to make healthcare and education decisions. From an RJ lens, this means that the right to have a child includes the legal ability to parent one's own child and make legal health and education decisions in raising their child. Legal recognition of a parent is also crucial for parent-child relationships and can impact parental stress and childhood development (Acevedo-Garcia et al., 2013). As a result, the legal definition of parent under the FMA has a great deal of influence and impact on whether a parent is or is not recognized as their child's parent at the time of the child's birth, as well as parental and child well-being in the future.

In 2020, legal proceedings were filed in Manitoba to challenge the definition of "parent" under Manitoba's FMA based on section 15 of the charter. The Public Interest Law Centre and Taylor McCaffrey LLP represented seven lesbian, gay, and bisexual families who had children using assisted reproduction and were not recognized under the FMA as legal parents of their children. Prior to this, the FMA and the definition of a legal parent was last updated in 1987. The FMA did not recognize non-biological parents who conceived children through assisted reproduction. Under this 1987 version of the FMA, "parent" was defined as "biological parent or adoptive parent of a child and includes a person declared to be the parent of a child." However, this definition of parent only includes the biological parent at birth, meaning other parent(s) would not be recognized without an adoption process. The parent who was not recognized at birth would need to go through a lengthy and expensive legal effort to be recognized as their child's parent through court proceedings or adoption. As a result, parents without a biological connection to their child faced discrimination and barriers to legal recognition as such.

For the families filing this proceeding, the non-recognition of legal parent status caused significant barriers and burdens for their families. The legal proceedings argued that the families and their children have been denied equal benefit of the law under section 15 of the Charter of Rights and Freedoms on the grounds of sexual orientation and family status. As envisaged by section 15 of the charter, every individual is equal before the law and is equally deserving of concern, respect, and consideration. As an equality rights case, these families, alongside other 2SLGBTQIA+ families, face discrimination on the grounds of family status and sexual orientation when they are not recognized as legal parents to their children without adoption or a court order. This case argued that the FMA, in its existing form, imposed barriers on 2SLGBTQIA+ families and was discriminatory under section 15 of the charter. At the time, other jurisdictions in Canada—including Ontario, Saskatchewan, Alberta, British Columbia, Nova Scotia, and Prince Edward Island—had already passed significant legislative reform on the use of assisted reproduction and legal parentage.

In making determinations under the charter, the courts often reach out to experts for evidence to support their case. The two co-authors of this chapter were invited to contribute an expert witness affidavit for this case, alongside other experts, based on their areas of research specialization in 2SLGBTQIA+ health. In supporting the legislation change, we argued that research evidence consistently finds legal and institutional barriers to be primary sources of psychological distress for 2SLGBTQIA+ people during the transition to parenthood as well as while raising their children. In the report, we presented research that supports the claim that legal recognition of all intended parents at the time of birth will promote the well-being of 2SLGBTQIA+ families.

Terminology

Cisnormative: A system of values and beliefs that unjustly favours cisgender people, in turn marginalizing trans people and rendering them invisible. This system of values treats trans people's needs and identities as less important than those of cisgender people.

Cissexism: The assumption that all people are cisgender and that cisgender people are "normal" and trans people are "abnormal," as well as normative assumptions about bodies (e.g., all women have vaginas, someone with a penis is male).

Heterosexism: The assumption that everyone is, or should be, heterosexual and that heterosexuality is inherently superior to its alternatives. It also refers to structural or organizational discrimination against people who are not heterosexual, or against behaviours not stereotypically heterosexual.

LEGAL PARENT STATUS AND THE RIGHT TO PARENT CHILDREN IN SAFE AND HEALTHY ENVIRONMENTS

Last updated in 1987, the FMA in Manitoba denied 2SLGBTQIA+ parents' equality in legal parentage. Under the FMA definition of legal parent, 2SLGBTQIA+ people who had children through assisted reproductive technologies would have to go through court processes to be recognized as their child's parent even if they were the intended parents. Thus, non-birthing 2SLGBTQIA+ parents faced a lack of legal parental recognition. For example, in a lesbian couple using in vitro fertilization to conceive, the non-birthing parent would have to go through a lengthy and expensive process to adopt their own child after birth (Ross et al., 2005). However, in the case of heterosexual couples conceiving using donor sperm, the intended father, who was not the donor, would still be recognized as a parent. For the lesbian couple, as well as gay, bisexual, and trans parents, Manitoba's laws around legal parentage result in a lack of equal treatment of intended parents, erasure of non-birthing parents, and additional financial burden. From an RJ lens, the law did not explicitly prohibit 2SLGBTQIA+ people from being legally recognized as parents, so technically everyone has the same rights, but because of how the definitions of legal parentage was written, non-birthing parents in particular couldn't access those rights. Overall, the legal proceedings argued that these are heteronormative, heterosexist, and discriminatory practices that have ongoing negative impacts on 2SLGBTQIA+ parent families.

Denial of legal parent status impacts a tenet of RJ, the ability of 2SLGBTQIA+ people to raise children in safe and healthy environments. 2SLGBTQIA+ families without legal parent recognition can face fears around being able to make important education and healthcare system decisions for their children, family and social supports, citizenship, travelling as a family, as well as legal custody in the cases of divorce and separation (Ross et al., 2005; Shapiro, 2020). These concerns around being able to raise their children in safe and healthy environments are a direct consequence of precarious legal status. Research has found that discrimination and second-class legal status causes physical, emotional, and financial harm to 2SLGBTQIA+ people, their families, and their children (Berkowitz, 2020; Pfeffer & Jones, 2020; Pollitt et al., 2020). In addition to second-parent adoption processes, other legal barriers include the need for donor contracts, worry about future custody battles, and the limitation that only two parents could be legally recognized (Ross et al., 2005). It has also been found that discriminatory and stigma-based stressors during and after the transition to parenthood can affect the level of support and social climates that 2SLGBTQIA+ families must navigate (Goldberg & Smith, 2011; Lick et al., 2012; Pollitt et al., 2020). Such family law issues impact 2SLGBTQIA+ family expansion, legal parent status, and the right to raise children in safe and healthy environments.

COURT RULING ON LEGAL PARENTAGE

In June 2020, seven couples filed legal proceedings to challenge Manitoba's laws around legal parentage rights. The charter challenge argued that the FMA was discriminatory on the grounds of sexual orientation and family status (under s. 15 of the charter) for requiring non-biological parents who used assisted reproductive technologies to obtain court orders to be declared the legal parent of their own child. In November 2020, the Court of Queen's Bench ruled that sections of the FMA on the definition of a legal parent are unconstitutional and violated the right to equality as guaranteed under the Charter of Rights and Freedoms. The court declared that the definition of "parent" and presumptions of paternity in the act violated the charter under section 15 "because they do not contemplate parentage through assisted human reproduction and therefore discriminate[d] on the basis of sexual orientation." The subsections of the FMA that were considered discriminatory were then declared invalid and suspended for 12 months. This court ruling gave the Manitoba government 12 months to revise the legislation. The Manitoba government announced that changes to the Manitoba's FMA will be made to include parentage legislation for children conceived through assisted reproduction. Lastly, the seven lesbian, gay, and bisexual families that filed the legal proceedings were declared legal parents and would not be required to go through an adoption or declaration process.

This constitutional challenge was a significant victory for 2SLGBTQIA+ parents who use assisted reproductive technologies; it is a victory for the right to parent children, have a child, and reproductive justice. Although much still needs to be done to ensure the right to raise children in safe and healthy environments for 2SLGBTQIA+ parent families, removing these legal barriers and burdens will impact the social, physical, and mental well-being of many families now and in the future.

REPRODUCTIVE JUSTICE AND FAMILY LAW

In this chapter, we focused on two key tenets of RJ as they apply to family law impacting 2SLGBTQIA+ parenting: (1) the right to have a child; and (2) the right to parent children in safe and healthy environments. We have shown that although prior legislation did not explicitly deny 2SLGBTQIA+ people the right to have a child, sexual orientation and gender identity impacted the ease with which 2SLGBTQIA+ people could exercise this right. In turn, denying legal parentage to some 2SLGBTQIA+ people impacted the safety and health of the environment for their children. Given that the conditions in which children are raised includes an environment that does or does not "keep people healthy and prevent injury, illness and premature death," legislation impacting the capacity for 2SLGBTQIA+ people to be recognized as legal parents is a public health issue. Taking a RJ approach to reproductive public health enables us to recognize that parenting and reproductive capacity are inherently interconnected to multiple intersections of power and oppression, including sexism, homophobia, racism, classism, health status, and access to healthcare.

KEY TAKEAWAYS

The key takeaways are as follows:

1. A RJ lens offers public health policy an approach that draws attention to intersectional forces of power that shape decision making in relation to reproductive health, including with respect to parenting and reproductive capacity.
2. Two of the key tenets of RJ are (1) the right to have a child, and (2) the right to raise children in safe and healthy environments.
3. In considering policies related to parenting and reproductive capacity, the right to have a child requires legal parent status for all intended parents.
4. The right to have a child and the right to parent children in safe and health environments are both informed by multiple intersections of oppression, including sexism, homophobia, racism, classism, and ableism.
5. In making public health policies, a RJ lens calls us to ensure not only that everyone has the same rights, but also that everyone is able to access those rights.
6. Applying a RJ lens to policymaking related to reproductive public health requires us to consider the people it will impact within multiple and integrative structural conditions (e.g., racism, sexism, heteropatriarchy, classism) that constitute their lived experiences, reproductive decisions, and parenting possibilities.

CRITICAL THINKING QUESTIONS

1. How does RJ help us to understand community needs? Reproductive capacity? Parenting decisions? Family decisions? Bodily autonomy?

2. What understandings can RJ bring to help us negotiate other realms of public health?
3. What other public health policies can a RJ lens inform?
4. What social, political, and economic inequalities can RJ help us to understand locally and globally?
5. How does the right to reproductive health and rights inform our lives and everyday realities?

KEY TERMS

reproductive justice
2SLGBTQIA+
family expansion
parenting
family law

SUGGESTED FURTHER READINGS

1. Cohen, C. J. (1997). Punks, bulldaggers, and welfare queens: The radical potential of queer politics? *GLQ: A Journal of Lesbian and Gay Studies*, *3*(4), 437–465.
2. Goldberg, A. E., & Allen, K. R. (Eds.). (2020). *LGBT-parent families: Innovations in research and implications for practice* (2nd ed.). Springer Nature Switzerland AG.
3. Ross, L. J. (2017). Reproductive justice as intersectional feminist activism. *Souls*, *19*(3), 286–314.
4. Ross, L., & Solinger, R. (2017). *Reproductive justice: An introduction* (Vol. 1). University of California Press.

CHAPTER 10

Strangers in Our Homeland: The Impact of Racism across Healthcare Policy and Delivery for Indigenous Peoples in Canada

Mikaela D. Gabriel

LEARNING OBJECTIVES

1. Gain a better understanding of current experiences of the intersectional dimensions of race, health, policy, and survival as it applies to Indigenous Peoples in Canada.
2. Explore Canadian healthcare gaps in the construction, implementation, and delivery of Indigenous healthcare policy across provinces.
3. Explore training and service delivery in healthcare for service providers treating Indigenous clients, as well as perspectives, narratives, and voices from Indigenous clients and outreach workers.

INTRODUCTION

In 1876, the Indian Act defined Indigenous Peoples as Canada's wards of state, ensuring many things—most notably, paternalistic control and responsibility for their healthcare (Eshet, 2015). Unsurprisingly, Indigenous health has gone sharply downhill ever since. To gain a better understanding of current experiences of the intersectional dimensions of race, health, policy, and survival, this chapter will provide a holistic review of policy, procedures, and the voices of Indigenous Elders, youth, and service providers searching for representation and safety in healthcare.

There's a lot of ground to cover, but let's give it a try.

HISTORY IN HEALTH

It would be more difficult to find a time in Canadian history when governmental systems were *not* trying to harm Indigenous Peoples. The earliest conception of colonial government in Canada has sought to decimate Indigenous populations through biowarfare (e.g., smallpox and cholera); the construction of, and forced starvation experiments in, residential school systems; forced sterilization of Indigenous women; and evolving methods of child extraction from communities, including still-ongoing birth alerts for Indigenous mothers. All depict a persistent and undeniably systematic assault on Indigenous well-being (Eshet, 2015; Royal Commission on Aboriginal Peoples, 1996). This is particularly easy to accomplish when the populations targeted are systematically dehumanized, their peoples and practices seen as inferior to those of Europeans; they have been seen as savage, uncivilized, and primitive, with sustained, systematic efforts "to continue until there is not a single Indian in Canada that has not been absorbed. They are a weird and wanting race" (Eshet, 2015, p. 51; National Archives of Canada, n.d.; Woolford, 2009). If put on a timeline, these genocidal measures would only cover a few generations. With such a rough beginning, there's little room to doubt why Indigenous Peoples are reluctant and distrustful to seek medical care from Western-based healthcare providers (Allan & Smylie, 2015; Barnett & Kendall, 2011; Browne et al., 2017; Lambert et al., 2014; de Leeuw et al., 2015; McCallum & Perry, 2018; Reading, 2015; Wylie et al., 2019). In an interview with this author, an Indigenous Elder described his own suspicions of Western systems: "Yeah, we have every right to be paranoid. There's a lot of people out here trying to kill us. Maybe not physically anymore, but spiritually" (Gabriel, 2021, p. 454).

It's not just in the doctor's office, however. Indigenous health barriers are "established through historical events, perpetuated in current policy, and expressed in behaviours that all interact in ways that inflict violence on Indigenous people" (Wylie et al., 2019, p. 1; Black & McBean, 2016). The foundations of survival, such as housing, food sovereignty and security, and clean drinking water are all at points of crisis, and have been for decades (Black & McBean, 2016; Fohlich et al., 2006; Lavoie, 2013). Just as Indigenous means of survival are severely under-supported, so too are the realities, histories, perspectives, stories, and practices kept from mainstream education and society, ensuring that Indigenous Peoples are understood to be Other, kept separate, as strangers; it takes a lot of advanced learning, and none of it mandatory, to fully understand Indigenous genocide in Canada. What is prominent, however, are negative stereotypes and damaging myths. In ensuring that Indigenous populations are unable to secure autonomy in healthcare, governmental bodies somehow have effectively managed to also "[shirk] their responsibility to ensure quality, comprehensive care" (Wylie et al., 2019, p. 16).

What's curious to consider is how the current state of Indigenous health inequity stands in perfect polarity prior to colonization. Traditional knowledge identifies health as a balance between spiritual, physical, emotional, and mental spheres; illness arises from imbalance (Absolon, 2010; Robbins & Dewar, 2011; Struthers et al., 2004). Both health and balance are restored through medicines and ceremonies, which promote a wealth of holistic health benefits, as well as connection to community; one Elder described the crucial value of ceremony, as "smudge to Anishinaabe people is just like drinking water, it's something that we need" (Gabriel, 2015, p. 160). Such medicines and ceremonies ensured living in connection with humanity's first mother, Mother Earth, and as a result, all beings, plants, and ecosystems are connected; hence the commonly used term *All My Relations* (Absolon, 2010, 2016). This intimate knowledge of ecology was so effective that over 25% of modern prescription pharmaceuticals are rooted in traditional medicines (Hill, 2003). However, colonization has ensured distance from traditional territories, barriers to cultural practices, and lack of sovereignty in managing ecological resources. Our mother is ill and so are we; every effort to right it is hindered by colonial structures.

POLICY

Let's start at the top: health policy in Canada. The healthcare of Indigenous Peoples sits at a vulnerable crossroads of Canadian policy, with Indigenous Peoples seldom truly included. While the federal government is fiscally responsible for the healthcare of Indigenous Peoples, each province and territory must determine the rules and regulations of healthcare delivery; this is where the seismic gaps in cultural integration and relationships occur (Indian Act, 1985; Lavoie et al., 2015; Wylie et al., 2019).

Since each province and territory is left to determine their unique relationship with Indigenous communities, great variability and a "jurisdictional patchwork" result, bringing with them great gaps (Lavoie, 2013, p. 5). At the time of writing, Yukon is the only territory that recognizes the importance of partnership with Indigenous Peoples for health and well-being and supports relationships and traditional practices in healthcare; Ontario the only province that has an Indigenous advisory council in regional healthcare; Nova Scotia and British Columbia have stipulations that must reflect the populations served, but this does not specify how it applies to Indigenous Peoples (Lavoie, 2013). While political parties play ruling musical chairs over time, one party's policies, intended to support Indigenous groups, are often dropped quickly when the music stops (Henderson et al., 2018; Wylie et al., 2019). Meanwhile, ongoing underfunding of basic structures and supports on reserves perpetuate health issues (Browne, 2017; Lavoie, 2013; Truth and Reconciliation Commission of Canada, 2015; Wylie et al., 2019, p. 2). No concrete guidelines for culturally safe and community-informed practices with Indigenous Peoples exist nationwide; in the spaces where they should be, instead, interprovincial inconsistencies, structural violence, and lack of follow-through from community recommendations grow like weeds. Despite the government's responsibility for Indigenous healthcare, lacking a national, unified approach only results in a minefield of variation, where community voices are often lost in the fray.

CHALLENGES IN SERVICE DELIVERY

It should come as no surprise that similar gaps exist in service delivery for Indigenous Peoples. While smaller, rural communities may form stronger relationships and include culturally based care delivery, they're noted to be underfunded and in need of increased infrastructure, resources, and specialization (Eby, 2007; Josewski, 2012; Wylie et al., 2019). While stereotypes of Indigenous Peoples largely living on reserves exist, statistical trends note that almost half of the total Indigenous population live off reserve and are increasingly urban, in search of employment and educational opportunities (Statistics Canada, 2016). On arrival to cities, however, we begin to see a much different story. Urban-based care centres typically lack sufficient culturally safe training, understanding, and empathy; without these, many staff members are ignorant to the realities and barriers Indigenous Peoples face (Browne, 2017; Browne et al., 2017; de Leeuw et al., 2015; NAHO, 2003; Reading, 2015; Wylie et al., 2019). They're even treated differently; a homeless outreach and housing worker described the vast treatment differences for his Indigenous clients when seeking services:

> I've seen it firsthand ... as long as I'm with my client, they'll treat my client with respect, but when I'm gone, I'll just stand around the corner and see how they talk, it's like they're lower, like my client felt like a foreigner, like "We were the first people here on this land and we're being treated like scum, basically," whereas a non-Aboriginal would be treated like the president of the United States. (Gabriel, 2015, p. 177)

It's no wonder that Indigenous clients are noted to have higher service discontinuation rates; they report fear of further harm, racial misunderstanding, and discrimination (Barnett & Kendall, 2011; Boot & Lowell, 2019; Lambert et al., 2014; Wylie et al., 2019). While cultural safety training is recommended, there's typically a lack of resources and training to make sure it's implemented (Boot & Lowell, 2019).

So, what are the other options? Seeking safety in community, of course. When presented with the option between a Western-based healthcare provider that lacks cultural understanding and an Indigenous community-based service provider, the latter will seem as a better option to receive inclusive and holistic care. However, as urban Indigenous rates continue to grow at four times that of the non-Indigenous population (Statistics Canada, 2016), these services are being spread thin in an effort to meet the demand. When these systems are overwhelmed, the quality of care is impacted; after all, something's got to give. A community youth described how urban Indigenous service providers offer a host of resources, but this comes at the cost of relationship. As he described,

> Downtown, they call you a number. They get hundreds of clients every day, that sort of interpersonal bond that you build with your clients isn't exactly there. Up north—it's very personal. It's a very personal bond that you have with you and your workers or your agency or a friendship centre, it's a very personal thing. Out here it's a lot different. Out here you're viewed as the number of the day, the quota. You have a need that got to be met, OK that's all of this, it's the best we can do for you. (Gabriel, 2021, p. 490)

While integrating cultural approaches, perspectives, and practices into Indigenous healthcare is a method that has been promoted as "one of the most successful strategies for creating a welcoming health care system" (Wylie et al., 2019, p. 12), urban push can strain relational capacity in community services past their limit, stretching thin the core support for meaningful healthcare.

Let's consider more from the voices of healthcare providers themselves. In a study that interviewed physicians and care staff working with Indigenous populations, staff participants encouraged personal investment and relationship building (Wylie et al., 2019). There's that word again: *relationship*, something that has been sorely missing in equitable, supportive ways across all intersections of Western-Indigenous interactions. To ensure comfortable, supported patients, the key was identified as "long-term, consistent, trusting relationships with people [health providers] that they respect." There is, of course, dissent in the ranks for relational investments with Indigenous patients. Some promote and understand the importance of relationality, while others can't seem to find the time, "As a family doctor shared, some physicians go 'wow, you are pretty complicated. I don't really want to get involved with you.' And so that exacerbated the whole doctor shortage" (Wylie et al., 2019, p. 11).

In direct contrast to the siloed approaches of Western healthcare providers, an Indigenous Elder described the differences in approaches and methods: "sadly, a lot of Western approaches are very either clinical or, if not, their engagement is very superficial as to the boundaries of client and worker ... our people are not interested in that, so that's the reality" (Gabriel, 2021, p. 437). From a different angle, Indigenous service providers themselves describe the ever-familiar blockades of Western governmental mandates that limit the ability for them to extend care in culturally rooted ways. This Elder continued to describe the treatment differences and culture clash across Western and Indigenous care provision:

> we try to provide essential things but with funding it's very much based on a whole different model ... organizations that are non-Indigenous, they have their service delivery models and they're very cookie-cutter. It's the same delivery model across the board, and then when they tend to see ours, they tend to be a little surprised that what we tend to provide is a lot different. (Gabriel, 2021, p. 438)

Indigenous services promote the community's holistic needs, including having flexibility to meet their unique circumstances. It will surprise no one that, of course, there would be blockades to such holistic care. This Elder continued to note how important service evaluation is to non-Indigenous funding bodies:

> they couldn't prove the financial benefit for a drop-in centre. They couldn't come up with a model that could satisfy the funders, to justify the funding. At most Friendship Centres ... they've turned into different service models, they'll focus on a particular service now, [or] make an appointment and come in, so very different compared to how things were 20 years ago where everything was a drop-in centre type of approach ... for our people was a huge loss. That's what people are still looking for is that sense of community and that place to belong and to have that place to go. (Gabriel, 2021, p. 438)

Keen readers would guess it: the more non-Indigenous policies and practices promote only Western-based approaches, the more barriers ensue. This incessant and unyielding clash in culture and treatment continues to create more and more barriers; not only do cultural services need to be seen as necessary, but Indigenous service providers need the freedom to provide what flexible treatments are right for the people.

But wait: a glimmer of hope appears. Some changes in representation are slowly being made. One outreach worker described observing some initial shifts in Western care facilities:

> I think the changes are already happening. Things are already a lot more respectful from non-Native organizations. We go to a lot of corner drop-ins at [location], and they give us space to smudge. They don't ask questions, like "what are they doing in there? What's that smell?" They know what's happening ... because they have a lot of Natives who stay there, they have a place for us to smudge too. It's not outside like a hospital would be, it's a place in the building, so there's a lot more awareness of Native culture even in non-Native places and organizations. (Gabriel, 2015, p. 183)

While these steps are important and hopefully improving, much, much more is needed than an individual approach; these changes need to be as systemic as the ignorance that bore their necessity. With expansive projected growth and increasing migration to cities, it is becoming too expensive and disastrous to *not* understand the healthcare and lived realities of Indigenous Peoples. Inevitably, a crossroads will be reached: either integrate our care, or let us do it ourselves. But, of course, that would require further Indigenous autonomy. And what government wants *that*?

INDIGENOUS AUTONOMY IN POLICY

While Indigenous community members, workers, researchers, and Elders promote the importance of Indigenous autonomy across levels of healthcare, one Elder pointed out that knowledge of this system is crucial: "we're talking about policies to reform a system ... the reality is that the system doesn't want to reform. It has no intentions, never did, it never will" (Gabriel, 2021, p. 455). He also described how important allyship is on this journey: "policies need to change and we need allies again and help, but the allies need to listen and we know what we need and what we want to create whatever we need to create" (Gabriel, 2021, p. 455).

Surprise! Changes to policy for Indigenous healthcare do not come easily. As noted, Indigenous Peoples and culture were seen as inherently inferior to those of

Europeans; this formed the grounds for constructing the residential school system. Its ghost continues to haunt the metaphorical halls, as culture is somehow still seen as a blockade by Western practices and is not well understood or appreciated for its role in health or "progress" (Cooper, 2011, p. 14; George et al., 2019). Once criminalized and targeted for genocide, this culture continues to be legally tolerated; however, it remains problematized, unappreciated, and removed when drafting policy for services with Indigenous Peoples. This cultural erasure is an interesting notion, considering communities continue to express that culture *is* treatment, a successful approach supported by research (Akena, 2012; Barwin, 2012; Boot & Lowell, 2019; Brady, 1995; Cooper, 2011; George et al., 2019; Lambert et al., 2014; Priest et al., 2012; Sherwood, 2013; Smylie et al., 2006; Vass et al., 2011). One would think that listening to the people regarding their own needs and treatment would be a good move, most especially when autonomy and the rights of self-governance "are essential for the health of [Indigenous] peoples" (George et al., 2019, p. 15; Black & McBean, 2016). Maybe it's that pesky ghost again?

Canada isn't alone in its colonial practices, of course, but still lags behind when it comes to health integration and autonomy. The Australian government easily recognized that "without self-determination it is not possible for Indigenous Australians to fully overcome the legacy of colonisation and dispossession" (George et al., 2019, p. 18). When culturally safe, supportive, and integrated approaches are present in care environments, interventions can reduce miscommunication, misinformation, and confusion, providing more effective care (Boot & Lowell, 2019). Simple consultation falls flat and is just another extension of paternalistic care. Even if consultation is completed, though, there is no assurance of follow-up and community wellness; these measures must engage communities as both community based and community driven (Anderson et al., 2007; Fisher et al., 2018; George et al., 2019; Lavoie, 2014; Mitchell & Macleod, 2014).

MOVING FORWARD?

This chapter has reviewed the multisystemic and intersectional mire that exists when trying to support Indigenous survival in Canada. Not balanced health and well-being—simply survival. It seems that there is no end to the barriers for Indigenous Peoples, no end to the reach and roots of colonialism. While commonly promoted as "historical issues," there's no doubt about its systemic, societal, and personal persistence. So, let's look now at how we might be able to tackle these aspects.

On a systemic level, ongoing opposition can no longer continue if we're looking for a meaningful, sustainable end. National structure for Indigenous rights in determining health policy must be collaboratively created and sustained. Education and understanding of Indigenous history and its long-term ramifications is well past mandatory; when done sufficiently, this will contextualize Indigenous health inequities and disparities, enrich societal understanding of Indigenous Peoples, and maybe, just maybe, work to dismantle racist viewpoints that demean Indigenous culture and society and create stereotypes (could education be the fourth Ghostbuster?). On a social and service level, mandating cultural safety training for service providers can better equip them to meaningfully engage their Indigenous clients, and additional supports such as trauma-informed care can offer skills and strategies to promote safe methods of relationship building. Providers must strive to ensure working partnerships with the Indigenous communities they serve, through working connections and workshops with nearby communities, knowledge exchanges, partnerships, or mentorship programs. Managers in healthcare and service settings should ensure that cultural safety is a core component of care staff training, alongside trauma-informed care; additionally, hiring increased Indigenous staff for representation, connecting with Elders for patient/client requests for diverse service approaches, and flexibility with smudging in indoor spaces should be supported and encouraged. These are simply some steps to have safe services that are better familiarized with Indigenous health inequities and better equipped with tools to challenge them. At any rate, it couldn't hurt to have more knowledge and more training; maybe then the burden of safety could be lifted from Indigenous service providers alone.

It can be hard for us, on a personal level, to believe we can make much of a difference. But deepening our understanding of the world around us, and the policies that impact our lives, can help guide us toward wise action, activism, and informed choices toward an equitable and compassionate society. So, let's start with just you, just now. Take time to reflect on the next pages, which provide questions for critical thinking: *How did I get here? Who was here before me? What do I need to learn?*

As we reflect, though, let's also look to the voices of the community themselves. When asked what benefit may exist at the intersections of traditional knowledge and policy, Indigenous community youth identified how existing policies challenge Indigenous culture: "I want people to recognize that the way that that policy is set up is intentionally divisive when it comes to Indigenous culture and us expressing ourselves" (Gabriel, 2021, p. 502). Additionally, youth highlighted how important it is for policymakers to participate in cultures to deepen their understanding: "Having that understanding with them, having that personal appreciation, I think can do wonders then for the people who this policy's affecting" (Gabriel, 2021, p. 514). This youth described how better understanding can enrich the policy to population process:

> I think it would set a standard in Canada of education and it would trickle down through people, a standard of having more profound respect and not being ignorant or being racist. I also think if everyone had this standard of more appreciation, that proper funding could be allocated and more work could be done to greatly impact a lot [of people] ... I think their lives could be immensely greater if people just understood better where they came from and why. (Gabriel, 2021, p. 516)

Even after genocide, some youth voices ring clear: share this with us. Join us. Maybe you'll understand why we've been trying to protect it for so long. Maybe it could help you, too.

When considering the intersections of race, health, policy, and care, we cannot forget the core crux: racism, which "pervades all levels and structures of Canadian settler society, with institutional and individual—government, front-line and emergency services, community supports, law enforcement, education, work life, and more" (Thistle, 2017, p. 27). As stated, Indigenous worldviews hold that *all* are my relations. All beings—humans, flora, fauna—are connected and must care for each other. Division and dehumanization will bring continued imbalance and illness, where some of us must struggle for autonomy and survival.

If only our neighbours knew us a little better. If only they could see the delicate, persistent thread that connects us: in being here, together, we have the same home. We come from the same mother. If that's true, then maybe we're not so different after all. Maybe we might realize that person is no stranger; that's my relation.

CRITICAL THINKING QUESTIONS

1. *How did I get here?* What is my story, my family's story, in connection to this land? Am I a settler? Am I an Indigenous person visiting for work or school? Locating yourself in the history of Canada can better help reframe your perspective to include Indigenous Peoples' truths.
2. *Who was here before me?* What tribes and peoples took care of the land I now live on, before I called it home? Do I live on land that was traded fairly or unfairly? Where are there communities nearby?

3. *What do I need to learn?* It's hard to know every detail of Canada's unjust history, even if our classrooms had prepared us. So, ask yourself: Do I know what the Sixties Scoop is? How does it relate to the Millennium Scoop? How recently have birth alerts been going on? While we don't know what we don't know, there is always room for further learning and increasing resources for deepening our knowledge. How can you deepen yours?

KEY TERMS

Indigenous health
racism
colonialism
culture
community

SUGGESTED FURTHER READINGS

1. Thunderbird Partnership Foundation. *Trainings, handouts, teachings, and a wealth of resources on Indigenous wellness and care.* https://thunderbirdpf.org/
2. King, T. (2017). *The inconvenient Indian illustrated: A curious account of Native people in North America.* Doubleday Canada.
3. Eshet, D. (2015). *Stolen lives: The Indigenous Peoples of Canada and the Indian residential schools.* Facing History and Ourselves.
4. Paul, D. N. (2000). *We were not the savages: Collision between European and Native American civilization.* Fernwood Publishing.

CHAPTER 11

The Critical Importance of Addressing Gender and Racial Inequities in the Public Health System

Christina Salmon and Andrea Tricco

LEARNING OBJECTIVES

1. Explain the history and the effect colonization has had on the current systems of inequity in public health.
2. Identify the intersection of race and gender.
3. Describe recommendations to support Black and Indigenous women and make critical system improvements in public health.

INTRODUCTION

The COVID-19 pandemic has amplified the inequities in the public health system for certain members of the population. Those who socially identify themselves as women have disproportionately been impacted due to being the main caregivers for children, parents, and other family members, as well as the highest proportion of front-line staff for public health (Hou & Schimmele, 2020; Shamseer et al., 2021; United Nations, 2020). Gender is a multidimensional and non-binary concept, and inequity multiplies when the intersections of being Black and Indigenous are added (Yu et al., 2013). Now more than ever, a public health feminism (PHF) approach is required.

PHF has been defined as "holistic and multidisciplinary activities, based on theoretical pluralism, multiple perspectives, and collective actions with the aim of improving the health of gender-subordinated groups" (Hammarström, 1999). PHF uses gender as an analytical category to examine health inequities by focusing on the connection between disadvantage, health, and the distribution of power

(Rogers, 2006). PHF is crucial to understanding the multifactorial and intersectional lens that has a substantial effect on health outcomes, inequity, and oppression. In this chapter, we examine the barriers and social constructs that women (particularly those who are Black and Indigenous) face in public health settings and provide suggestions for critical system improvements. We also demonstrate why it is imperative to drastically overhaul the current patriarchy and systemic racism embedded in the public health system.

The historical and current narrative is that unfair social structures result in health disparities and lead to poor outcomes, such as lack of Black and Indigenous women in leadership roles. However, this framing of inequity fails to consider how this system continues to benefit some over others, which has severe consequences. Change is possible through tangible support of women in public health environments, intentional actionable career pathways that enable Black and Indigenous women's leadership, breaking barriers through systemic change, and equity in healthcare access. It is our collective responsibility to recognize, learn and unlearn, address, advocate, and, as John Lewis stated, "make good trouble" (Associated Press, 2020).

GENDER INEQUITY

The COVID-19 pandemic has created an immense workload and burden for women, many of whom have had to take on additional household responsibilities in addition to being primary caregivers for children and dependents (McKinsey & Company, 2021). Women carry more cognitive and emotional workload than men (Hogenboom, 2022), and this has been amplified during the pandemic (Minello, 2020), leading many women to struggle with their mental health, including experiencing burnout (Sriharan et al., 2020). Compared to men, women are more likely to advance equity, diversity, and inclusion efforts personally and professionally and be allies to Black and Indigenous women (McKinsey & Company, 2021), which can carry with it great emotional weight. It is for many of these reasons that more women have been forced to leave the workforce than ever before (McKinsey & Company, 2021; US Bureau of Statistics, 2022a, Table A-1). Racialized women—especially Black women—have likewise experienced more job loss during the COVID-19 pandemic (Tucker, 2022; US Bureau of Statistics, 2022b, Table A-2; US Bureau of Statistics, 2022c, Table A-3), and BIPOC women presently disproportionately have jobs deemed essential during the pandemic (McKinsey & Company, 2021). The confounding factors of caregiving responsibilities while also being mandated as essential and front-line workers have led to staggering job losses for women (McKinsey & Company, 2020).

During the pandemic, women who work in academia have fallen substantially behind their male counterparts (Shamseer et al., 2021). Evidence shows that women published fewer pre-prints and journal publications (Andersen et al., 2020), registered fewer new projects (Frederickson, 2020), and led fewer COVID-related studies (Amano-Patiño et al., 2020) than men (Gabster et al., 2020; Viglione, 2020). Women were also cited less in the media regarding their COVID expertise (Rajan et al., 2020). However, men's productivity substantially increased during this time (Fazackerley, 2020).

THE INTERSECTION OF RACE AND GENDER

The term *intersectionality* was first coined by 1989 by Kimberlé Crenshaw and defined "as a way to help explain the oppression of African-American women" (Crenshaw, 1989, 1991). There is abundant evidence to demonstrate poor health outcomes for racialized women because of a multitude of barriers due to the intersection of race and gender. Black, Indigenous and people of colour (BIPOC) women also experienced far higher rates of COVID-19 in Canada, including higher rates morbidity and mortality, which is closely tied to the social determinants of health (Government of Manitoba, 2021).

Indeed, according to Franke, "structural racism is a form of racism that is embedded in the laws, policies, institutions, and practices that provide advantages to certain racial groups while disadvantaging others" (Franke, 2018). It is a deliberate system that upholds the existing hierarchy through creating multiple barriers for those designated to be at the bottom. As Dorothy E. Roberts states, "race is not a biological category that naturally produces health disparities because of genetic differences. Race is a political category that has staggering biological consequences because of the impact of social inequity on people's health" (Williams et al., 2019).

Despite the many obstacles to disempower Black and Indigenous people and their cultures, histories, contributions, and expertise, they have stayed rooted in their identities and continuously fought for equity for centuries. However, racism continues to have a deep and significant impact. Black and Indigenous people have experienced extensive hardship because of colonization, which is an intentional system to exploit, marginalize, assimilate, and commit cultural genocide. The outcomes have had a confounding intergenerational impact, including health disparities (Bethune et al., 2019; Dryden & Nnorom, 2021) and poor health outcomes. The murder of George Floyd in Minneapolis in 2020 and the continuous recovery of unmarked gravesites of Indigenous children from residential schools have shed a mainstream and highly publicized spotlight on the inequity that Black and Indigenous people face. This recent public spotlight has unfortunately created a narrative that racism is a novel phenomenon, which is inaccurate and fails to acknowledge the intentional system that is in place to allow it to continue. This evidence of glaring disparities in health outcomes, incarceration, child welfare, leadership positions in public health, and socio-economic status has been vocalized and published by public health scholars for decades.

Systemic racism has also significantly impacted racialized women in public health leadership positions. Racialized women are promoted at far lower rates than men to manager levels and above, with a 75% drop off between entry level and C-suite leaders. Despite more women being promoted to directorships in public companies, the proportion of women executives is low in Canada (18.2%) and has not changed since 2015. Only 8 out of 2,200 board positions were held by Indigenous women (MacDougall et al., 2021). Furthermore, a recent study examined race and gender in healthcare leadership positions across Canada (Sergeant et al., 2022). Overall, of the 2,658 leaders identified, 49.9% were women and only 3.8% were BIPOC women. At the ministry level, none of the 78 leaders were BIPOC women. When this hierarchy is upheld with very few racialized women in public health leadership positions,

> it continues the uphold systemic and institutional racism; micro and macro aggressions from those in the same position in the dominant group; and internalized racism in those of the less dominant group. To avoid sanctions or to move up the hierarchy, members of less-dominant groups tend to show deference to members of the dominant group, a process that reinforces and perpetuates this hierarchy, whereas people at the top often deny that a group-based hierarchy exist. (Sidanius & Pratto, 1999)

It is therefore imperative to understand that success is not solely a result of a person's abilities; the intersections of race and gender profoundly impact one's ability to achieve a leadership position in public health. Privilege is of paramount importance in this intentional system.

The countless historical and current consequences of systemic racism, including health disparities and outcomes, access to education, access to healthcare, mental health, and leadership opportunities pervade all aspects of public health. These social determinants of health have had a devastating effect on racialized women.

IMPACT OF WHITE CIS MALE PATRIARCHY

Our social identities are compounded by systems of privilege, power, and oppression, leading to inequities and discrimination. The white cisgender male without a visible disability is still deemed the norm in public health despite all the evidence to show the harm to women and racialized people that results. This is especially the case for leadership positions, where characteristics of good leaders are often ascribed to men. Individuals who hold the power to make decisions that drastically effect public health institutions did not ask for this unearned advantage (McLean, 2018). This power is also not a result of higher worth, but instead these positions are acquired and held because of aspects of social identity that were not chosen. These demographics continue to uphold inequitable systems, such as being a settler, white, cisgender, and able-bodied. Several barriers preventing Black and Indigenous women from attaining leadership positions were outlined in a recent article (Morgan, 1996; Sergeant et al., 2022); these included a lack of networking opportunities and a racist and gender-biased institutional culture. The push of some organizations within public health to return to "normalcy" post-COVID is an intentional way to cover the cracks that have surfaced and to continue a system that has allowed patriarchy and racism to reign. A post-COVID-19 pandemic recovery requires a PHF lens, and several recommendations are highlighted in the next section to help public health organizations achieve an equitable recovery.

RECOMMENDATIONS

Recommendation #1—Distribution of Power

To avoid tokenism, institutions must ensure that leaders who are racialized are included on the highest level of the executive leadership and, furthermore, that they have the same authority to make decisions as others who are included at the table (Glass & Cook, 2020; Hirshfield & Joseph, 2012). Policies and practices must exist and be enforced within human resources departments to protect Black and Indigenous staff. These policies must be co-designed with Black and Indigenous women and focus on HR policies (e.g., diversity of HR staff, cultural safety training for hiring committee, diversity on application review and hiring committee, equity audits, use of inclusive language in job postings), education (e.g., mandatory equity, diversity, and inclusion (EDI), anti-racism, and anti-oppression training for all staff), work-life balance (e.g., prohibiting work and emails after 5 p.m., and on weekends, shortened workdays), childcare (e.g., providing financial support and flexible hours to working parents), non-gendered parental leave, and upholding Indigenous ways of knowing. Inclusion must be woven and mandated into all processes, procedures, and care to result in diversity. Reverse quotas (e.g., only 50% membership of white cis men) can be used so that there is not only one or two diverse leaders in the institution, which leads to tokenism that places Black and Indigenous women in harm's way. Those currently in power need to own their privilege and complicity in achieving and upholding their powerful positions and not see it as separate from the system of inequity that continues to keep those who face inequity at the bottom. As stated by Stephanie Nixon (2019),

> These systems were designed to oppress, and they are sustained, intentionally by some and unintentionally by others, who are on top of the coin. It is not the intent of one's actions that matters but the impact, and the impact of oblivion among people on the top can be deeply harmful, dehumanizing and violent to people on the bottom.

Through their lived experience, Black and Indigenous women who carry various intersections are the experts to overhaul the current public health system due to centuries of their lived experience of being at the bottom.

Recommendation #2—Gender Inequity, Anti-Oppression, and Anti-Racism Education

Education is a component of learning and unlearning, as spoken by the Honourable Justice Murray Sinclair (2010, p. 9), who stated,

> We ... believe that it will be education, again, that will be the tool that best addresses all of that, for education will create knowledge and from knowledge will come understanding. From understanding will come respect—both self-respect for Indigenous people and mutual respect for all.

Since 2020, there has been an immense push for EDI training in institutions. EDI training is invaluable, but it is not nearly enough on its own to dismantle the pervasive system in public health leadership and healthcare. These trainings have included focusing on the self (e.g., identifying unconscious bias) to demonstrating systemic racism. EDI trainings have most often fallen on the shoulder of Black and Indigenous EDI leaders, which carries with it an immense emotional weight to not only educate those in power but potentially trigger personal traumas and cause harm. Often the individuals who take on the burden of providing the EDI trainings are underfunded and understaffed, which ultimately leads to burnout. These trainings have frequently been mandated for staff in leadership positions who, as mentioned earlier, are disproportionally non-BIPOC individuals who have no lived experience of racism, nor have they ever been held accountable for dismantling systemic inequities. EDI training is an important first step, but it must be used in combination with other strategies; it is not sufficient on its own. EDI training should be mandated for all staff (not just leaders), and the individuals responsible for the training should be adequately supported and funded (e.g., additional stipend provided on top of salary for those leading and participating in this important work). It should not be the sole responsibility of the EDI trainers and Black and Indigenous staff to deconstruct systemic racism in the organization; that should fall on all leadership of the organization collectively.

Recommendation #3—Evidence and Ongoing Monitoring

Intervention effectiveness should be further examined, especially for those initiatives that will support Black and Indigenous women within the organization. The organization should set realistic, tangible EDI goals and benchmarks using a PHF lens. Ongoing monitoring is required to document the progress that organizations have made towards their goals and this needs to be transparently reported and publicly shared. Funding and additional support must be allocated to conduct this ongoing monitoring; this requires a substantial investment from the organization so that it is not tokenistic and demonstrates an actionable commitment. Strategy sustainability and effectiveness should be examined annually at the minimum and scaled up accordingly. Strategies need to be designed and executed by leaders at the top and be incorporated in all levels of the organization.

Recommendation #4—Unification, Mentorship, and Sponsorship

Everyone must be united to achieve a public health system that is equitable for everyone. Diverse role models—especially Black and Indigenous women—are required to demonstrate inclusion of everyone. Since so few Black and Indigenous women hold public health leadership positions, a system for succession planning, peer mentoring, and support programming can fill the gap until more are hired into such positions. Everyone must be committed to lifting others up—those of all genders and races, not just people who resemble those consistently in power. Mentorship and sponsorship are required to promote and support Black and Indigenous women, so the focus is on lifting others while they themselves are lifted.

Committing to mentoring and sponsoring Black and Indigenous women, including allocating required organizational resources, should be a goal and an accountability of all public health leaders.

Recommendation #5—Accountability

Leaders who are white cis males without a disability must be held accountable for their demonstrated commitment to anti-racism, anti-oppression, and gender equity efforts, as they are the ones who disproportionally currently hold the most decision-making power. This can be achieved through performance appraisals on hiring metrics, demographic-based staff promotion, and handling of inequity perpetrated by direct staff. All public health organization leadership must be held accountable for their leadership hiring practices and there needs to be ongoing, transparent, and public reporting on benchmarks. Managers have a profound impact on hiring practices, promotions, and the well-being of their staff. For their direct employees, they are also a crucial obstacle or pathway to moving up and gaining more power within the organization. It is therefore imperative that middle management is held accountable by senior leadership through clearly mandated expectations. If an organization has a set of expectations and values that are not successfully downloaded to middle managers, those managers will have little incentive to uphold them (Cohen & Gavett, 2019). Public health organizations must be held accountable for improving the health outcomes of racialized patients and their hiring of Black and Indigenous women to leadership roles.

CONCLUSION

It is our collective responsibility to ensure we address and dismantle the barriers that have prevailed for far too long. In the wise words of Archbishop Desmond Tutu, "If you are neutral in situations of injustice, you have chosen the side of the oppressor." We must take actionable steps to embrace the work that is needed to continuously strive for social justice and to dismantle the white supremacist patriarchy that has had such a profoundly detrimental effect on racialized women's health outcomes and ability to attain leadership positions. Black flourishing and Indigenous joy should be paramount to the future of humanity, and we must undo notions of established power that believe that equity feels like oppression. Benefiting from the oppression of others is not power but instead a deliberate process to retain that power. Public health should be a paramount system in which to address this due to the profound effect it has on general population health outcomes.

The aim is to create a public health system that is abundantly inclusive and equitable, incorporating PHF-based co-design in all aspects, from hiring practices and education to childcare, along with a consciousness of Indigenous ways of knowing, and the social determinants of health. Risks must be courageously welcomed to dismantle the harmful system that has predominated for far too long. Individuals must openly and intentionally practise critical allyship to transform public health institutions (Richardson & Murphy, 2018), placing Black and Indigenous women in long-overdue and much-needed public health leadership positions and working together in partnership to transform the current system.

CRITICAL THINKING QUESTIONS

1. What will happen if we return to the pre-COVID public health system?
2. Why is a public health feminism lens crucial to addressing the lack of Black and Indigenous women in leadership roles?
3. Why is it critical to implement the recommendations outlined by the authors?

KEY TERMS

gender
race
Indigenous
Black
leadership
COVID-19
critical allyship

SUGGESTED FURTHER READINGS

1. Nixon, S. A. (2019). The coin model of privilege and critical allyship: Implications for health. *BMC Public Health, 19*(1), 1637. https://doi.org/10.1186/s12889-019-7884-9
2. McKinsey & Company. (2021, September 27). *Women in the workplace 2021.* https://www.mckinsey.com/featured-insights/diversity-and-inclusion/women-in-the-workplace
3. Ford, C. L., & Airhihenbuwa, C. O. (2018). Commentary: Just what is critical race theory and what's it doing in a progressive field like public health? *Ethnicity & Disease, 28*(Suppl 1), 223.

CHAPTER 12

Reclamation of Matriarchy and Kinship Systems

Miranda Lesperance

LEARNING OBJECTIVES

1. Understand the concept of Indigenous kinship, particularly from an Anishinaabe lens.
2. Recognize that some societies are matriarchal and that patriarchy still negatively affects these societies.
3. Strength-based methods and approaches, like storytelling, are appropriate and valid.

I am sitting here in the dark of the early morning hours writing the introduction and conclusion to this book chapter. I am up before my children wake for the day and the hustle and bustle of their day takes over mine. It is the morning of September 30—the first National Day for Truth and Reconciliation in what is now known as Canada. For many years, this day has been known as Orange Shirt Day in the Indigenous community. It was named and practised for Phyllis Webstad. She had the new orange shirt that her Grandmother gave her taken away from her on her first day of attending residential school (Webstad, 2021). I am still processing how I feel about this new national holiday and what it will mean for myself, my children, family, and kin.

On the one hand, it is excellent to see settlers learning about and participating in activities about this country's deep colonial history, yet I can't help feeling sad and weary. I am grieving for my Grandparents who attended residential school. I am mourning for my parents that attended Indian day school. I am forlorn because childhood could have been better for us. I am tired of delivering lectures on the health impacts of colonization and colonial policies. I am tired of seeing the nasty comments and reactions on social media. I am exhausted from hearing about my kin going missing, injured, trafficked, or dying prematurely.

But with all of these feelings, I also feel gratefulness and deep admiration for my kin who held me up this week. This week and many weeks before this one, particularly during a global pandemic. I am fortunate to be surrounded by a kinship system that understands what it is like to move through this world with many intersections: as a pansexual Indigenous woman, mother, academic scholar, community member, and daughter of survivors of the residential school systems. I've had incredibly supportive exchanges about self-care from my caregiver kin who know what it is like to be sad and weary while trying to break harmful parenting cycles. I've had words of encouragement from my fellow Indigenous academics who know what it is like to work in institutions that perpetuate colonial attitudes. We cheer each other on to keep going. I have family and community members who ensure that my family and I are included in the reclamation and resurgence of our traditional and cultural practices. I sit beside water when working out complex thoughts. I have bird friends that I periodically look up from my laptop to watch. I have the trees that share oxygen with me when I go in the forest for mental health breaks. I do not believe I will make it through this first National Day of Truth and Reconciliation—or this book chapter, PhD dissertation, global pandemic, week, month, and year—without my kinship support. My children and I are truly thankful for the support that we (hopefully) effectively reciprocate.

I've come across many definitions of kinship over the years. Some are settler interpretations, and some are from other Indigenous nations. One of the most cited is the concept of *wahkohtowin* in Cree (Wildcat, 2019). While the idea of kinship is common among Indigenous Peoples, it is described in potentially different ways, and caution must be exercised when discussing this concept in and between other nations. In addition, non-Indigenous academia sometimes questionably applies nation-specific concepts in a pan-Indigenous fashion, which I would like to avoid in my research.

In my nation, Ojibwe, and language, Anishinaabemowin, I've come to understand that kinship comes from the root word *inawendiwag*, which translates to "they are related to each other." You would call your kinsperson or relative *inawemaagan*. I've never before had to spell this word on paper, nor did my family. Hence, I turned to the Ojibwe People's Dictionary (Nichols & Nyholm, 1995) for this purpose. I've also heard this concept referred to as *abi inawendiwag*, which includes the word *abi*, which translates to "occupying a certain place." I like this addition because it adds more action to the concept, ensuring that it retains a dynamic, ever-changing, evolving quality while maintaining respect. In colonial

English, you could say "all my relations," and it includes not just human relations, but also relations from other species or earth elements, as I've alluded to when describing my gratefulness above.

Unfortunately, these matrilineal kinship networks were severely impacted by settler colonialism. Just yesterday, my family and I spoke about how we have lost many teachings related to matriarchy in my community. Some of our teachings say that children follow the clan system of our fathers (patrilineal), and some say that children follow the clan system of our mothers (matrilineal). We discussed being uncertain which teaching is closer to tradition and which is influenced by the settler colonial and religious state. I left the conversation still not knowing for sure, but with a remaining belief that matriarchy and kinship relationships were significant and continue to be.

Since Europeans first colonized North America, there has been a war on Indigenous matriarchy and kinship networks in Canada. Indigenous lands and peoples have been subjected to cultural genocide, violence, land appropriation, oppression, and legislated policies like the Gradual Civilization Act and the Indian Act (Allan & Smylie, 2015). Residential schools have been the most damaging colonizer-legislated policies to assimilate Indigenous Peoples into dominant white culture. Residential schools were used to remove Indigenous children from their homes, away from their parents, to attend government-sponsored religious boarding schools. The children were forbidden from practising their culture or speaking their language (Truth and Reconciliation Commission of Canada, 2016). The "schools" were intended to disrupt the relationships between the children, their parents, and their communities, as evidenced by former prime minister John A. Macdonald saying in his official report of the debates of the House of Commons of the Dominion of Canada (1883),

> when the school is on the reserve the child lives with its parents, who are savages; he is surrounded by savages, and though he may learn to read and write his habits, and training and mode of thought are Indian. He is simply a savage who can read or write. It has been strongly pressed on myself, as the head of the Department, the Indian children should be withdrawn as much as possible from the parental influence, and the only way to do that would be to put them in central training industrial schools where they acquire the habits and modes of thought of white men.

After many generations of children were ripped from their families to fulfil Macdonald's mission and legacy, whistleblowers like Dr. Peter Bryce (Hay et al.,

2020) advocated for First Nation children to stay in their communities. First Nation children were then forced to attend Indian day schools, which were schools located in the communities where children lived with their parents. However, children were still expected to assimilate into Euro-Canadian culture (Walls & Whitbeck, 2012). Although the children remained in the community with their families, the residential schools damaged many families and abuse was still rampant in the day schools. My own family, and most other First Nation families, were scarred by these "schools." My Grandfathers were part of the tail end of the last generation to leave my community for school. The Department of Indian Affairs, as it was called at the time, then built a day school in the community. My Grandmothers and parents attended the day school; I was the first generation not to attend, although I still had to go to school in a town nearby.

The Sixties Scoop was another mechanism used to assimilate Indigenous children by removing them from their families and kinship networks and forcing them to be re-homed and parented by non-Indigenous parents (Alston-O'Connor, 2019). This mass removal of children spanned over 20 years—a lot of Indigenous children did not have the opportunity to be supported by larger family and kinship networks. Many of these scooped children report a loss of identity, even when they did not know they were adopted into non-Indigenous families (Legacy of Hope, 2017). Even in more recent times, the number of Indigenous children in foster care is higher than any other group in Canada (Trocme et al., 2004). This phenomenon is now known as the Millennial Scoop (Blackstock, 2015) and it is shameful that Indigenous children continue to be removed from their families. Indigenous child welfare agencies have formed to minimize the number of children removed from families and communities. They now use "kinship adoptions," foster care or adoptions by family/community members, which have helped children find lasting homes (Ryan et al., 2010) and, therefore, keep the children in the community and maintain their kinship ties.

Sometimes colonial policies destroyed the matriarchy and kinship networks before an Indigenous woman could begin to or continue having children. There are documented cases of government-mandated and privately mandated programs that medically sterilized First Nation women deemed too incompetent to have children (Dyck, 2013). The definition of what is "unfit" is uncertain and inconsistent. Still, the stories from women who have been forced or coerced into sterilization for various reasons exist, including women deemed "sexually promiscuous" or "mentally incapacitated" (Black et al., 2021). There is currently a class-action lawsuit representing approximately 100 Indigenous women forced or coerced into sterilization. Alisa Lombard, a partner at Semaganis Worme Lombard, an Indigenous-owned law firm, leads this lawsuit. Alisa presented before the Standing Senate Committee on Human Rights, stating, "wealth is life, children, family, and culture for my clients. The decision on whether to gain in this wealth was stolen from them, and we must all remember that in our work" (Senate of Canada, 2019).

The chapter on Indigenous women in the Statistics Canada *First Nations, Métis and Inuit Women* report shows that between the years of 2010 and 2011, Indigenous women had a fertility rate of 2.2 children compared to 1.6 children for all Canadian women (Statistics Canada, 2016). This fertility rate, combined with the health effects resulting from the colonial policies described above, is a public health issue of epic proportions in Canada. The marginalization of Indigenous Peoples and communities has resulted in significant inequalities in health determinants compared with Canada's general population (Greenwood et al., 2018), and this disparity has affected Indigenous women more than Indigenous men (Statistics Canada, 2016). It will continue to impact generations of Indigenous mothers, who may struggle to raise holistically healthy children. Families have lost the traditional way of parenting. Some mothers pass on the effects of the physical, emotional, verbal, and sexual abuse that they were exposed to due to the processes and impacts of colonization (Muir & Bohr, 2019). The loss of parenting skills perpetuates adverse health outcomes and poor coping methods in mothers and children. Van Herk et al. (2011) demonstrate that mothering is a protective factor for children's early development. Many colonial policies have impacted the ability of Indigenous mothers to bond with their children and exercise healthy parenting skills.

There is overwhelming evidence that Indigenous mothers may not have optimal health and subsequently may have unhealthy coping methods. The factors that affect First Nation mothers in Ontario include age, psychological and biological disorders, smoking, and alcohol and substance use (Sharma et al., 2016). First Nation women are more likely to be young mothers than non-Indigenous mothers, and young mothers are less likely to graduate high school and more likely to have a lower income. They live in overcrowded housing that requires repair (Garner et al., 2013). Indigenous women have some of the highest rates of substance use in Canada, and substance use in pregnancy and parenting is a significant concern (Guèvremont & Kohen, 2013). Smoking rates before, during, and after pregnancy are also much higher in Indigenous women than in the general population (Wright et al., 2020). Indigenous mothers in Canada face higher rates of all types of abuse and intimate partner violence compared to non-Indigenous mothers, and it can likely be explained by socioeconomic position (Daoud et al., 2013). Indigenous mothers are more likely to be lone parents than non-Indigenous mothers. This statistic leaves them disadvantaged when accessing provincial and federal parental benefits only available to two-parent families (Hull, 2013). Children and mothers, separated from each other due to colonial policies, have shown depressive symptoms, eroding their ability to parent and increasing their vulnerability to harmful coping methods (Walls & Whitbeck, 2012). Again, I am cognizant of many unhealthy coping strategies in my own family. Other family members and I are left with breaking unhealthy chains and a sense of responsibility to reclaim our traditional methods, including re-establishing our matriarchal kinship networks to support each other.

As demonstrated above, there is a lot of academic, peer-reviewed literature establishing the "problems" that plague First Nation mothers. However, there is very little academic, peer-reviewed literature substantiating the reclamation of Indigenous matriarchy practices and a sense of pride that is clearly shown in practice and captured in grey literature. Nevertheless, there are documented cases of individuals, organizations, and communities reclaiming Indigenous matriarchy and utilizing strength-based traditional parenting methods (Lavell & Lavell-Harvard, 2006). This reclaimed knowledge is then shared with their kinship networks (Anderson & Lavell-Harvard, 2014). Fortunately, their kinship networks and the existing grey literature are more readily accessible and applicable to First Nations mothers, who need access to social programs, further education, and the support of their families and communities to improve their holistic health (Minthorn, 2018). This improvement in the health of mothers impacts the health and parenting of future generations and thereby the kinship network and community at large.

There are, however, other academics out there celebrating Indigenous reclamation and strength-based intersectional approaches (FNIGC, 2020). Moreover, it is not just all doom-and-gloom, problem-based research. Indigenous scholars recognize that Indigenous folks have strengths that need to be highlighted, including within the academy itself. I am greatly looking forward to sharing an article published in 2022 called "Indigenous Motherhood in the Academy" (Minthorn, 2022) because it examines the intersections of being a mother with a role in scholarship and the academy. In general and outside of academia, however, we know that community researchers are gathering strengths that address specific "deficits" that Indigenous Peoples face with methods that already exist in Indigenous individuals, families, and communities (Kirmayer et al., 2011). For example, acknowledging traditional health and birthing practices leads to proper programming within the community and in urban health facilities (O'Driscoll et al., 2011). These researchers, and other Indigenous mothers, inspired me to use my PhD dissertation to highlight how female First Nation mothers, all with different intersecting identifiers, are actively reclaiming culture and relying on kinship networks to eschew colonial labels.

My research focuses on colonizer labels (both historical and contemporary) applied to First Nation women and the children for which they care. It is evident from the Jesuit and fur trader archives that I combed through that First Nation women have been subject to these labels presumptively since the time of first contact. For example, one Jesuit record justified the indoctrination of children by stating that First Nation mothers showered "their children with wonderful affection; but they preserve no discipline, for they neither themselves correct them nor allow others to do so" (Canadian Research Knowledge Network, n.d.). This quote demonstrates that even our love and affection for our children was weaponized against us. Current society also places labels on our women. My PhD research shows that these labels come from healthcare providers, service providers (such as those at child welfare agencies), Indigenous and non-Indigenous community members, and other non-Indigenous mothers. Such labelling is also evident in most of the current scholarship on Indigenous women and mothers, as referenced above, which reduces each woman to their "affliction," whether it be substance use or lone parenting.

While I did not precisely pinpoint Kimberlé Crenshaw's theory of intersectionality (Crenshaw, 1991) in my PhD research, I did draw on my understanding of how my participants' intersecting identities affect how each of them interacts with their surrounding world. My participants identified as mothers, grandmothers parenting grandchildren, and foster and adopted mothers. There was a relatively good sample of women of different ages, socioeconomic classes, and geographic locations in what is now known as Canada. Some of these women also belonged to the 2SLGBTQIA+ community. Despite their intersecting identities, the central overlapping theme was pride in their culture and traditions and their families and kinship networks.

Participating women touched on how their parenting of their children had been affected by the parenting that they received. They acknowledged that the individual and collective trauma in our homes and communities is understandable yet unacceptable. These women also talked about how important it was to stop the cycle and reduce the detrimental impacts on the children that they parent. Most women said they turn to cultural practices and traditions to ground themselves and remind themselves that their ancestors also handed down "intergenerational strength" (Lesperance, 2022). The few women who did not yet turn to cultural practices expressed a "desperate need to reconnect" and were actively building their kinship networks in the urban and off-community locations where they lived.

The mentioned cultural practices were varied and unique to each woman. There was some overlap in practice, but each woman had a specific tradition that resonated with them. For example, to connect with relations, there were stories about going on the land, whether it was on the lake neighbouring the community or a particular tree in an urban centre. One participant said that she "always goes to the water to speak to ancestors and creation," while another "finds solace and comfort in their urban medicinal garden" (Lesperance, 2022).

There were stories about making and playing drums, attending ceremonies like sweat lodges, and making themselves and their children powwow regalia. One participant talked about "how [their] children loved making drums with [her], and they played together." Some women worked traplines with their families, and some made beautiful art and adornments. A participant said that "she loves gifting her creations to friends and family," and other participants were able to make a viable business selling their creations (Lesperance, 2022). But, again, the overall feeling when the women spoke about these cultural practices was pride.

There were stories about how women found and established kin networks that supported their desire to reconnect to culture and understand the collective experience and impact that colonization and colonial policies have had on their families. Some women mentioned that it could be a struggle to find these networks in their more urban communities, particularly those located within other Indigenous nations different from their own. Still, it was worth it and helpful when found and practised. Group cultural activities, like beading circles and hide-tanning camps, were indispensable in establishing kin networks both in community and in urban centres. One woman reported that she "had never felt more alive and supported" than when she was at hide-tanning camp. There is a collective effort to sustain these established kinship networks by scheduling more group activities in person or using video chat software or various social media sites. Many women spoke about how these virtual meetings kept them connected during the pandemic when it was not always possible or safe to meet in person (Lesperance, 2022).

I am incredibly grateful to have gathered these women's stories to highlight how they are reclaiming kinship and reconnection to culture and tradition. Their stories have inspired me to continue the same work with my children and share my experiences with my kinship networks. Through these kin networks, we all can re-establish our connection to each other, our ancestors, and the natural world, thereby restoring balance to our day-to-day lives that continue to be significantly influenced by settler colonialism. This healthy balance will lead to the overall health of individuals and communities, or mino bimaadiziwin—the good life.

Dibiki giizis, the sun, is rising now that I am finished writing this conclusion today. A flurry of messages between my cousins and I about the start of our day have already been exchanged. My children will be rising soon, and I will start making breakfast and shuffling us into our day. A student from the course I am teaching this semester invited us to today's powwow on Anemki Wajiw (thunder mountain). So, while my children's peers will be wearing orange shirts and learning about truth and reconciliation, my children and I will be again surrounded by kin, laughing and dancing to the healing sound of the Grandfather drum.

Mii i'iw, chi miigwech.

CRITICAL THINKING QUESTIONS

1. Why do you think settler societies can be against or indifferent to matriarchal and kinship systems?
2. What does it mean for Indigenous motherhood(s) to be governed by patriarchal ideals/norms?
3. How do storytelling and other strength-based approaches differ from mainstream Western-colonial methods? What benefits are there to this style of information sharing?

KEY TERMS

kinship
Indigenous matriarchy
residential schools
mothering
reclamation

SUGGESTED FURTHER READINGS

1. Anderson, K. (2011). *Life stages and Native women: Memory, teachings, and story medicine*. University of Manitoba Press.
2. First Nations Health Authority & Office of Provincial Health Officer. (2021). *Sacred and strong: Upholding our matriarchal roles—the health and wellness journeys of BC First Nations women and girls*.
3. Senklip Harvey, K. (2019). *Kamloopa: An Indigenous matriarch story*. Talonbooks.

CHAPTER 13

Engendering a Feminist Ethic of Care to Training a New Generation of Public Health Researchers: Reflecting on 4theRecord

Sarah Flicker, Nadha Hassen, Jessica Fields, and 4theRecord Research Team, with Amanda Galusha, Anjalee Srinivasan, Caitlin Arizala, Emily Sutton, Jessica J. Mencia, Julia Ferguson, Kethmi Egodage, Kezia Arinka, Nadia Bevan, Reece Rabanal, Seventy Hall, Vaishnavy Puvipalan, and Zarin Tasnim

LEARNING OBJECTIVES

1. Define a feminist ethic of care.
2. Provide examples of how to enact a feminist ethic of care in public health research.
3. Explain the challenges and opportunities of adopting a feminist model to training a new generation of researchers.

INTRODUCTION

4theRecord is a research team focused on understanding how COVID-19 has changed the ways that queer and racialized young women and non-binary folks think about risk. Often asked to put their bodies (and labour) on the front lines of the pandemic response, these youth have also experienced increased surveillance, scrutiny, policing, and violence that has made taking even salutary risks very challenging.

As the investigator team sought to study these relationships in Melbourne, Toronto, and New York City, we wanted to do so in a way that honoured our commitments to feminism and anti-racist praxis. Moreover, we wanted to celebrate and affirm the positive possibilities of risk-taking! We welcomed diverse queer and/or racialized young people onto the research team in an explicit effort to train a new generation of public health scholars in practices that disrupted the status quo (Moss et al., 1999; Wilson et al., 2021). Drawing on a feminist ethic of care (Gilligan, 1993; Noddings, 2013), we centred the lived experience and realities of team members to draw on our collective strengths and prepare ourselves to take big risks and dream up alternative possibilities. Here, we share our approach to enacting and threading a feminist ethic of care through our international, interdisciplinary, and intergenerational research team. We were not always successful in our efforts. We present these process reflections as part of a commitment to "staying in the mess" of reflexive praxis (Finlay, 2002; Salmon & Steinberg, 2007). We offer this paradigm for how public health research can be done from a standpoint that strives to confront sexism and racism in its implementation.

THEORIZING A FEMINIST ETHIC OF CARE

bell hooks (2014, p. 1) famously offered a broad and blunt definition of feminism: "simply put, feminism is a movement to end sexism, sexist exploitation, and oppression." Feminism is about calling attention to the ways that gender (and other identity structures) organize(s) our daily lives and then challenging the resulting inequities. Sara Ahmed (2017) takes up hooks' legacy and, in the introduction to *Living a Feminist Life*, writes that feminism fills her with hope and energy, because "it brings to mind loud acts of refusal and rebellion as well as the quiet ways we might have of not holding on to things that diminish us" (p. 1). This enthusiasm for celebrating the possibilities of feminism is part of what brought us together as a research group.

Rather than relying on a specific set of methods, a feminist research practice is distinguished by its application of feminist principles (Beckman, 2014; Harding, 1987). White and colleagues (2001) identified four important principles of feminist research: "inclusiveness and diversity, the importance of social and historical context, combating power and privilege, and social activism" (p. 267). Beckman (2014) offers an expanded list that also includes "listening to women's voices and experience," "reflexivity," and attending to social relationships during the research process through an "ethic of care." Blakely (2007, p. 62) argues that caring, in this context, involves

> caring for the research (or the issue/topic itself), the research participants, what becomes of the research (including the eventual narrative, research notes, all of the data), and the researcher and the research team.

Others have drawn on this work (Gringeri, Wahab, & Anderson-Nathe, 2010; Mauthner & Edwards, 2010) to argue that a feminist ethic of care acknowledges the links between personal and professional lives. We take up this expansive vision for an ethic of care and draw on the work of disability justice scholar and activist Leah Lakshmi Piepzna-Samarasinha (2018) to consider

> What does it mean to shift our ideas of access and care ... from an individual chore ... to a collective responsibility that's maybe even deeply joyful? ... What does it mean to wrestle with these ideas of softness and strength, vulnerability, pride, asking for help, and not—all of which are so deeply raced and classed and gendered? ... This is about some of the ways we are attempting to dream ways to access care deeply, in a way where we are in control, joyful, building community, loved, giving and receiving, that doesn't burn anyone out or abuse or underpay anyone in the process. (p. 33)

STUDY BACKGROUND

Our larger research project takes a mixed-methods approach to understanding risk in young women's and non-binary people's lives. Following an initial screener, eligible participants were sent a link to a demographic survey that queried their experiences of COVID and risk taking. Survey completers were then sent unique links to a digital life history calendar (Bay-Cheng, 2009, 2017). They were prompted to create personal COVID timelines and post about risks taken and averted in their personal, professional, and romantic lives. Those interested were interviewed synchronously over Zoom by an undergraduate youth peer researcher (YPR). Ultimately, results will be shared through an interactive travelling exhibit that we are tentatively calling the Gallery of Risk.

To better reflect the community that we sought to engage and explicitly welcome those who commonly experience marginalization, our research team prioritized hiring, training, and supporting young women and non-binary folks who identify as racialized and/or queer. Four graduate research assistants (RAs) were brought into the project who met these criteria. (A fifth RA from Melbourne joined later.)

The RAs recruited eight enthusiastic YPRs who also identified as racialized and/or queer. YPRs and RAs took the lead on participant recruitment, outreach, and interviewing. In addition, they participate in cleaning up auto-generated transcripts, drafting fieldnotes, coding, and analyzing the data.

To get the team ready for these tasks, we invested in several months of training. RAs worked closely with principal investigators (PIs) to plan 10 training modules. Topics ranged from ethics to recruitment to trauma-informed interviewing.

In addition, each YPR engaged in two practice interviews and two coaching sessions with an RA, who reviewed their practice interviews. As analysis is ongoing, our team continues to meet regularly in large and small groups.

METHODS

Each module was recorded on Zoom. We took copious notes during regular planning and debrief meetings. All team members were invited to fill out reflection surveys in December and March. To draft this chapter, we reviewed these data sources and searched for moments when a feminist ethic of care was invoked. Nadha (an RA) drew quotes, stories, and examples from each of these moments to draft an outline. It was circulated to the entire team for feedback, discussion, and further comment. Sarah (co-PI) then fleshed out the chapter. It was recirculated for review. We used a shared Google Doc to collectively comment and contribute.

We write in a collective voice and include the entire RA and YPR team as co-authors, as an explicitly feminist practice to honour the diverse contributions and labour of all involved (Ahmed, 2017; Liboiron et al., 2017; McKittrick, 2021); direct quotes are attributed to particular team members as necessary.

This chapter was a collaborative effort. PIs, RAs, and YPRs came together to share our reflections about how we strove to infuse our public health research practices with a feminist ethic of care. Together, we want to create new methodological space and possibilities for imagining a different kind of academic community: one where diverse young people can bring their whole selves into critical conversations about health, well-being, and future possibilities. In the next section we point to several moments where this ethic came to light in our process.

ENACTING A FEMINIST ETHIC OF CARE

(A) Setting the Stage for Shared Leadership, Risks, and Growth

Empowering the RAs to lead the recruitment and hiring of the YPRs was one of our first opportunities to practise the principles of shared leadership. This task helped RAs get to know each other and work together to meet a goal. It exemplified the commitment to create conditions for team members to take risks, learn new things, flex their skills, succeed, and (sometimes) fail. While 10 positions were initially offered, eight YPRs ultimately joined the team.

RAs then worked closely with PIs to plan the training sessions and practise their mentorship skills. RAs were encouraged to take on several leadership roles, including co-planning and facilitating trainings, meeting with YPRs one-on-one to offer feedback on practice interviews, and later leading teams that spearheaded different online and community recruitment tactics.

RAs reflected that this experience of tiered mentorship has been the highlight of their participation on the project. Zarin (RA) noted: "My favorite part of this experience has been hiring and training the YPRs.... It was a great learning experience for me to mentor [younger] researchers." Similarly, Jessica M. (RA) reflected, "It's been really rewarding getting to know them as researchers/collaborators, but also as people ... being able to be a mentor figure to the YPRs and give them a good research experience meant a lot to me. I'm really grateful ... that I got to work with them." Nadha (RA) too shared that "working with a group of racialized and/or queer young people and seeing them come into their own has been incredible—from reading their applications ... to seeing them fly." As queer and racialized feminists, they all felt deeply connected to the politic of supporting a new generation of similarly situated scholars and opening opportunities in a way that felt authentic to our shared values.

Similarly, the YPRs were all extremely vocal about the value of having role models that looked and felt like they did. As Caitlin shared,

> I really enjoyed how the team of RAs and lead investigators empowered the YPRs to leadership. Seeing [RAs] who are fellow BIWOC researchers really gives me confidence that I'm meant to be in this space! ... [I] feel like my identity as a queer, disabled, WOC is held, valued, and given space to grow on this team!

(B) Imagining the Community that We Wanted to Create

Early in the YPR training, the PIs asked everyone what kind of community we wanted to build. Together, we collectively imagined a beautiful and caring space through brainstorming concrete commitments and each suggesting one for consideration. These were transcribed, posted in our shared online space, and returned to periodically over the course of our time together.

We generated principles that included the following:

- "Spend time talking to each other ... [make] space to become friends"
- "Assume the best; when people fall down, extend generosity and care"
- "Divide work as equitably as possible, allowing people to play to strengths"

Other notable points included "practice care and compassion," "step in to help each other," "let us know up front if you're not able to compete or take on a task," "respect one another as individual, autonomous people who have different views and frames of reference" and "celebrate good ideas."

Taken together, these principles affirmed our interest in infusing a feminist ethic of care into our daily practices and resisting patriarchal and hierarchical notions of workplace dynamics. We explicitly made space for recognizing each other as more than just colleagues—as human beings. This set a strong foundation for collaborative teamwork. Moreover, we attempted to counter the underlying expectation and assumption that researchers and scholars (including and especially racialized, queer, female, and non-binary folks) must excel at everything or routinely take on the burdens of inequitable workloads.

When RAs and YPRs reflected on the degree to which we have been successful in upholding our values, there was unanimous agreement that indeed we had. Many offered poignant examples of when these principles had come to life for them. For instance, over the course of the semester, several team members who struggled with physical or mental health challenges talked about how the team was, as Emily (YPR) explained, "always understanding and extremely kind in their response ... I was extremely grateful for these rules and that all people on our team fully believed and practised them." Similarly, Caitlin (YPR) recounted about how when she fell ill with COVID, "the entire team extended compassion and support. I feel like this work environment is rooted in support, care, advocacy, and respect." This sentiment was echoed by many other YPRs who appreciated both the room to step out when they needed a break and the chance to step in to support one another.

The pleasure of unanimous agreement should not mute the fact that tensions did still arise, even as we practised an ethic of care. Consistently, however, these principles provided us with a prism for considering how we wanted to work through challenging moments. For instance, at first, YPRs who interviewed participants were expected to take responsibility for cleaning their own transcripts. However, what quickly became apparent was that those YPRs who were more available during popular interview slots were having to do double (sometimes triple!) the work—not only were they spending more time preparing for and conducting interviews, but the time-consuming transcription work was also piling up. When we realized that we were falling behind with transcription and discussed the matter collectively, we were able to fall back on our principle of an equitable division of labour. During a team meeting, Kethmi (YPR) suggested that "maybe if people with less interviews could help with transcription that would be helpful." This suggestion, coming from a YPR to their peers, encouraged the team to rethink our processes and create new systems for distributing the workload.

(C) Centring the Voices/Opinions of Black, Indigenous and/or People of Colour (BIPOC) and Women and Confronting Racism and Sexism Explicitly

A hallmark of this process included providing space for open discussion about difficult issues. Team members appreciated that preparatory assigned readings were almost exclusively written by women who identified as Black, Indigenous and/or People of Colour (BIPOC). In addition, YPRs noticed and appreciated that efforts were even taken to bring in young queer and BIPOC women for ancillary roles (e.g., graphic design). In her reflections, Reece (YPR) commented that even as a junior member of team, she felt supported: "There was never any power dynamic, and we were all treated equally."

Despite the care that went into planning, not everyone felt the same. When the PIs (Jessica F. and Sarah) first invited the RAs to plan YPR training, they were met with some resistance. There was a lot of confusion and ambiguity around roles and accountability structures. In their efforts to flatten hierarchies, Jessica and Sarah had inadvertently reinscribed them. When Sarah checked in with Nadha about how things were going, the two ended up having a deep and frank discussion about the challenges. The conversation quickly turned to the politics of what it meant to have two white PIs leading a project that focused on racialized women's experiences and delegating tasks to racialized RAs.

Sarah and Jessica F. reflected deeply on this conversation. As white women who have worked in solidarity with racial justice movements for a long time, we were both acutely aware of the politics of race, our considerable privilege and power, and the challenges associated with dismantling systems of white supremacy in the academy. We wanted this project to run differently and reaffirmed our commitment to enacting a feminist ethic of care. We quickly worked with RAs to reorganize the distribution and flow of work. Together, we created a final training schedule and decided to work in pairs (of RA and investigator) to take turns leading each session. We also intentionally brought in all the other scholars on the team (some of whom are racialized) to co-lead sessions and centre their experiences.

Rather than shy away from these hard conversations, Sarah decided to lean straight into them. In a very early YPR session, she assigned a paper written by co-investigator Ciann Wilson that talks about how her lab of (mostly) racialized students has experienced and resisted white supremacy in the academy (Wilson et al., 2021). In conversation with Ciann, Sarah invited the YPRs to consider

> to what extent did you see yourself in some of the experiences? ... how can we engage in this project of disrupting white supremacy and

> heteronormativity and patriarchy in the academy? Like, what can we ... do as a collective together, especially in this research project, to create a different kind of space?

Several of the RAs and YPRs reflected (both at the time and through subsequent conversations) that this was a pivotal moment for them. They felt seen, understood, and safe to name the quotidian microaggressions they experience. Few had ever been invited to name these infractions in an academic space and to consider how to challenge the status quo. During the conversation, Anjalee, a YPR, reminded the group that

> representation ... doesn't mean anything if you're not following it up with inclusion ... even our space right now, we can't just view it as a check mark, that we accomplished that, okay, we got the diverse representation, we need it. How do we ... actually, like, interact with people? How do we value their experience?

Anjalee points out that while naming systemic inequities does not necessarily redress them, addressing the challenges directly can help open the door for a refusal to remain silent and complicit. As more trust is built among team members, we have continued to create space for challenging conversations and centring the voices of BIPOC women in the project.

(D) Sharing Power and Space and Responsibility

We began every meeting with a land acknowledgement. Sarah began this practice when she co-facilitated the first YPR meeting. As an international project situated in university spaces, we wanted to acknowledge our links to settler colonialism. Rather than offer a rote reading, she instead shared a beautiful video created by a local Indigenous community member who shared the history of Toronto as a meeting place.

As part of each subsequent session, each YPR and RA took a turn leading a brief land acknowledgement activity and an icebreaker. This practice helped us centre respectful engagement with Indigenous lands and knowledges. It invited everyone into the conversation to learn about different territories, histories, and traditions. As people stepped into this activity, they became extremely creative. Some offered in-depth history lessons of the Indigenous Peoples in their territories. Some shared their own settler journeys and narratives in relation to the land. Others shared documentaries or other video clips. It was a fun way for us to get to know and learn about each other and our various geographical spaces and relationships.

Sometimes, when time was tight, these felt like long detours. The urge to cut them short was sometimes strong. Planners found it hard to balance competing priorities. We regularly asked ourselves how we could make time for both the work that must get done (e.g., training to interview!) as well as the important work that should get done (e.g., relationship building, decolonizing our processes). Our team spanned multiple countries and time zones and, like many other projects that were born during the COVID-19 pandemic, we were never able to meet in person. And so, carving out space for these informal learning and storytelling opportunities was key to creating shared norms and values. In subsequent feedback sessions, folks shared that these moments were some of people's favourite points of connection during our training. The goodwill generated through community building and care was foundational for our success in getting the other work done. Emily (YPR) succinctly summarized this idea when she reflected,

> My favorite part has been the inclusive and safe environment built by our team leaders.... I felt each member cared extremely deeply for each other, which allowed for beautiful work to be produced and a safe environment for all to express their thoughts.

(E) Leaving Space for Vulnerability

Over the course of our training, we sought to teach YPRs new research skills and give each other opportunities to try out new competencies. We wanted to both build everyone's confidence but also encourage a humble growth-learning mindset. Interviewing is a skill that is most certainly honed with practice.

During training, several YPRs voiced feeling extremely excited but also nervous and overwhelmed by the prospect of conducting interviews with human beings with complex lives. Jules (YPR) shared that,

> Before every interview I conducted, whether it was for practice or with a participant, I was incredibly nervous... I think it's getting better as I complete more interviews! Rather than only being stressed about future interviews, these days I am so excited to connect and learn from more participants!

Jules also mentioned how helpful it was to receive constructive feedback on her practice interviews. These sentiments were echoed by others, including Anjalee, Vaish, and Kezia, who also noted their growing confidence over time.

Given the sensitive nature of some of the questions that we are asking (and topics being broached), many of the YPRs expressed their concerns about how to manage difficult conversations and navigate disclosures of depression, violence, or self-harm. Raising these fears demonstrated their deep commitment to participant well-being and doing a good job. It also provided the team with an impetus to offer further training and coaching. We brought in a trained psychotherapist to provide several sessions and help our team think through these complexities.

However, despite these best efforts, the impacts of white supremacy and sexism in academia could be felt as Kethmi (YPR) noted,

> As a woman of colour, it's a bit hard to feel truly comfortable with the skills I've developed. I'm always wondering whether I'm missing something or whether I'm doing something wrong—even if there's no inclination that there is anything off about the interview. There's always this underlying pressure that I have to be perfect.... It's hard to trust myself when your whole life as a woman you have to feel perfect to feel successful.

As interviewing progressed, we developed practices of taking care of each other. As a team, we encouraged everyone to reach out if they needed support. If, as a YPR was preparing for an interview, they were particularly troubled or worried or triggered by content, they could ask for help from another YPR, RA, or investigator. Importantly, they could reach out afterwards, too. At first, YPRs were shy to come forward, but one of the surprising outcomes was how taking this step encouraged others to do the same. Several YPRs shared that they were so happy to offer an ear and felt more encouraged to ask for help once they had offered it. Ironically, encouraging vulnerability (and support-seeking behaviour) led to increased community strength.

(F) Taking Care of Each Other—Accessibility, Self-Care and Well-Being

Meeting virtually did not diminish our ability to care for each other. When Nadha (RA) was particularly unwell, others on the team reached out to offer support. Reflecting on this experience, she offered, "I feel like being seen and heard really matters when doing research and in work settings, because we're all dealing with so much." Similarly, Emily (YPR) shared how Zoom and virtual participation made her involvement possible and minimized her needs for other kinds of accommodations to manage her disability. Another YPR, Kethmi noted that

> I think there's always a pressure to prove yourself as a woman ... I learned to prioritize my well-being and rely on the support of my team when I needed because I don't have to kill myself to prove my worth.

By making space and allowances for the team to show up as they could, while emphasizing communication and respect for the work and each other, we sought to challenge the notion of perfection. With so many moving parts, it was essential that the team felt they could be up front about their capacity to complete tasks in a timely manner.

(G) A Commitment to Doing Better

Despite our best efforts, we got lots wrong. It took us a while to find the right communication systems. Between email and Slack and SharePoint and Google documents, some things still fell through the cracks. Working online meant that we were never all in the same place at the same time (except virtually) and so all interactions had to be intentional and planned. In December, we decided we needed to hire more administrative help and welcomed an incredible new team member to help us get organized. It took us even longer to properly define everyone's work expectations and roles. As we grow into each other and learn more about team strengths and dynamics, we are committed to growth and change. When we asked everyone about what we could do differently, there was a desire for even clearer expectations around roles, responsibilities, communication, and timelines. This is always an ongoing process that requires regular check-ins and course corrections. As a feminist project that is interested in flattening hierarchies and adopting consensus models of decision making, finding the right balance between structure, fluidity, and responsiveness can be tricky.

Moreover, some tasks associated with our project are inherently more fun than others. Folks involved in leading the social media team have shared that they like working on Instagram posts more than they like cleaning transcripts. Others have enjoyed front-line interviewing. It seems no one loves transcribing. Nevertheless, we decided to address this challenge collectively. As Jessica M. (RA) recounted,

> For example, with the transcriptions people were having a difficult time getting things done. The conversations around this were honest as to why people were having a hard time getting them done and what could be done. It was a team effort instead of viewed as an individual failing.

CONCLUSIONS

As we embarked on data collection last winter, our team was ready. These young researchers have proven themselves to be a group of brave, empathetic, creative problem solvers who have excelled at recruiting and interviewing their peers. Despite a few bumps along the way, we maintain our desire to infuse our project with a feminist ethic of care.

Most recently, we have been engaging in individual performance evaluations with each team member. Several YPRs have commented on the "niceness" of the investigator team. As PIs, Sarah and Jessica have repeatedly tried to gently remind the group that we were not taking this approach because we want to be nice or kind. Rather, we see this approach as a political project of doing research differently and manifesting a feminist ethic of care.

The commitment to doing academic work differently takes time and emotional labour. Mauthner & Edwards (2010) have argued that this approach can be particularly difficult to enact in neoliberal institutions that push feminist senior scholars into managerial roles. We have felt this challenge. Nevertheless, calling out sexism and racism is a necessary first step to addressing these inequities. As Ahmed (2017) notes, "giving the problem a name does not make the problem go away. To give the problem a name can be experienced as magnifying the problem" (p. 34). Naming the explicit instances when those systemic issues play out within an academic project is even more challenging. Even within our project, while we have named our successes and challenges explicitly, there is always more that is unsaid, more that cannot be named (just yet), and as such, more work to do.

Nevertheless, we are proud that we all now have a model of how a feminist ethic of care can be enacted in the workplace. It is a model that we can bring forward as team members go on to become public health leaders, researchers, and practitioners of tomorrow.

ACKNOWLEDGEMENTS

We want to thank the rest of the 4theRecord team, including Alanna Goldstein, Ciann Wilson, Deana Leahy, Jen Gilbert, Laina Bay-Cheng, and Seventy Hall. We appreciate the generous funding provided by the Social Sciences and Humanities Research Council of Canada—for Transnational Perspectives on COVID-19's Impact on Youth Sexuality, Risk and Relationships project (Ref. No. NFRFE 2020-01107) as well as support from all participating universities.

CRITICAL THINKING QUESTIONS

1. Why were the authors committed to hiring research assistants that came from the same communities as research participants? Do you think diversity and representation matter on research teams?
2. What does it mean to be able to "bring your whole self" onto a research team?

3. What does a feminist ethic of care mean to you? How might you go about infusing a feminist ethic of care into a public health research project that you are working on?
4. What challenges might arise when trying to balance your political commitments with the realities of timelines and budget constraints? How might you address these in your work?

KEY TERMS

feminist ethic of care
leadership
community
sexism
racism
youth

SUGGESTED FURTHER READINGS

1. Bay-Cheng, L. Y. (2009). Beyond trickle-down benefits to research participants. *Social Work Research, 33*(4), 243–247.
2. Fields, J. (2016). The racialized erotics of participatory research: A queer feminist understanding. *Women's Studies Quarterly, 44*(3/4), 31–50.
3. Liboiron, M., Ammendolia, J., Winsor, K., Zahara, A., Bradshaw, H., Melvin, J., Mather, C., Dawe, N., Wells, E., Liboiron, F., Fürst, B., Coyle, C., Saturno, J., Novacefski, M., Westscott, S., & Liboiron, G. (2017). Equity in author order: A feminist laboratory's approach. *Catalyst: Feminism, Theory, Technoscience, 3*(2), 1–17.
4. Wilson, C. L., Singh, A. K., Beals, A. M., Sharma, R., Hunt, B., Furman, E., Darko, N. A., Fante-Coleman, T., Liu, V., & Kivell, N. (2021). Dialogues of disruption: Confronting oppression in the academy. *Global Journal of Community Psychology Practice, 12*(3), 2–25.

CHAPTER 14

Chronicles of Public Health Doctoral Students: Overcoming the Ivory Tower through a Revolution of "Self-Care" for a Better Future

Corey McAuliffe, Ifrah Abdillahi, Karima Joy, Astrid Escrig-Pinol, Apondi J. Odhiambo, and Renée Monchalin

LEARNING OBJECTIVES

1. Explore the patriarchal and colonial underpinnings of public health higher education in Canada.
2. Through a public health feminist lens, hear from the stories of former and current public health PhD students whose voices represent the often-ignored voices in public health.
3. Explore solutions to revolutionary "self-care" from critical and intersectional perspectives.

> *The fundamental problem is not that some are excluded from the hegemonic centers of the academy but that the university (as a specific institutional site) and academy (as a shifting material network) themselves cannot be disentangled from the long historical apparatuses of genocidal and protogenocidal social organization.*
> *(Rodríguez, 2012, p. 812)*

Across Canada, the United States, and globally, there is significant consensus that universities are predominantly Eurocentric, "rooted in colonial, apartheid and Western worldviews and epistemological traditions" and therefore continue "to reinforce white and Western dominance and privilege" (Heleta, 2016). As colonial sites, universities are upheld through structural and systemic racism, embedded processes in "laws (local, state, and federal), policies, and practices of society and its institutions that provide advantages to racial groups deemed as superior, while differentially oppressing, disadvantaging, or otherwise neglecting racial groups viewed as inferior" (Dryden & Nnorom, 2021). Racism is complex, varied, and not a universal experience. For example, anti-Black racism is a distinct form of racial evil rooted in European colonization of Africans and legacies of transatlantic slave trade (Grimes, 2018). Underscored in Lawson's (2020) reflection on institutional racism at Canadian universities, she observes that commitments to concepts like *people of colour* "presume or insist upon the monolithic character of victimization under white supremacy." Further scholarly work focuses on the relationship between state-sponsored Indigenous genocide and anti-Blackness (King et al., 2020). Disrupting monolithic characterization of group experiences of white supremacy means noting particularities within these experiences of anti-Blackness and anti-Indigenousness.

Universities throughout history have functioned as hubs for the capitalist and religious goals of the settler state, reflecting its histories of enslavement, dispossession, exclusion, forced assimilation, and integration (Grande, 2018). Universities continue their legacies as places of colonialism (Tuhiwai Smith, 2012). From this standpoint we acknowledge the underpinnings of Canadian academic public health programs. Despite the goal of public health aiming to "protect and promote the health of all Canadians" (Canadian Public Health Association, 2020), public health programming, services, and policy miss the mark on protecting and promoting health of Black, Indigenous, racialized, refugee, immigrant, two-spirit, non-binary, trans women and/or gender-diverse, neurodiverse, disabled, and other marginalized/oppressed women in Canada (Allan & Smylie, 2015; Jee-Lyn et al., 2015; Kielsgard & Brown, 2021; Sharpe, 2020; Yakubovich & Maki, 2021). Given these exclusions, the authors of this chapter, who represent many of these groups, gather here to give voice to positions and perspectives that often lack support in the academy and healthcare system.

To protect and promote the health of *all* Canadians through a public health feminisms approach, university programs training public health professionals must create safe and supportive spaces for students who represent marginalized/oppressed groups. However, when speaking of anti-Black racism, we must be mindful that "the fully racialized social and epistemological architecture upon which the modern university is built cannot be radically transformed by 'simply' adding darker faces, safer spaces, better training, and a curriculum that acknowledges historical and contemporary oppressions" (Kelley, 2016). Experiences of marginalization/oppression within universities further occur through gatekeeping, "the process by which an arbiter influences high performers' transition between and ascension within developmental stages" (Knotek et al., 2020). Within higher educational settings, DeAngelo et al. (2021) discuss the role of faculty in grooming and gatekeeping students of colour into future faculty along what they term *the professoriate pipeline*. The authors note the important role faculty play in acting as arbiters along the spectrum of the academic profession, from entry into doctoral programs to entry/promotion within academic professional spaces (DeAngelo et al., 2021). In their role as arbiters, racist faculty operate under a deficit-oriented cognitive frame, reinforcing "negative and oppressive stereotypes that marginalize Black, Latinx, and Native American students" (DeAngelo et al., 2021). Accordingly, when faculty hold these deficit ideologies, they are more likely to label racialized and Indigenous students as unprepared and inadequate to justify and mask structural inequities faced along the pipeline.

To transform the academic complex, the university must be decolonized. Decolonization is not a metaphor; rather, it aims to unsettle and dismantle settler colonialism (Tuck & Yang, 2012). To dismantle and decolonize universities and public health programs, the authors critically reflect and share their experiences disrupting the silence that allows these dysfunctions to persevere. Despite academia's deeply colonial history, the university is an important site of transformation (Gaudry & Lorenz, 2018a). In recognizing this, we, a group of academics from the same doctoral cohort, aim to acknowledge precarity and dangers in these institutions and consider how we can unsettle and dismantle settler-colonial public health university programs through public health feminist perspectives. In doing this, public health programming, policy, and services in Canada can better protect and promote the health of *all* Canadians.

In the passages below, women academics from a multitude of identities (Black, Indigenous, multiracial, international, disabled) share their experiences of structural and systemic racism and oppression within the university setting. While our stories may appear individualized, these experiences are common and often normalized within academia. The following anecdotes speak to experiences of gatekeeping, relational power dynamics, violent interactions with faculty, tokenism, strategies to stay safe, and challenges related to international status, access to healthcare, and accessibility services.

GATEKEEPING AND THE (UN)MAKING OF BLACK SCHOLARS

What does it mean when someone says you have *potential*? What is *potential*? In academia, the concept of potential is often evoked but rarely unpacked. Potential is conjured when thinking of hope, promise, and prospects of success. As graduate students, our potential is our currency. It is the invisible tokens we collect and dispense to gain access and entry into spaces and relationships that transform potential into tangible material and social resources (jobs, networks, promotions, awards, and publications).

For example, in 2022, government grants like the Tri-Council Doctoral Fellowships offered material benefits of $15,000 to $50,000 per year for a period of 12 and 48 months. However, social and professional benefits extend far beyond award duration. Each year, a select number of students who receive these coveted awards gain legitimacy from the academy, alongside a stamp of approval signalling to other selection boards and future employers they are a *worthy* investment. These awards often list an initial selection criterion of "research ability and potential" representing up to 50% of the score. The indicators for this criterion include quality of research proposal, relevant training, research experience and achievements, and quality of contributions. These seem like innocuous expectations, but to gain research experience, training, and demonstrate quality of contribution, a student needs alignment with faculty and mentors who act as conduits to networks, trainings, conferences, publication opportunities, and sustained financial support. Support of this kind is crucial to the graduate student experience, as it affords students conditions to focus on their studies rather than working in multiple short-term, precarious, and exploitive employment situations. Having support of invested faculty offers an invitation into professional circles, grants, publications, conference subsidies, and access to costly software, offering greater opportunities to secure similar awards. Now, in Canada, only 2% of post-secondary educators are Black, leaving Black students often to be supervised by non-Black academics. This also increases competition to secure rare opportunities to be aligned with the few Black scholars at each university.

In my own graduate experience, I struggled to find invested faculty and mentors, particularly in the doctoral program. During those first years, I spent much time and emotional energy navigating structural barriers and endless hurdles. A lack of faculty aligned with my research interests meant I had few options for supportive supervisors, forcing me to work and write about issues inauthentic to my worldview. The deep connections academics must have, to engage in aligned research, are often informed by our lives and lived experiences. As a Black, Muslim, second-generation immigrant with diasporic identity, I did not see myself represented in my program, creating an uncomfortable situation of parroting ideas I could not organically speak to. Because no faculty looked like me or saw the world from my perspective, my ideas were scrutinized, dismissed, and outright ridiculed. I felt undermined, subjugated, and often defeated by the hegemony of whiteness that surrounded me.

One interaction with a white faculty member left me traumatized after she insisted I would fail her course if I did not sign up for writing assistance. On one assignment, she claimed I had so much *potential*, noting I was intellectually sophisticated but needed writing support. The support she insisted I gain wasn't out of legitimate need or poor performance; rather, it was a means to diminish my capacity and invisibilize my contribution. Again, there was that illusive yet always present idea of *potential*. Potential became like an intellectual purgatory, where I will always be becoming, forever on a road to somewhere but with no expected time of arrival and diminishing prospects for actualization. The moment of intellectual alchemy always just over the horizon, beyond the vast plain of my potential. Yet in reality, this professor's systemic exclusion, and that of other gatekeepers, is a clear flashing sign reading "Stop! That's far enough for you." Despite this, I and other students like me forge forward. Like many of us who experience exclusion, gatekeeping, and oppression, we are defiant. Thus, I prefer defiance to the often-overused term of *resilience*. Defiance is grounded in my agency and willful rejection of white supremacy. I refuse and reject weapons its agents form against me. Instead, I stand my ground in defiance, occupying the centre of my own narrative.

POLICIES AND INSTITUTIONAL PRACTICES

My graduate school experiences were shaped and impacted by rigid and oppressive policies and practices I was oblivious to. I assumed my student experience would be smooth and aligned to complete the program within a shortened timeframe. One of the most critical institutional practices is supervision, greatly influencing the time to degree completion. Graduate supervision guidelines at Canadian universities identify that one (or more) faculty members must take primary responsibility to guide and assist a student's learning and process to successfully complete their degree. Therefore, supervisors, *should* play a significant role in the life of a graduate student. However, supervision as an institutional practice can be problematic when there is a disjuncture between supervisorial guidelines and a student's experience. The constitution of the dissertation committee can be equally problematic, as students are responsible to identify committee members whose research goals and expertise align with their own. For new immigrants and international students, this is challenging.

Poor student-supervisor relationships, communication issues, and a lack of commitment from committee members negatively impacted my experience, productivity, and ability to complete the program expeditiously. I experienced long wait times for feedback, alongside a lack of guidance, mentorship, and support to access funding, publication, and teaching opportunities. The lack of compassion and remorse from my supervisor further normalized this culture of inaccessibility and lack of communication. The power dynamics between students and supervisors, and absence of clear policies and resolution guidelines, left me with little recourse and a fear of punishment (e.g., intentional delay of completion), forcing me into silence. The lack of appropriate institutional policies and practices is problematic, creating a hostile, oppressive, and violent environment. A review of supervisory and dissertation committee policies and guidelines outlining steps students, faculty, staff, and departments should take to resolve conflicts and address challenges is needed.

THE ERA OF RECONCILIATION AND DECOLONIZATION

Following the release of the Truth and Reconciliation Commission's (TRC) Calls to Action (2015), changes across the country came into effect within Canadian post-secondary education. For many institutions, this led to required Indigenous history courses for all students and creating space for Indigenous students and faculty in programs (Gaudry & Lorenz, 2018b). While intentions *may* be good, what often happens are experiences of tokenism, isolation, and dismissal of ways of knowing and doing. As Gaudry and Lorenz (2018b) remind us, "Canadian universities have, for the majority of their existence, operated as a tool of de-indigenization, a legacy that now runs counter to many of the public statements on reconciliation found in institutional plans across Canada" (p. 221). Often students who represent marginalized/oppressed groups, such as Indigenous students, are called to participate in additional work, not asked of others. Yet when these students are asked to voice their opinion, they are often dismissed.

On my first day of the public health program, I remember the excitement of a new school year filling the air. My peers and I arrived at a theories of health class. We were a small cohort, sitting at tables in a circle. As the professor reviewed the syllabus, noticeably absent were Indigenous theorists. A peer raised her hand and very politely asked if we would be exploring any Indigenous theories—a fair question, as universities across the country had been claiming to rise to TRC recommendations. In fact, I felt the only reason I was accepted into this elite program was because of my Indigenous identity. In response to the question, the professor raised their voice and yelled three times while hitting the desk, "We are only focusing on DOMINANT theories! We are only focusing on DOMINANT theories! WE ARE ONLY FOCUSING ON DOMINANT THEORIES!" The class fell silent. As students, we had all just met, and we refrained from looking at each other. Being the only known self-identified Indigenous student, I stayed silent, as past educational experiences demonstrated this was no place to speak up. I was grateful to be there—*ironic, right?*—and I did not want to jeopardize my enrollment. I was grateful my peer spoke up about this Indigenous absence; however, the class refrained from bringing this up for the entirety of the term. I received the lowest mark of my graduate degree—just enough to pass.

Staying silent as a method of safety continued throughout my degree. In the event of any negative student experience, advice from Indigenous mentors and family was "put your head down and finish the program," "don't push back or else you will never graduate." This was hard, as part of me felt lucky to be there, and I did not want to jeopardize my enrollment. At the same time, I felt responsible to "bush whack" for future students (Absolon, 2011). With support of Indigenous faculty and faculty of colour, I was able to strategically "bush whack" my way through academic thorns. For example, during my comprehensive exams, I was met with resistance due to Indigenous and Black theories I chose, as they pushed margins of Western public health frameworks. I was threatened with failing if I used my selected theories, but with support from Indigenous faculty and faculty of colour, I did so *keemoochly* (Cree word meaning "in secret" and/or "strategically"). This term was an expression taught to me by a prominent Cree scholar over tea. Indigenous knowledges and ways of doing continue to be pushed underground, and it is our responsibility to strategically (keemoochly) bring them into the Western academy. Choosing to do this work, with threat of failing, was decolonization and/or "bush whacking" within itself.

RELATIONSHIPS WITHIN THE UNIVERSITY

Relationships with supervisors, faculty, and administration are fraught with inherent asymmetries and power dynamics. By nature of being a student, one holds less power, requiring vigilance and caution when navigating relationships that impact access to resources or future work. When abuses of power occur without accountability, students are often left to withdraw. Given the competitive and individualistic academic culture, these dynamics require scrutiny as student mental health is trivialized. Many of the abuses of power I encountered have no system for reporting or requesting accountability. During my in-person qualifying exam, one examiner asked how a framework I was using would be applied to her personal trauma. None of the other examiners interjected to this inappropriate question. It felt like a psychological landmine, and my future was on the line. Afterwards one person normalized the interaction, saying, "great students elicit lively debates." I was left alone and powerless. On another occasion, at a conference, a gatekeeper gave me an obscenely low presentation evaluation with no justification. This grade felt malicious and far from instructive. I could have shrunk in shame, thinking this evaluation said something about me or my work; however, in an act of resistance, I forwarded the evaluation to administration to flag it as inappropriate. In response, they acknowledged the injustice and said they would discuss changing their evaluation style for future conferences. While distressed, I took on the labour of trying to effect change to benefit future students—a form of hidden and unacknowledged labour. Both incidents were setbacks to completing the program, requiring me to seek mental health support at my own expense. The lack of accountability for those in positions of power causes serious harm to student dignity and safety.

RELATIONSHIPS: VIOLENT REACTIONS FROM FACULTY

As a student, I was encouraged to share my work with colleagues and faculty to help support growth and learning. Accordingly, I shared my dissertation at a departmental seminar, prior to my defence, with hope of receiving challenging questions to advance my findings. Unexpectedly, I encountered a hostile and violent reaction from a tenured faculty member who was personally triggered by my research. The interaction, which was not disrupted by other faculty members, made me question if I was blowing things out of proportion. However, after the seminar, I received calls from my co-supervisors to check to see if I was okay. One had felt unable to disrupt due to her non-tenured position, while the other did not want to appear patronizing by "saving me." After our discussions, I approached the seminar moderator, who promptly told me, "Yah, I had to debrief with another faculty member afterwards. That was intense!" While he apologized for not stepping in, this behaviour had been allowed in front of many students with no recourse or public apology. The lack of accountability led to mental and emotion distress for me and other students who witnessed this attack. The only critical learning in that seminar was watching how power structures and disregard for those not on "equal" footing play out in destructive and detrimental ways.

INTERNATIONAL STUDENT EXPERIENCE

As a privileged white woman of European origin, I have experienced many advantages in comparison to non-white international students, who, in addition to gender-based discrimination and violence, are subject to abject racism. Over the course of seven years as an international student in Canada, there have been many shared struggles with other international students, especially with women who have English as a second language (ESL) and who come from a working-class background.

While aspiring to attract high-achieving international students, Canadian universities fall short at supporting them once arrived. While English proficiency is a requirement for most programs, once accepted there are additional hurdles. For example, many professors penalized me for not having native-level English, explicitly lowering grades on assignments and tests. While an A+ student throughout my academic journey, once in Canada, and despite having a near-native English level, it was never enough compared with anglophone colleagues. I made use of all available university resources: ESL courses, writing workshops, writing support centres, peer editing support, and more. Despite this, language-based discrimination resulted in a lower GPA, directly impacting future scholarships, grants, and jobs. Being unable to achieve the impossible native-English bar resulted in sleepless nights alongside increased anxiety and stress. Mental and emotional suffering negatively impacted my health, relationships with professors and peers, social life, and academic performance.

As a woman from a working-class background, I also experienced stress from being charged international fees (almost triple domestic student fees). To pursue my doctorate, I was fortunately awarded a four-year scholarship, as I would have been unable to support myself on the program's funding package. Just prior to the program I received permanent residency, which reduced my fees to those of domestic students; however, while my permanent residence was officially approved, I had yet to receive the card. A month into the program I was informed I would be charged international fees for the first semester, as my change of residency status was not accepted without the card. With a full course load, I applied to jobs frantically, taking on a 30-plus-hour/week job to afford tuition and accommodations. I received no additional financial support from the university, leaving me on the verge of dropping out. Moreover, after taking the job, I was unable to disclose my work given the program's policy banning full-time students from working over 10 hours/week. Thus, in addition to struggling with feeling inadequate due to language-based discrimination, I was working almost full-time to stay in the program, leading to increased anxiety and exhaustion.

Why do professors penalize non-native English speakers and universities financially discriminate against international students? From a decolonial feminist perspective, one might argue our knowledges are devalued for not belonging to the hegemonic culture, forever relegated as less than our peers. While white and European, and thus a privileged subject of Western ethnocentricity, I experienced discrimination and was denied several opportunities for not belonging to the dominant English-speaking culture. Moreover, given my class background, I had no family or savings, constantly living in a state of precarity. In my identity, the intersection of gender, class, and language was a source of suffering, which undoubtedly clouded my experience as a student and worsened my mental, emotional, and physical health. During my studies, I invested substantial time and money in care (therapy, physiotherapy, massage therapy) to protect myself from the systemic oppression I faced and to try to heal from the violence I experienced.

INTERNATIONAL STUDENT HEALTHCARE

Taking care of your mental, physical, and emotional health comes at a high cost for many students, especially international students who do not have access to the same services as domestic students. Moreover, international students (in some provinces) must pay for healthcare insurance offered through the university, receiving less coverage than provincial programs and creating further out-of-pocket expenses. In addition to the financial burden, international students must also learn to navigate the Canadian healthcare system, a steep learning curve. We have to learn what is or is not included, services offered, how to make a claim, get reimbursed, and so on. There was little support offered with this process. Achieving proficiency at navigating the healthcare system and overcoming barriers within this process (e.g., language, discrimination) is emotionally draining, especially when already suffering from health issues. Moreover, this experience is compounded with a financial burden, adding stress, particularly for those with limited or no financial support. From a decolonial feminist standpoint, the emotional and financial stress international students go through to access care in Canada can be interpreted as rooted in practices of exclusion, limiting our ability to access the system in the same way as domestic students. Practices of exclusion have tangible impacts on our health. Moreover, from personal experience, barriers I faced sometimes resulted in me giving up on seeking care and leaving issues untreated.

ACCESSIBILITY

Living with a predominantly invisible, episodic disability has highlighted for me many of the systemic challenges faced by scholars who live within a wide spectrum of disability, accessibility needs, and intersecting identities. Since I developed my condition/disability later in life, my doctoral program was the first experience in which I studied with a disability. This experience was further impacted by my intersectional identity as an international student, highlighting my need to quickly learn how to navigate a new health system (as discussed by my peer above) to quickly identify a team of specialists.

Within the university, I experienced distress when trying to access university supports. It was my first exposure to being "forced" into identifying and being labelled as "disabled," while having to provide proof of it. Due to this barrier, it took me nine months to accept a label with which I did not yet identify. Moreover, early on, I had a meeting with a professor who encouraged me to hide my condition, forewarning me that sharing my experience would negatively impact my career. This further supported my concern with being labelled to access services and kept me silent when I most needed supports.

As a postdoctoral fellow, still within the Canadian university system, I developed a more severe secondary condition, which led to a three-month medical leave, influenced by stress due to defending my dissertation, starting a new job cross-country, and losing the majority of supports I had built, all amid a global pandemic. While my experience as a postdoctoral fellow has been different than as a student (including experiential knowledge and protective financial employment policies), I still received the same advice—"do not share your health status with anyone unless necessary"—and if I did, I would put my career and reputation in jeopardy.

With my return to work, I began to ask professors to help me identify a potential academic mentor dealing with similar health challenges. I hoped to find someone with experience to help me discern ways to best support myself. The starkest yet most apt response I received was, "No one is doing it well. We're all digging our own graves. Maybe you could be the person who figures it out." This statement has weighed heavily on me ever since. To stay well and keep my condition from requiring me to take another medical leave, I cannot work the 60-plus weekly hours demanded of many high-level academic positions. Moreover, I often do not qualify for accommodations (e.g., reduced work hours as a preventative measure), as one needs to be in an active flare/relapse or unwell enough to qualify. As a public health professional, this structural constraint prioritizes my need to "prove a level of disability" rather than to have ownership of keeping myself well. These experiences have led me to reflect and critically question my continued participation in a system where achieving well-being feels like a perilous battle.

DISCUSSION

Colonization is not an event in the distant past, but an ever-present evolving structure (Wolfe, 2006) that does not recognize and aims to eliminate other forms of knowing (Kuokkanen, 2008). Many universities are colonial institutions that reflect the country's history of enslavement, dispossession, exclusion, forced assimilation, and integration (Grande, 2018). Canadian academic public health programs, as demonstrated above, are complicit in processes of colonization, elimination, and exclusion and do not serve as safe learning spaces for Black, Indigenous, multiracial, international, and disabled students.

When considering alternative approaches to effect change within a public health feminist lens, feminist ethics (FE), also referred to as feminist ethics of care or care ethics, offers guidance on how to imagine paths forward. Ethics, defined as the study of moral reasoning and behaviour, aiming to critique and amend practices and beliefs on the best approaches to life (Lindemann, 2006), are often produced by Anglo-European elite men who exclude diverse voices, leading to problematic and unrepresentative biases (Walker, 2007). FE is a corrective approach to traditional androcentric, rational, ahistorical, and idealized ethics (Liaschenko & Peter, 2006; Lindemann, 2006). Contemporary approaches to FE are critical, moral, intersectional, anti-essentialist, political, and contextualized (Hankivsky, 2014; Liaschenko & Peter, 2006), guided by a relational ontology, valuing human interdependence and dynamics (Ribbens McCarthy, 2012). Care is a central concept in this approach (Tronto, 1993). According to Fisher and Tronto (1991, as cited in Tronto, 1993), care is defined as "a species activity that includes everything we do to maintain, continue, and repair our 'world' so that we can live in it as well as possible." Overall, FE offers a multi-scalar approach to problematizing care labour and relationality, highlighting human interdependence, how society organizes and responds to care responsibilities, and social, political, and economic mechanisms that devalue these responsibilities (Robinson, 2015). In the context of public health feminisms and education, FE raises awareness that care is constantly negotiated between individuals/groups and among micro and macro stakeholders in an unjust and unfortunate political context (Hankivsky, 2014).

Care labour is generally invisible, devalued, and unpaid, leading to less motivation to engage with students or consider their well-being. Social locations are connected to how we can accept or deflect responsibility (Walker, 2007). It is not uncommon for academics to deflect responsibility for student mental health as not in their realm of influence, claiming their responsibility is solely teaching students. This attitude delineates mental health as an individual responsibility, takes no responsibility to care for students, and rejects accountability for personal roles in perpetuating harmful dynamics. While no one individual can bear the responsibility to change these toxic systems and dynamics, we can no longer afford to produce and perpetuate a version of public health laced with uncaring and irresponsible values prioritizing profit over well-being.

An outcome of oppression, injustice, and trauma is for individuals to be shaped by shame, precarity, grief, and anger. Students internalize that they are unsafe or that problems are personal weaknesses, which influences their nervous systems, mental and physical health, and ability to participate in academia. Perpetuating these dynamics maintains the status quo and generates collective grief and trauma. Students experiencing normalized oppression may not have resources to heal and break the cycles. Thus, whose responsibility is it to break these cycles that perpetuate harmful dynamics? True to foundations of public health reasoning, how can we acknowledge our interdependence, invest in community building and well-being, and create systems that promote health and dignity for all?

CONCLUSION

Having space and time to come together as a group of former and current doctoral students from different intersecting identities was one of the first opportunities for us to acknowledge and recognize how our academic experiences overlapped in what felt like a toxic, unsupportive, and Othering environment. To challenge this condition and envision a new way forward, we are voicing our stories in hopes that others who feel marginalized/oppressed will know they are not alone and that these are structural, not individual limitations. This practice of coming together disrupts oppressive structures, allowing for the process of healing to occur. Below, we have outlined ways in which we accessed supports and put in place practices to not only get through and survive, but to do our best to be defiant and thrive.

The challenges of graduate school are varied. Navigating the turbulence is a personal journey. Thus, one strategy is to establish a distinction between work and living space. Even if it is a small partition, separate these two aspects. The graduate experience can feel all-consuming. Separation can help to create time for work and rest, to survive the process. Moreover, create a support team, connecting with peers or exploring options on student health plans. This involves time and resources—however, seeking out supports offers a perspective outside of academia that helps to prioritize mental, physical, emotional, and spiritual well-being. Finding support through those who can witness and validate your experiences is critical. University studies can feel isolating and lonely. Creating peer sessions to support one another (writing clubs, review groups, etc.) is a way to connect, gain insights, and socialize. Furthermore, some students benefit from identifying academics outside of their program from whom to gain mentorship and advice. Cultivate these networks by drawing upon professors from previous programs, past work colleagues, and new spaces derived from current passions. Routinely connect with these people to get their thoughts and advice on a range of topics, from research to career discussions.

In reading this, you likely now recognize that many academic settings are in unsupportive environments. Thus, as a coping mechanism, try to conceptualize the school as a wild and unsafe jungle. The jungle holds all sorts of joy and harm. One never knows what to expect and what creatures will be encountered. For some, it may feel safest to stay silent and unthreatening. Remain vigilant that danger exists—it is a safe, protective assumption. Blending in offers an opportunity to dodge unnecessary confrontations or harms while protecting your energy. We recognize this does not equate to being free of harm, as there is still a need to cope with jungle animals jumping out of trees. To be clear, while this is not an ideal metaphor to live by, as self-enrichment is best done in safe and supportive learning environments, it taps into the unpredictable and unsafe nature of the status quo and offers some buffer against harm, demoralization, and injustice. We recognize that these workaround practices and coping mechanisms employed to survive put responsibility on individual students while obscuring and normalizing systems of oppression and institutional practices within academic settings. Therefore, long-term solutions warrant an overhaul of social structures, including laws, policies, and institutional practices organizing the realities of students. Strong mentorship, leadership, and student advocacy programs are crucial in advancing equity and social justice in academic settings. Overall, we encourage you to seek community with colleagues, as we have, and make it a priority to stay connected to those who are dear in your life.

CRITICAL THINKING QUESTIONS

1. How do you define self-care? How do you incorporate it into your daily routine to stay balanced?
2. If you are reading this chapter as a part of an educational program, do you see yourself within the syllabus and course materials? How does this impact your well-being as a student?
3. What mentorship, leadership, and student advocacy programs and bodies are available for you in your current program? Do you access any of these supports? Why or why not?

KEY TERMS

decolonization
doctoral students
ethics of care
university
well-being

SUGGESTED FURTHER READINGS

1. Annamma, S. A., Ferri, B. A., & Connor, D. J. (2016). *DisCrit: Disability studies and critical race theory in education*. Teachers College Press.
2. Hankivsky, O. (2014). Rethinking care ethics: On the promise and potential of an intersectional analysis. *American Political Science Review, 108*(2), 252–264.
3. Lee, J. J., & Rice, C. (2007). Welcome to America? International student perceptions of discrimination. *Higher Education, 53*, 381–409. https://doi.org/10.1007/s10734-005-4508-3
4. Lawson, E. S. (2020). Anti-Black racism on the sidelines: The limits of "listening sessions" to address institutional racism at Canadian universities. *Canadian Review of Sociology, 57*(3), 491–494. https://doi.org/10.1111/cars.12296
5. Tronto, J. (1993). *Moral boundaries: A political argument for an ethic of care*. Routledge.

CHAPTER 15

Public Health Feminism and Housing: Status Quo or Transformational?

Melissa Perri and Patricia O'Campo

LEARNING OBJECTIVES

1. Reflect on gaps created in public health and housing practices with respect to the unique challenges faced by women of all backgrounds.
2. Understand how consideration of the ideas within feminism's myriad movements facilitate a comprehensive analysis of public health issues.
3. Learn how to engage with and integrate feminism to inform the design of effective and inclusive housing solutions.

INTRODUCTION

The recent emergence of public health feminism (PHF) represents a unique opportunity to merge theory and practice in addressing health disparities that occur across society. Along with this opportunity, it is important to acknowledge the potential limitations of PHF in its current form and draw on multiple feminist theories to better understand and design solutions to major public health challenges. Comprehensive integration of varying forms of feminism can address the multidimensional challenges that are often driven by the structuring of society. Ensuring an all-encompassing approach to public health will aid in understanding and addressing fundamental causes of health disparities among members of society while unpacking dimensions of these disparities on micro, meso, and macro levels. This chapter identifies how forms of feminism that focus on assessing and dismantling forms of oppression can benefit the development and future application of PHF. Throughout, we define *gender* as the roles and expectations attributed to individuals, which are influenced by societal, institutional, and interpersonal ideologies that shift over time and place (Phillips, 2005). We take up housing as a case example to demonstrate how multiple systemic oppressions and feminist perspectives shape everyday public health challenges. Housing can be used to illustrate how systems are gendered, as seen through common housing-related regulations, programs, and policies. When compared to men, women face unique challenges attaining and maintaining adequate housing simply because of their gender. We explore this further below. We benefit from the perspectives we've been exposed to in our work with those with lived experience of lifelong oppression. While we have listened to and worked with those individuals on issues of critical importance in public health, we cannot represent nor speak for them but, rather, convey what we understand to be the ongoing systemic oppressions that prevent public health equity from being realized. We end the chapter with implications for PHF to inform strong solutions for mending gendered inequities.

OBJECTIVES

The objectives of this chapter are twofold, to demonstrate: (1) the potential for public health feminism to prioritize the unique challenges faced by women of all backgrounds, and (2) how myriad feminist movements facilitate a comprehensive analysis of public health issues such as housing insecurity and inform the design of effective and inclusive solutions. We take up housing as a case example to carry out these objectives.

GENDERED INEQUITIES

Sex, defined as the biological attribute assigned to an individual at birth based on their physiological features, is often considered in public health research due to its overreliance on a biomedical model of health (Short, Yang, & Jenkins, 2013; van Hagen, Muntinga, Appelman, & Verdonk, 2020). Gender, defined above, is often absent. The lack of focus on gender is driven by the hegemonic structuring of our patriarchal society. Gendered systems produce harmful health and social impacts and perpetuate health disparities for women and gender minorities given their disregard for factors such as: disproportionate experiences of sexual, physical, emotional, and financial violence; caring for children; experiences of gendered stigmatization; unequal pay distribution; and increased employment precarity (Hansen, 2017; Hansen & Roberts, 2012; Lykes, 1985; Perri, Metheny, Matheson, Potvin, & O'Campo, 2021; Perri & O'Campo, 2021). Research has highlighted the disproportionate health consequences faced by women of varying social identities when compared to cisgender men when engaging with such institutions (Hansen, 2017; Hansen & Roberts, 2012; Lykes, 1985; Perri et al., 2021). These harms are multifaceted and often overlapping, particularly for women who experience a multitude of oppressions (e.g., racism, ableism, sexism, heteronormativity) (Collins, 2019; Collins & Bilge, 2020; Hansen, 2017). For example, women and gender-diverse people who are racialized, have disabilities, and/or are immigrants face an increased likelihood of being unemployed and face disproportionate health risks when engaging in employment (Mawani, 2018; Smith & Mustard, 2010; Premki, 2018). The lack of focus on gender within employment sectors negates consideration of the health and social implications of gender discrimination, caregiving, and unequal wage losses. Similarly, the lack of focus on gender within immigration policies influences experiences of violence for women (e.g., needing to be married for two years prior to gaining permanent residency in the US), thus excluding these women from accessing essential services (Crenshaw, 1991).

PUBLIC HEALTH, GENDER, AND HOUSING

Public health focuses on improving the health of populations through disease prevention and health promotion efforts at the levels of the individual, neighbourhood, municipality, or nation. In the last century, public health played critical roles in the successful management and surveillance of infectious diseases (e.g., sanitation, vaccination) in high-income countries. In North America, public health currently faces novel challenges surrounding the rise of chronic diseases and growing health inequity, requiring innovative and inclusive strategies. Over the years, as public health has attempted to emphasize the social determinants of health, it has expanded to consider interventions going beyond biomedical healthcare to include social (e.g., education) and systemic (e.g., racism) issues. Given public health's focus on individuals, it has succeeded in incorporating a focus on the intermediary social determinants of health but not the upstream structural social determinants of health (CSDH, 2008). Public health actors aim for equity when designing, implementing, and evaluating public health preventative and treatment-oriented interventions. However, research highlights how neglecting to address components of our public systems that foster inequity facilitates the production of health disparities and manifests issues relating directly to public health (Braveman et al., 2011; Phelan, Link, & Tehranifar, 2010). Furthermore, critiques surrounding the medicalized approach to public health research and programming remain. Medicalized perspectives and solutions relevant for social issues range but have been connected to the conceptualization of the sick role—a passive body who is dependent on medical institutions—and broader forms of social control (Conrad, 1975, 1992; Conrad & Scheider, 1980). Despite the prominent nature of these critiques, limited attention has been placed on gender and how such common medicalized public health processes facilitate the production of women as "passive recipients," compared to the characterization of cisgender men as "active proponents." (Bell, 1987; Bell & Figert, 2010, 2012; Riessman, 1983). The gender-blind nature of the medical and public health spheres has led to further arguments stating that relevant processes have been used to control women and their actions and desires (Bell, 1987; Bell & Figert, 2010, 2012; Riessman, 1983). Examples of this control can be seen through how masculine ideologies have shaped the discovery and treatment of gender-specific experiences such as pregnancy, childbirth, or menstruation (e.g., relating to one's femininity and the construction of women as sex and reproductive objects) over time (Bell, 1987; Bell & Figert, 2010, 2012; Riessman, 1983). Of relevance to this chapter, notions of femininity and womanhood remain within housing systems and related experiences. Poverty and experiences of homelessness for women create gendered stigma surrounding their expectations as women—both societally, surrounding notions of motherhood, childcare, and maintaining the home, and through interpersonal relationships, where women are forced into using their bodies to maintain some sense of security (Bell, 1987; Bell & Figert, 2010, 2012; Conrad, 1975, 1992; Conrad & Scheider, 1980; Riessman, 1983).

Access to stable, safe, and quality housing has been rendered a human right and a fundamental need for health and well-being (Rolfe et al., 2020). However, the provision, regulation, and maintenance of housing in both public and private markets are largely determined by those with power (e.g., developers, politicians, banks) and are gendered processes. Yearly, hundreds of thousands of individuals living across North America face housing insecurity and/or homelessness. For example, reports from Canada from 2016 highlighted that over 200,000 Canadians experienced homelessness yearly (Gaetz, Dej, Richter, & Redman, 2016). There is a vast amount of research identifying the relationship between precarious or poor-quality housing (e.g., the physical structure of a home; toxins, mold, overcrowding) and negative health outcomes for individuals. These experiences are augmented among women who face multiple forms of oppressions. Those living in lower socioeconomic neighbourhoods are disproportionately impacted by poorer quality homes and the subsequent health outcomes associated with these homes (Singh, Daniel, Baker, & Bentley, 2019). Research demonstrates that racial segregation contributes to the divide and experiences of housing insecurity particularly among Black communities. Akbar and colleagues demonstrate that rent prices in neighbourhoods that transitioned from all white individuals to predominately Black individuals rose 50% over a decade across America (Akbar, Li, Shertzer, & Walsh, 2019).

Similar divides are seen when analyzing eviction rates within neighbourhoods across Canada. Indigenous and 2SLGBTQIA+ women, girls, and gender-diverse people, for example, have been found to experience eviction at disproportionate rates compared to those who do not identify as such (Schwan, Vaccaro, Reid, Ali, & Baig, 2021). Housing programs and policies often ignore the needs and realities of women (e.g., disproportionate experiences of poverty) due to their gender-blind or neutral development and implementation (treating all individuals as if they have the same needs) and because of this, perpetuate gendered harm such as physical violence (e.g., remaining in violent relationships for shelter), stigma, and alienation. Such programs and policies often include co-gender habitation and strict regulations surrounding living with children who identify as men. A recent pan-Canadian survey conducted with five hundred women, girls, and gender-diverse people with lived/living experience of homelessness or housing insecurity documented that all these factors contributed to barriers faced in accessing housing services (Schwan et al., 2021).

What Is Oppression?

As we have noted throughout this chapter, public health identifies and formulates solutions to health inequities (e.g., differences by income in cardiovascular mortality, homicides, COVID-19 infections, or access to healthcare) or social outcomes (e.g., differences by gender or age in violence victimization, poverty, housing stability). These inequities are actually the endpoints of historical, political, social, and economic processes locally, nationally, and globally (Brisbois, O'Campo, & Kamalanathan, 2018), and they are expressed in many forms, such as sexism, racism, and neoliberal policies to support the upward redistribution of wealth, cultural genocide, and employment exploitation that all have one common mechanism: oppression. Oppressive processes are key to creating and maintaining these inequities and include "institutionalized procedures and practices of domination and control" (McGibbon, 2021, p. 30). Taking a critical feminist perspective is important to not only acknowledge those who are harmed by oppression but to call out and identify those who deliver and benefit from it. Naming oppression, defined as "discrimination backed up by systemic or structural power (e.g., public policy, economic regimes, education, legal, health and media decision-making and governance systems)" (McGibbon, 2021, p. 34), allows us to identify the common sources of power we must focus on if inequities are to be eliminated.

FEMINISM

Feminism's end goal is social change and gender parity or equity in alignment with ending other forms of oppression. As described earlier in this book, feminism represents continually evolving movements fuelled by the multilayered experiences of oppression faced by women. It focuses on analyzing and dismantling systems of power relating to gender and its influence on the production of knowledge, meaning, and experiences (Collins, 2019). Feminism's alignment with critical emancipatory epistemology stems from its focus on power and how this manifests into multiple dimensions of oppression for women of multifaceted identities (Collins, 1989, 2015, 2019). In addition, feminism is aligned with social constructionism, which proposes that an individual's understanding of reality is shaped by systems of significant symbols (e.g., culture), which are, in turn, associated with individuals' pre-existing social and historical ideologies and experiences, influencing both human behaviour and meaning-making processes (Crotty, 1998; Edley, 2001). These forms of power are understood within the feminist theoretical landscape as structurally driven, through hegemonic ideologies and institutions.

Over the years, inclusive forms of feminism have evolved through movements, responses to oppression, and critical assessments of communities whose experiences were not captured by early writings about the theory. Leveraging the full spectrum of feminist thought and its associated theories is essential if public health is to successfully address current challenges driven by the gendered nature of existing health and social systems. Mainstream feminism, which is often described as driven by white, upper-class, corporate feminists, is not inclusive of the realities of all women (Grande, 2003). As put forth by Grande (2003), "what has long passed as 'mainstream' feminism is perhaps more appropriately termed 'whitestream' feminism" (Grande, 2003, p. 330). This form of feminism serves and speaks to the experiences of white, middle/upper-class women and their ethno-political and capital interests (Grande, 2003). As taken up by Phipps (2021), the communal mainstream feminist concept of "wounded identities," which creates the "woman as an identity based on injury" who need to "speak out" against modernity and the related structuring of society, ignores the heterogeneous realities of all women. This unified perspective ignores the white, heteronormative, colonialist, ableist, and classist political systems that govern society as we know it (Phipps, 2021). Further critiques of mainstream feminism build on this, expressing how it detaches itself from grand narratives, such as colonialism and racism, and acts to protect white, cis, straight, upper-class women from acknowledging their role as colonizers (Grande, 2003). Relying solely on these theories thus risks augmenting harm for those already made vulnerable by existing systems of power. An abundance of work put forth by critical race feminists and feminists of colour speaks to the need to integrate critical feminist thought that acknowledges the differences in identity, oppression, subjectivity, and meaning among all women (Mama, 2011; Maluf, 2011; Milevska, 2011; Mitra, 2011; Pirtle, 2022; Silverstein, 2017; Tuck & Yang, 2012). We believe this approach is essential in conceptualizing and expanding PHF.

Beyond Liberal Feminism

We noted earlier that the dominance of mainstream or white feminism in PHF, to the discursive exclusion of other and older feminisms—such as feminisms from the Global South, Indigenous feminisms, Marxian feminism, and intersectional feminism—risks PHF replicating the inequities generated by the dominance of white and wealthy perspectives in the design and implementation of public health initiatives. Indigenous and decolonial feminisms have been active for centuries, in response to the impacts on Indigenous populations of settler colonialism, and in North America since the late 1400s (Arvin & Morrill, 2013; Upadhyay, 2021). Indigenous and decolonial feminism challenge notions of racial and gender hierarchy that originate from colonization and its ideologies justifying and shaping the forms of domination of racialized peoples (e.g., slavery, cultural genocide) and exclusion of gender non-binary and/or trans people (Upadhyay, 2021). Of particular relevance to public health, the formation of racial and gender hierarchies was assisted by health sciences.

Intersectionality was first coined in the 1980s by Kimberlé Crenshaw as a critique of early feminist theory and anti-racist politics (Collins, 1989; Crenshaw, 1989; Tyson, 2003). Intersectionality "investigates how intersecting power relations influence social relations across diverse societies as well as individual experiences in everyday life" (Collins, 2019, p. 4). Building on the work of Black feminist thought, Crenshaw expressed that mainstream feminist theory invisibilized and further marginalized the experiences of Black women (Cho, Crenshaw, & McCall, 2013; Collins, 1989; Crenshaw, 1989; Nash, 2008; Tyson, 2003). Intersectional considerations are key to PHF if we are to be inclusive of those who are most marginalized. Ideologies core to intersectionality have been driven by many key Black feminists (Combahee River Collective, 1981), all of whom argued that patriarchy, racial oppression, capitalism, and heteronormativity interlocked and drove experiences and the embodiment of oppression for Black women (Clarke, 1981; Collins & Bilge, 2020; Combahee River Collective, 1981; Kandiyoti, 1988).

Despite the influence of decolonizing feminism on nations globally—especially in the Global South—over the last five hundred years and intersectional feminism in the recognition of the multiple oppressions sometimes generated by mainstream feminists, the prominence, visibility, and inclusion of Indigenous feminisms within "whitestream" feminism has been consistently marginalized (Arvin & Morrill, 2013; Upadhyay, 2021). For example, the dominant description of the history of feminism's four waves makes no mention of decolonizing or intersectional feminism's existence before or along with the feminism "waves" or their influence on gender or gender parity.

Feminist political economy emerged in response to the gaps created when economists failed to fully consider how markets are influenced by women and influence women's roles and perceptions surrounding the domestic arena (Syed, 2021; Vosko, 2002). Feminist political economy reveals the tensions in employment and pay, such as unequal pay for work among men and women, the sources of unpaid labour performed by women, and the consequences of these tensions for men's and women's lives (Syed, 2021). Feminist political economists highlight the myriad sources of unpaid labour that women perform, such as having a larger share of domestic and childcare responsibilities in households where both partners are employed, and women having a larger share of the caregiving work at home and in society (Roberts & Zulfiqar, 2019; Roseman, Barber, & Neis, 2016). Paid caregiving work, primarily performed and expected by women, is also less valued and therefore caregivers earn low wages, reinforcing and sustaining patriarchal societal structures. Expectations of gendered "work" and disparities associated with economic security are further relevant for those found at the intersections of class, race, sexual, or colonial oppression (Roberts & Zulfiqar, 2019; Roseman, Barber, & Neis, 2016).

PUBLIC HEALTH FEMINISM

Given the sparse literature on PHF, including limited descriptions in this volume, we surmise the concept promotes an interdisciplinary approach that combines fundamental principles and ideologies from mainstream and liberal feminism and public health. PHF should enable stakeholders to assess gendered notions prevalent within public health and broader structural systems, providing tools to consider the unique needs of and alleviate health disparities for women. In addition,

Hammarström (1999) highlighted the utility of feminist theory within the field of public health, given the former's ability to foster the development of new research and gender-informed frameworks, increase agency among women, and its strengths in producing gender-sensitive programs and policies. It is not clear that the feminist component of PHF has kept pace with evolving feminism literatures and, therefore, has the potential to be exclusive of the those who identify as women with diverse histories or who experience multiple marginalizations (Mama, 2011; Maluf, 2011; Milevska, 2011; Mitra, 2011; Pirtle, 2022; Silverstein, 2017; Tuck & Yang, 2012). The novelty of PHF provides an opportunity to inform the practice to ensure it dismantles oppression in all its forms, promotes equity, and remains effective for all. For example, PHF could help mend issues relating to existing messaging about the need for the COVID-19 vaccine, which is a one-size-fits-all approach and disregards the need for women-specific evidence and messaging. Women of child-bearing age or who are pregnant have higher vaccine hesitancy compared to men of the same age and must therefore have easy access to tailored information about vaccine safety for pregnancy and fertility (Murphy et al., 2021). Understanding, surveilling, and intervening in major public health threats are core public health functions. And while evidence abounds around how patriarchy and gender discrimination cause harm and even death, public health repeatedly fails to engage with these threats as evidenced by failure to fully fund services related to domestic violence globally or programs and services that are designed to be gender blind. By adopting a PHF approach, major threats to women can be made explicit and receive focused resource allocation.

PUBLIC HEALTH FEMINISM AND HOUSING: A CASE EXAMPLE

While women have different needs and challenges in securing safe and stable housing compared to men, we risk oversimplifying the problem of housing security and affordability as being experienced uniformly by all men or all women. We must also consider historical legacies (e.g., colonization or slavery) and contemporary systemic hierarchies and discrimination by gender, social class, and race, among other factors (e.g., immigration from low-income to high-income countries) that create privilege for some, especially those who are male and white, and deprivation for others who are women and racialized. Using intersectionality and Indigenous feminist approaches, we highlight below how leveraging a myriad of critical feminisms can help uncover the multidimensional aspects of public health challenges, such as housing insecurity.

Intersectionality centres those experiencing the greatest levels of oppression: Black women. Our example focuses on that group. Evidence supports the relevance of an intersectional approach to understanding the unique oppressions experienced by Black women seeking to secure safe and affordable housing. This starts with the historical practices of redlining or banks systematically refusing loans to Black people, falsely claiming that the loans would be at high risk of failure and simultaneously depriving Black people of wealth accumulation and home ownership, both key avenues to securing safe and affordable housing. Evanston, Illinois, became the first North American municipality to create a reparations program in 2020 for Black families who experienced intergenerational deprivation from historical redlining (Adams, 2021). Nonetheless, recent data demonstrates continued discrimination of Black women, as they have the highest rates of unapproved mortgages (Adams, 2021; Cheng, Lin, & Liu, 2015). Black women have also been reported to face disproportionate forms of landlord discrimination when compared to white women. Forms of power and oppression are also relevant in navigating the existing housing affordability and availability crisis across North America as Black women, compared to Black men and of course white people, pay the highest interest rates in order to obtain a mortgage (Cheng, Lin, & Liu, 2015). Residential segregation is another mechanism by which Black people and other racialized populations were prevented from securing high-quality housing, even when they possessed the financial means to do so. Segregation became illegal after the passage of the 1968 Fair Housing Act in the US, yet residential segregation by race remains unacceptably high in the 21st century (Sharkey, 2013). An intersectional lens allows a clearer understanding of the specific forms of state-sanctioned systemic discrimination in policies and practices that keep Black and racialized women from securing safe and high-quality housing.

Indigenous feminist approaches to housing could not take place without discussions of land appropriation and the need to address treaty violations and land settlements. Self-determination for housing solutions would have to be honoured if using a decolonizing approach. Indigenous approaches to well-being, informed by the medicine wheel, take the full person into account, and address myriad concerns, not just an individual need for a home. The need to eliminate racial and gender hierarchies and white privilege should be part of discussions when designing solutions to housing challenges to ensure that we address power abuses and oppression and mitigate the damaging impacts of race and gender discrimination.

REFLECTIONS OF OUR EXPERIENCES

From the perspectives of a student and a professor, both authors have had very few opportunities within the classroom or curriculum to engage with the forms of feminism presented in this chapter. We both believe it is imperative to engage with critical forms of feminism that are attentive to the multifaceted dimensions of oppression. As a student, Melissa Perri, a cisgender, white settler woman, is actively unlearning the ways in which liberal feminism dominates courses, readings, and research. She is also actively attempting to engage in critical allyship that reorients her understanding of oppression and aims to facilitate collective action and provide power to those with expertise. She encourages students to be critical of theory they are taught within institutions and to continue to be mindful of how our own positionality influences how we incorporate theory within our work and ideologies. Patricia O'Campo, a racialized cis woman with a mixed Japanese and Indigenous North American background, has lived experience of some of the types of oppressions described in this chapter. She seeks to include the perspectives of women experiencing multiple types of oppression in her community-based partnerships, as their voices are too often erased or ignored in research. In her teaching on issues of women and housing, she uses myriad feminisms to promote ideas around gender transformation and its value in creating housing solutions for women.

BRINGING IT ALL TOGETHER

We argue here for a PHF that is inclusive of the myriad movements happening globally surrounding the rights of women of varying social identities. We believe it is unacceptable if PHF only integrates mainstream liberal feminism as doing so would augment harm for many women across varying communities and would provide an inaccurate understanding of the multi-dimensional forms of oppression faced. Tenets relating to forms of feminism that focus on highlighting and dismantling systems of oppression must be integrated within PHF moving forward. Using three examples of feminisms that all centre experiences of oppression for women of multifaceted identities, we demonstrate how useful an inclusive PHF could be in understanding and addressing common public health challenges such as housing insecurity for women. Without a comprehensive understanding of the unique needs of women, public health and housing programming and policies will continue to perpetuate harm for these groups.

However, the development of PHF may also come with its own limitations. Western and forms of feminism that are not decolonized view gender as binary, ignoring the unique needs of those who do not identify on this binary spectrum. PHF must move beyond this and incorporate theoretical ideologies which speak to and aim to alleviate experiences of oppression among gender-diverse people.

Broader considerations surrounding accessibility of knowledge of varying forms of feminism must also be made for the effective future implementation of PHF. Both students and educators must strive to incorporate different feminist works within knowledge-generating spaces and advocate for all-inclusive curricula and discussion.

This chapter does not provide all the answers to how PHF can be adapted and implemented to eliminate the perpetuation of harm. However, we provide insight into gaps that might be created if a narrow approach to feminism is used. In addition, we identify additional feminisms that have the potential to radically transform the practice and impact of public health on the equity and well-being of populations.

CRITICAL THINKING QUESTIONS

1. Which feminisms do you think are relevant for public health and why?
2. What are the consequences to population health and equity of adopting a narrow feminist focus within public health?
3. How can public health feminism inform strategies to address social and health inequities beyond housing insecurity?
4. How would public health change if a decolonizing feminist approach was adopted?
5. Which feminisms are you familiar with and about which feminisms do you need to find out more information?

KEY TERMS

intersectionality
gender
decolonial feminism
feminist political economy

SUGGESTED FURTHER READINGS

1. Schwan, K., Vaccaro, M., Reid, L., Ali, N., & Baig, K. (2021). *The Pan-Canadian Women's Housing & Homelessness Survey.* Women's Housing and Homelessness Network.
2. Tuck, E., & Yang, K. W. (2012). Decolonialization is not a metaphor. *Decolonization: Indigeneity, Education & Society*, *1*(1), 1–40.
3. Nixon, S. A. (2019). The coin model of privilege and critical allyship: Implications for health. *BMC Public Health*, *19*(1637), 1–13.

CHAPTER 16

Public Health Feminist Futures and Moving Forward

Renée Monchalin

LEARNING OBJECTIVES

1. Understand how the chapters are interwoven for a public health feminist future.
2. Explore public health feminist praxis through (1) uncovering, disrupting, and dismantling public health programming, policies, education, and services; and (2) making space and moving over.

INTRODUCTION

Critical Perspectives in Public Health Feminisms begins to unpack public health policies, programs, and education in Canada, exposing the intersectional layers of how the field is embedded within patriarchy and colonialism. The critical perspectives in this edited collection, while diverse in their understandings and approach to defining what public health feminisms is or could be, aims to offer readers in the field tools to peel back the colonial and patriarchal layers of public health. Acknowledging that while public health programming, policies, and services in Canada aim to "protect and promote the health of all Canadians" (Canadian Public Health Association, 2020), there is much room for transformation.

Though the topics explored within this volume do not cover all areas in the field, this book's purpose was to begin to bring forward and make space for perspectives with(in) public health discourse that we do not often hear from in the mainstream. For many authors, including myself, this is the first time many of us are speaking to the injustices and exclusionary nature in the field. Many of the chapters highlight the silencing that takes place in public health programming, education, policies, and services experienced by Black, Indigenous, racialized, refugee, immigrant, neurodiverse, (dis)abled, two-spirit, non-binary, trans and/or gender-diverse, and/or other marginalized/oppressed women. This silencing is both forced upon and adapted as a safety measure in the field. In the era of reconciliation and "decolonization," and to remedy this historic and ongoing silencing in public health, the symbolic act of tokenism is often adapted. This then reinforces and maintains the status quo in public health programming, education, policies, and services. For true transformation to occur, it is important that public health feminism is not viewed solely as a theory that will reinforce and maintain the status quo, but rather as praxis, as action is intrinsic to the success of public health feminisms.

PUBLIC HEALTH FEMINISM AS PRAXIS

In Paulo Freire's (1970) *Pedagogy of the Oppressed*, *praxis* is defined as the "reflection and action upon the world in order to transform it" (p. 36). For some authors, this edited collection was described as an act of praxis. For example, in describing embroidery's long relationship with politics, power, and resistance, cover artist Matsuko Friedland shares that their artwork "was itself a practice of public health feminisms." The white fabric represented "the existing foundation of public health on which we build public health futures: predominantly white, timeworn, and in desperate need of replacement or repair" and "the colours represent[ed] diverse populations, [which serves] to recognize some of the groups who continue to be disproportionately affected by negative health outcomes." Friedland concludes by sharing that they hope their art piece can be "used as a tool" to ignite interest in public health feminisms. To support students and researchers with analytical tools that may help reveal and unpack how public health in Canada is embedded within patriarchal and colonial ways of knowing and doing through public health feminist praxis, I offer two insights that draw from the author discussions and concluding thoughts in this collection.

To transform public health through public health feminist praxis, two things must be done: (1) *uncover, disrupt, and dismantle*; and (2) *make space and move over*.

First, to *uncover, disrupt, and dismantle* the field of public health, public health feminism as praxis can be used to reveal and unpack how public health in Canada is a direct reflection of the country's very own beginnings, that of patriarchy and colonialism. As Kelly shares in chapter 2 surrounding the experiences of being a Métis public health nurse: "The exclusionary practices within our public health systems that suppress anything other than cisgender, heterosexual, white, able-bodied, neurotypical experience require our commitment to uncover and disrupt." This work is later supported by Ross in chapter 5 surrounding abortion stigma and reclaiming Indigenous knowledges: we must "dismantle systemic inequities and structures of oppression found in public health models to create a safer and healthier future for all." As public health scholars, policymakers, and front-line workers, we hold a responsibility to uncover, disrupt, and dismantle public health systems that have excluded the experiences of Black, Indigenous, racialized, refugee, immigrant, neurodiverse, (dis)abled, two-spirit, non-binary, trans and/or gender-diverse, and/or other marginalized/oppressed women. We must not be afraid to ask the hard questions that have been proposed in chapter 1: Why are things the way they are in public health practice, policy, programming, and education? What are public health decisions rooted in, and who do they *actually* serve? What are the implications for marginalized and/or oppressed groups of women and their communities?

The second action I offer as a result of the perspectives in this collection to transform the field public health through public health feminist praxis is to *make space and move over*. This requires that public health spaces create equitable, meaningful, supportive, and safe opportunities for Black, Indigenous, racialized, refugee, immigrant, neurodiverse, (dis)abled, two-spirit, non-binary, trans and/or gender-diverse, and/or other marginalized/oppressed women in public health leadership positions. These individuals carry many of the intersectional experiences described throughout this book and are the experts on their lived experience; such expertise is required to overhaul and transform the current public health system in Canada. For example, Amri and colleagues in chapter 3 underscore the gender inequities and inequalities in Canadian global health. They propose questions to investigate global health institutions' gender makeup and to make space and move over for those whose experiences are commonly "swept under the rug":

> Are women represented, and if so, do their voices include intersecting identities and are they able to freely express these perspectives to shape organizational decisions that ensure gender-equitable policies? ... Do these institutions reflect on power and privilege with the aim to overcome differences?

Making space and moving over to ensure public health feminist praxis is transformative but must go beyond the tokenistic nature that currently exists in public health programming, education, policy, and service decision making. Public health feminist praxis calls for collaboration, inclusion, and supportive environments that listen to those who hold intersectional experiences to overhaul and transform public health. Further acknowledging the gender and racial inequities in public health systems, while providing practical recommendations to support Black and Indigenous women to improve public health programming, Salmon and Tricco in chapter 11 state,

> Change is possible through tangible support of women in public health environments, intentional actionable career pathways that enable Black and Indigenous women's leadership, breaking barriers through systemic change, and equity in healthcare access. It is our collective responsibility to recognize, learn and unlearn, address, advocate.

COMING TO A CLOSE, FOR NOW ...

By exposing how patriarchy and colonialism are embedded in public health services, policies, education, and programming, *Critical Perspectives in Public Health Feminisms* provides an innovative approach that aims to explore what it means to protect and promote the health of *all* Canadians. This edited collection brings together insights from public health scholars, policymakers, and front-line workers who are at the intersections and who are experts in their fields and their experiences. By making space, moving over, and listening to these voices that often go ignored, public health's colonial and patriarchal origins will be uncovered, disrupted, and dismantled. It is then that public health in Canada will become transformed to protect and promote the health of *all* Canadians. Through this collection of voices, our hope is that others' experiences in the field of public health are validated and that they feel supported to speak their truth and continue to shape the future of public health through a public health feminist approach.

References

COVER ART BY MATSUKO FRIEDLAND

Crenshaw, K. (1989). Demarginalizing the intersection of race and sex: A Black feminist critique of antidiscrimination doctrine, feminist theory, and antiracist politics. *University of Chicago Legal Forum, 1989*(1), 139–167.

Day, L. F., & Buckle, M. (1907). *Art in needlework: A book about embroidery* (3rd ed.). B. T. Batsford.

Fulu, E., Leung, L., & Viana, M. (2021, June 28). Feminist movements are key to public health equity. *BMJ Opinion*. https://blogs.bmj.com/bmj/2021/06/28/feminist-movements-are-key-to-public-health-equity/

Galea, S. (2021). The arts and public health: Changing the conversation on health. *Health Promotion Practice, 22*(Suppl 1), 8S–11S. https://doi.org/10.1177/1524839921996341

Jones, C., Monchalin, R., Bourgeois, C., & Smylie, J. (2020). Kokums to the Iskwêsisisak: COVID-19 and urban Métis girls and young women. *Girlhood Studies, 13*(3), 116–132. https://doi.org/10.3167/ghs.2020.130309

Kielsgard, T. R., & Brown, L. X. Z. (2021). Trans, autistic and BIPOC: Living at the intersections of autism, race, and gender diversity. In *Working with autistic transgender and non-binary people: Research, practice and experience* (pp. 71–85). Jessica Kingsley Publishers.

Parker, R. (1989). *The subversive stitch: Embroidery and the making of the feminine*. Routledge.

Pratt Institute. (2021, January 11). *Craftivism: An introduction*. LibGuides at Pratt Institute LIS. https://prattlis.libguides.com/craftivism

Queer in the World. (n.d.). What is the Philadelphia pride flag, and what does it stand for? https://queerintheworld.com/philadelphia-pride-flag/

Raphael, D., Bryant, T., Mikkonen, J., & Raphael, A. (2020). *Social determinants of health: The Canadian facts* (2nd ed.). Ontario Tech University Faculty of Health Sciences and Toronto: York University School of Health Policy and Management. https://thecanadianfacts.org/

Segalo, P., & Fine, M. (2017). Threading life stories: Embroidery as an engaged method. In *Emancipatory and participatory methodologies in peace, critical, and community psychology* (pp. 107–117). Springer International Publishing.

Wharry, G. (2021, July 19). Stitching a life: The power of craftivism. *Geraldine Wharry*. https://www.geraldinewharry.com/getinspired/embroidery-craftivism-stitching-a-life-slow-fashion-feminism-political-craft

CHAPTER 1: PUBLIC HEALTH FEMINISMS, AN INTRODUCTION, BY RENÉE MONCHALIN

Ackerman, K., & Stettner, S. (2019). "The public is not ready for this": 1969 and the long road to abortion access. *Canadian Historical Review, 100*(2), 239–256. https://doi.org/10.3138/chr.2018-0082-3

Allan, B., & Smylie, J. (2015). *First peoples, second class treatment: The role of racism in the health and well-being of Indigenous peoples in Canada*. Wellesley Institute.

Baijius, W., & Patrick, R. J. (2019). "We don't drink the water here": The reproduction of undrinkable water for First Nations in Canada. *Water (Switzerland), 11*(5), 1079. https://doi.org/10.3390/w11051079

Banerjee, A. (2021, April 1). How the pandemic has shown social justice needs to be central to public health education in Canada. *University Affairs*. https://www.universityaffairs.ca/opinion/in-my-opinion/how-the-pandemic-has-shown-social-justice-needs-to-be-central-to-public-health-education-in-canada/

Berkhout, S. G., & Richardson, L. (2020). Identity, politics, and the pandemic: Why is COVID-19 a disaster for feminism(s)? *History and Philosophy of the Life Sciences, 42*(4), 1–6. https://doi.org/10.1007/s40656-020-00346-7

Canadian Public Health Association. (2017). *Public health: A conceptual framework*. https://www.cpha.ca/sites/default/files/uploads/policy/ph-framework/phcf_e.pdf

Canadian Public Health Association. (2020a). *What are the social determinants of health?* https://www.cpha.ca/what-are-social-determinants-health

Canadian Public Health Association. (2020b). *What is public health?* https://www.cpha.ca/what-public-health

Carbado, D. W., Crenshaw, K. W., Mays, V. M., & Tomlinson, B. (2013). Intersectionality: Mapping the movements of a theory. *Du Bois Review, 10*(2), 303–312. https://doi.org/10.1017/S1742058X13000349

Collins, P. H. (1998). *Fighting words: Black women and the search for justice*. University of Minnesota Press.

Crenshaw, K. (1989). Demarginalizing the intersection of race and sex: A Black feminist critique of antidiscrimination doctrine, feminist theory and antiracist politics. *University of Chicago Legal Forum*, 139–168.

Crenshaw, K. (1991). Mapping the margins: Intersectionality, identity politics, and violence against women of color. *Stanford Law Review*, *43*(6), 1241–1299.

Eidinger, A. (2022). Feminism. *The Canadian Encyclopedia*. https://www.thecanadianencyclopedia.ca/en/article/feminism

Hammarström, A. (1999). Why feminism in public health? *Scandinavian Journal of Public Health*, *27*(4), 241–244. https://doi.org/10.1177/14034948990270040601

Harper, R. (2018). *Why gender-based violence is a public health issue*. University of Alberta, School of Public Health. https://www.ualberta.ca/public-health/about/this-is-public-health/this-is-public-health-articles/2018/november/why-gender-based-violence-is-a-public-health-issues.html

hooks, b. (2015). *Feminism is for everybody: Passionate politics*. Routledge.

Jones, C., Monchalin, R., Bourgeois, C., & Smylie, J. (2020). Kokums to the Iskwêsisisak: COVID-19 and urban Métis girls and young women. *Girlhood Studies*, *13*(3), 116–132. https://doi.org/10.3167/GHS.2020.130309

Kelly, F. (2008). Confession of a born again pagan. In *From truth to reconciliation: Transforming the legacy of residential schools* (pp. 11–42). Aboriginal Healing Foundation Research Series.

Lisnyj, K. T., & Dickson-Anderson, S. E. (2018). Community resilience in Walkerton, Canada: Sixteen years post-outbreak. *International Journal of Disaster Risk Reduction*, *31*(May), 196–202. https://doi.org/10.1016/j.ijdrr.2018.05.001

Loreto, N. (2020). *Take back the fight: Organizing feminism for the digital age*. Fernwood Publishing.

Master Class. (2022). *Redefining feminism*. https://www.masterclass.com/classes/redefining-feminism-with-gloria-steinem-and-noted-co-instructors

me too. (2022). *History & inception*. https://metoomvmt.org/get-to-know-us/history-inception/

Monchalin, L. (2016). *The colonial problem: An Indigenous perspective on crime and injustice in Canada*. University of Toronto Press.

Monchalin, R. (2020). Novel coronavirus, access to abortion services, and bridging Western and Indigenous knowledges in a postpandemic world. *Women's Health Issues*, *1*, 5–8. https://doi.org/10.1016/j.whi.2020.10.004

Native Women's Association of Canada. (2020). *The impact of COVID-19 on Indigenous Peoples: Submission to the UN Special Rapporteur on the rights of Indigenous Peoples.* https://www.ohchr.org/Documents/Issues/IPeoples/SR/COVID-19/IndigenousCSOs/Canada_Native_Women_Association_of_Canada.pdf

Shaw, D., & Norman, W. V. (2020). When there are no abortion laws: A case study of Canada. *Best Practice and Research: Clinical Obstetrics and Gynaecology, 62*, 49–62. https://doi.org/10.1016/j.bpobgyn.2019.05.010

Stote, K. (2022). From eugenics to family planning: The coerced sterilization of Indigenous women in post-1970 Saskatchewan. *Native American and Indigenous Studies, 9*(1), 102–132.

Tulchinsky, T. H. (2018). John Snow, cholera, the Broad Street Pump; waterborne diseases then and now. *Case Studies in Public Health*, 77–99. https://doi.org/10.1016/B978-0-12-804571-8.00017-2

United Nations. (2020). *Policy brief: The impact of COVID-19 on women.* https://www.unwomen.org/sites/default/files/Headquarters/Attachments/Sections/Library/Publications/2020/Policy-brief-The-impact-of-COVID-19-on-women-en.pdf

United Nations. (2021). *Do you know all 17 SDGs?* United Nations: Department of Economic and Social Affairs, Sustainable Development. https://sdgs.un.org/goals

Yellowhead Institute. (2020). *Anishinaabe pandemic prophecies.* https://yellowheadinstitute.org/2020/04/24/fn-pandemic-prophecies/

CHAPTER 2: A REALLY GOOD BROWN NURSE, BY LEANNE POITRAS KELLY

Chrisjohn, R., & Young, S. (1994). *Appendix B. Research and residential schooling: Ideas for First Nations individuals and communities. Chapter 8: The circle game* (p. 109). Report to the Royal Commission on Aboriginal Peoples, Government of Canada.

Cook, V. J., & Elwood, K. (2004). BCG adieu. *British Columbia Medical Journal, 46*(1), 12.

Dumont, M. (1996). *A really good brown girl.* Brick Books.

Green, J. (Ed). (2007). *Making space for Indigenous feminism.* Fernwood Publishing.

Government of Canada. (2013, April 22). *Common experience payments*. https://www.rcaanc-cirnac.gc.ca/eng/1100100015594/1571582431348
hooks, b. (1994). *Teaching to transgress*. Routledge.
Kelm, M. E. (1998). *Colonizing bodies: Aboriginal health and healing in British Columbia, 1900–50*. UBC Press.
Lazarus, M., & Wunderlich, R. (Directors). (1979). *Killing us softly: Advertising's image of women* [Film]. Cambridge Documentary Films.
Lux, M. K. (2016). *Separate beds: A history of Indian hospitals in Canada, 1920s–1980s*. University of Toronto Press.
Maracle, L. (1996). *I am woman: A Native perspective on sociology and feminism*. Press Gang.
Menchú, R. (1984). *I, Rigoberta Menchú: An Indian woman in Guatemala*. Verso.
St. Denis, V. (2007). Feminism is for everybody: Aboriginal women, feminism and diversity. In J. Green (Ed.), *Making space for Indigenous feminism* (pp. 33–51). Fernwood Publishing.
Weber-Pillwax, C. (2021). It's in the blood: Theory and praxis of lifelong Indigenous education. *International Journal of Lifelong Education*, *40*(4), 395–414.

CHAPTER 3: EXPLORING GENDER EQUALITY AND EQUITY IN CANADIAN GLOBAL HEALTH INSTITUTIONS, BY MICHELLE AMRI, BIANCA CARDUCCI, KATRINA M. PLAMONDON, MURIEL MAC-SEING, JEANNIE SHOVELLER, AND ERICA DI RUGGIERO

Abimbola, S., & Pai, M. (2020, November 21). Will global health survive its decolonisation? *The Lancet*, *396*(10263), 1627–1628. https://doi.org/10.1016/s0140-6736(20)32417-x
Amri, M. M. (2017). Global public health: Preparation and training. In A. N. Arya (Ed.), *Preparing for international health experiences* (pp. 205–211). Routledge.
Amri, M. M., & Drummond, D. (2021). Punctuating the equilibrium: An application of policy theory to COVID-19. *Policy Design and Practice*, *4*(1), 33–43. https://doi.org/10.1080/25741292.2020.1841397
Amri, M. M., Jessiman-Perreault, G., Siddiqi, A., O'Campo, P., Enright, T., & Di Ruggiero, E. (2021). Scoping review of the World Health Organization's underlying equity discourses: Apparent ambiguities, inadequacy, and contradictions. *International Journal for Equity in Health*, *20*(1), 70. https://doi.org/10.1186/s12939-021-01400-x

Amri, M. M., Siddiqi, A., O'Campo, P., Enright, T., & Di Ruggiero, E. (2020). Underlying equity discourses of the World Health Organization: A scoping review protocol. *Social Science Protocols, 3*. http://journals.ed.ac.uk/social-science-protocols/article/view/4383

Bilge, S. (2013). Intersectionality undone. *Du Bois Review, 10*(2), 405–424.

Cadesky, J. (2020). Built on shaky ground: Reflections on Canada's Feminist International Assistance Policy. *International Journal: Canada's Journal of Global Policy Analysis, 75*(3), 298–312.

Canadian Association for Global Health. (2021). *Canadian women in global health 2021*. https://cagh-acsm.org/en/programmes/femmes-en-sante-mondiale/canadian-women-global-health

Canadian Institutes of Health Research. (2017). *Shaping science for a healthier world: Strategy 2017*. https://cihr-irsc.gc.ca/e/48638.html

Canadian Institutes of Health Research. (2018). *Science is better with sex and gender: Strategic plan 2018–2023*. https://cihr-irsc.gc.ca/e/51310.html

Canadian Institutes of Health Research. (2021). *Global health 3.0: CIHR's framework for action on global health research 2021–2026*. https://cihr-irsc.gc.ca/e/52503.html

Canadian Medical Association. (n.d.). *Quick facts on Canada's physicians*. https://www.cma.ca/quick-facts-canadas-physicians#:~:text=Physicians%20in%20training,was%20estimated%20at%202%2C8606

Coe, I. R., Wiley, R., & Bekker, L.-G. (2019). Organisational best practices towards gender equality in science and medicine. *The Lancet, 393*(10171), 587–593. https://doi.org/10.1016/S0140-6736(18)33188-X

Collins, P. H., & Bilge, S. (2016). *Intersectionality*. Polity Press.

Crenshaw, K. (1989). Demarginalizing the intersection of race and sex: A Black feminist critique of antidiscrimination doctrine, feminist theory and antiracist politics. *University of Chicago Legal Forum, 1989*(1), 139–167.

Diehl, A. B., Stephenson, A. L., Dzubinski, L. M., & Wang, D. C. (2020). Measuring the invisible: Development and multi-industry validation of the Gender Bias Scale for Women Leaders. *Human Resource Development Quarterly, 31*(1), 249–280.

Dimitris, M., Gittings, M., & King, N. (2021). How global is global health research? A large-scale analysis of trends in authorship. *BMJ Global Health, 6*(1).

Downs, J. A., Mathad, J. S., Reif, L. K., McNairy, M. L., Celum, C., Boutin-Foster, C., Deschamps, M. M., Gupta, A., Hokororo, A., Katz, I. T., Konopasek, L., Nelson, R., Riviere, C., Glimcher, L. H., & Fitzgerald, D. W. (2016, December 21). The ripple effect: Why promoting female leadership in global health matters. *Public Health Action*, *6*(4), 210–211. https://doi.org/10.5588/pha.16.0072

Garry, A. (2011). Intersectionality, metaphors, and the multiplicity of gender. *Hypatia*, *26*(4), 826–850. https://doi.org/https://doi.org/10.1111/j.1527-2001.2011.01194.x

Global Health 50/50. (2020). *The Global Health 50/50 report 2020: Power, privilege and priorities*. https://globalhealth5050.org/wp-content/uploads/2020/03/Power-Privilege-and-Priorities-2020-Global-Health-5050-Report.pdf

Goodkind, S., Gartner, R. E., Jacobs, L. A., Branson, D., King, J., Meaux, S., & Miller, E. (2021). Making AIMS explicit: Establishing intersectionality criteria for gender equity analyses. *Social Work Research*, *45*(3), 169–186. https://doi.org/10.1093/swr/svab013

Government of Canada. (2017). *Canada's Feminist International Assistance Policy*.

Hankivsky, O. (2014). *Intersectionality 101*. Institute for Intersectionality Research & Policy, SFU. http://vawforum-cwr.ca/sites/default/files/attachments/intersectionallity_101.pdf

International Development Research Centre. (2021). *A more sustainable and inclusive world: Strategy 2030*. https://www.idrc.ca/sites/default/files/sp/strategy2030.pdf

Jones, C. M., Gautier, L., Kadio, K., Mac-Seing, M., Miranda, É., Omenka, C., Ouédraogo, S., Pérez, M. C., Turcotte-Tremblay, A. M., Tiné, S., & WGH Francophone Working Group (2018). Equity in the gender equality movement in global health [Letter]. *The Lancet*, *392*(10142), e2–e3. https://doi.org/10.1016/S0140-6736(18)31561-7

Kapilashrami, A., & Hankivsky, O. (2018). Intersectionality and why it matters to global health. *The Lancet*, *391*(10140), 2589–2591.

Kawachi, I., Subramanian, S. V., & Almeida-Filho, N. (2002). A glossary for health inequalities. *Journal of Epidemiology and Community Health*, *56*, 647–652. https://doi.org/https://www.ncbi.nlm.nih.gov/pmc/articles/PMC1732240/pdf/v056p00647.pdf

Larivière, V., Ni, C., Gingras, Y., Cronin, B., & Sugimoto, C. R. (2013). Bibliometrics: Global gender disparities in science. *Nature*, *504*(7479), 211–213. https://doi.org/10.1038/504211a

Merriman, R., Galizia, I., Tanaka, S., Sheffel, A., Buse, K., & Hawkes, S. (2021). The gender and geography of publishing: A review of sex/gender reporting and author representation in leading general medical and global health journals. *BMJ Global Health*, *6*(5), e005672. https://doi.org/10.1136/bmjgh-2021-005672

Moyer, C. A., Abedini, N. C., Youngblood, J., Talib, Z., Jayaraman, T., Manzoor, M., Larson, H. J., Garcia, P. J., Binagwaho, A., Burke, K. S., & Barry, M. (2018). Advancing women leaders in global health: Getting to solutions. *Annals of Global Health*, *84*(4), 743–752.

Nielsen, M. W., Bloch, C. W., & Schiebinger, L. (2018). Making gender diversity work for scientific discovery and innovation. *Nature Human Behaviour*, *2*(10), 726–734. https://doi.org/10.1038/s41562-018-0433-1

Ouédraogo, S., Gautier, L., Mac-Seing, M., Tine, S., Perez, M. C., Kadio, K., Chegno, R., & Jones, C. M. (2019). De-patriarchalising and levelling science for French-speaking women. *The Lancet*, *393*(10171), e23–e24. https://doi.org/10.1016/S0140-6736(18)32092-0

Plamondon, K., & Bisung, E. (2019). The CCGHR Principles for Global Health Research: Centering equity in research, knowledge translation, and practice. *Social Science Medicine*, *239*.

Plamondon, K., Shahram, S., & Ndumbe-Eyoh. (2022). Equity, power & transformative research co-production. In I. Graham, J. Salsberg, A. Kothari & J. Rycroft-Malone (Eds.), *Research co-production in healthcare* (pp. 34–53). Wiley-Blackwell.

Porter, A., & Bourgeault, I. (2017). *Gender, workforce and health system change in Canada*. CIHI. Presented at the Fourth Global Forum on Human Resources for Health, Dublin Ireland, November 2017.

Rice, C., Harrison, E., & Friedman, M. (2019). Doing justice to intersectionality in research. *Cultural Studies ↔ Critical Methodologies*, *19*(6), 409–420. https://doi.org/10.1177/1532708619829779

Rosser, E., Morgan, R., Tan, H., Hawkins, K., Ngunjiri, A., Oyekunle, A., Schall, B., Nacif Pimenta, D., Tamaki, E., Rocha, M., & Wenham, C. (2021). *How to create a gender-responsive pandemic plan: Addressing the secondary effects of COVID-19*. https://www.genderandcovid-19.org/how-to-create-a-gender-responsive-pandemic-plan-addressing-the-secondary-effects-of-covid-19/

Shannon, G., Jansen, M., Williams, K., Cáceres, C., Motta, A., Odhiambo, A., Eleveld, A., & Mannell, J. (2019). Gender equality in science, medicine, and global health: Where are we at and why does it matter? *The Lancet*, *393*(10171), 560–569. https://doi.org/10.1016/S0140-6736(18)33135-0

Squazzoni, F., Bravo, G., Grimaldo, F., García-Costa, D., Farjam, M., & Mehmani, B. (2021). Gender gap in journal submissions and peer review during the first wave of the COVID-19 pandemic. A study on 2329 Elsevier journals. *PLoS ONE*, *16*(10), e0257919. https://doi.org/10.1371/journal.pone.0257919

Tricco, A. C., Bourgeault, I., Moore, A., Grunfeld, E., Peer, N., & Straus, S. E. (2021). Advancing gender equity in medicine. *CMAJ*, *193*(7), E244–E250. https://doi.org/10.1503/cmaj.200951

United Nations. (2015). *Sustainable Development Goals.* https://sdgs.un.org/goals

United Nations. (2020). *Policy brief: The impact of COVID-19 on women.* https://www.unwomen.org/sites/default/files/Headquarters/Attachments/Sections/Library/Publications/2020/Policy-brief-The-impact-of-COVID-19-on-women-en.pdf

Whitehead, M. (1990). *The concepts and principles of equity and health.* World Health Organization Regional Office for Europe. https://citeseerx.ist.psu.edu/viewdoc/download?doi=10.1.1.196.7167&rep=rep1&type=pdf

World Economic Forum. (2022). *Global gender gap report 2022.* https://www.weforum.org/reports/global-gender-gap-report-2022

World Health Organization. (2011). WHO Gender Responsive Assessment Scale: Criteria for assessing programmes and policies. In *WHO gender mainstreaming manual for health managers: A practical approach.* https://www.who.int/gender/mainstreaming/GMH_Participant_GenderAssessmentScale.pdf

World Health Organization. (2019). *Delivered by women, led by men: A gender and equity analysis of the global health and social workforce.* https://cdn.who.int/media/docs/default-source/health-workforce/delivered-by-women-led-by-men.pdf

World Health Organization. (n.d.). *Women's health.* https://www.who.int/health-topics/women-s-health/

CHAPTER 4: STUCK IN A HIGH WIRE ACT: WAYS OF UNDERSTANDING IMMIGRANT WOMEN'S MENTAL HEALTH BEYOND BIOMEDICINE, BY NICOLA GAILITS, DENISE GASTALDO, IZUMI SAKAMOTO, CELESTE BILBAO-JOSEPH, GISELLE VAZQUEZ, AND LORI E. ROSS

Bhatia, S., & Priya, K. R. (2021). Coloniality and psychology: From silencing to re-centering marginalized voices in postcolonial times. *Review of General Psychology*, *25*(4), 422–436.

Carter, L., & Rossi, A. (2019). Embodying strength: The origin, representations, and socialization of the strong Black woman ideal and its effect on Black women's mental health. *Women & Therapy*, *42*(3-4), 289–300.

Donoghue, M. (2022). Resilience, discipline and financialisation in the UK's liberal welfare state. *New Political Economy*, *27*(3), 504–516. https://doi.org/10.1080/13563467.2021.1994538

Fricker, M. (2007). *Epistemic injustice: Power and the ethics of knowing.* Oxford University Press.

Gailits, N. (2023). *Making the invisible, visible: Reimagining immigrant mental health through the stories of Latinx women* [Unpublished doctoral dissertation]. University of Toronto.

Gailits, N., Gastaldo, D., Sakamoto, I., & Ross, L. (Forthcoming). Postcolonial narrative inquiry: Using deep seeing, deep listening, deep hearing, and deep feeling to combat epistemic violence and refocus the research process.

Gailits, N., Pastor-Bravo, M. M., Gastaldo, D., Bajwa, U., Bilbao-Joseph, C., Castro, C., & Godoy, S. (2021). Fighting for inclusion across borders: Latin American trans women's health in Canada. *International Journal of Transgender Health, 23*(1–2), 5–23. https://doi.org/10.1080/26895269.2021.1988877

Government of Canada. (2021). *Eligibility to apply as a federal skilled worker (Express Entry).* https://www.canada.ca/en/immigration-refugees-citizenship/services/immigrate-canada/express-entry/eligibility/federal-skilled-workers.html

Guruge, S., & Khanlou, N. (2004). Intersectionalities of influence: Researching the health of immigrant and refugee women. *Canadian Journal of Nursing Research, 36*(3), 32–47.

Immigration, Refugees and Citizenship Canada (IRCC). (2020). *Annual report to Parliament on immigration.* https://www.canada.ca/en/immigration-refugees-citizenship/corporate/publications-manuals/annual-report-parliament-immigration-2020.html

Jack, D. C., & Ali, A. (2010). *Silencing the self across cultures: Depression and gender in the social world.* Oxford University Press.

Kirmayer, L. J., Narasiah, L., Munoz, M., Rashid, M., Ryder, A. G., Guzder, J., Hassan, G., Rousseau, C., & Pottie, K. (2011). Common mental health problems in immigrants and refugees: General approach in primary care. *CMAJ, 183*(12), E959–E967. https://dx.doi.org/10.1503/cmaj.090292

Lakatos, P. P. (1992). *The effects of migratory grief on the adjustment of the adult Hispanic immigrant* [Unpublished doctoral dissertation]. California School of Professional Psychology.

Mills, C. & Fernando, S. (2014). Globalising mental health or pathologising the global south? Mapping the ethics, theory and practice of global mental health. *Disability and the Global South, 1*(2), 188–202.

Summerfield, D. (2012). Afterword: Against "global mental health." *Transcultural Psychiatry*, *49*(3–4), 519–530. https://doi.org/10.1177/1363461512454701

Vanderkruik, R., & Dimidjian, S. (2019). Perspectives on task-shifting depression care to peers for depressed Latina mothers. *Journal of Latinx Psychology*, 7(1), 22–38. http://dx.doi.org/10.1037/lat0000104

Viruell-Fuentes, E. A., Miranda, P. Y., & Abdulrahim, S. (2012). More than culture: Structural racism, intersectionality theory, and immigrant health. *Social Science & Medicine*, *75*(12), 2099–2106. https://doi.org/10.1016/j.socscimed.2011.12.037

Zaheer, J., Shera, W., Tsang, A. K. T., Law, S., Fung, W. L. A., Eynan, R., Lam, J., Zheng, X., Pozi, L., & Links, P. S. (2016). "I just couldn't step out of the circle. I was trapped": Patterns of endurance and distress in Chinese-Canadian women with a history of suicidal behaviour. *Social Science & Medicine*, *160*, 43–53.

CHAPTER 5: SPURRING THE WITCH HUNT: ABORTION, COLONIALISM, STIGMA, AND INDIGENOUS KNOWLEDGES IN CANADA, BY ARIE ROSS

Abortion Rights Coalition of Canada. (2017). *Position paper #92: Catholic Church and Abortion*.

Abortion Rights Coalition of Canada. (n.d.). *Abortion Rights Coalition of Canada*. https://www.arcc-cdac.ca/

Abortion Support Services Atlantic. (n.d.). *Abortion Support Services Atlantic*. https://atlanticabortionco.wixsite.com/website

Ackerman, K., & Stettner, S. (2019). "The public is not ready for this": 1969 and the long road to abortion access. *Canadian Historical Review*, *100*, 239–256. https://doi.org/10.3138/chr.2018-0082-3

Action Canada for Sexual Health and Rights. (2019). *Three decades since Morgentaler, stigma still restricts access to abortion*. https://www.actioncanadashr.org/news/2019-11-05-three-decades-morgentaler-stigma-still-restricts-access-abortion

Action Canada for Sexual Health and Rights. (n.d.). *Find sexual health services near you*. https://www.actioncanadashr.org/resources/services

Agecoutay, C. (2022, February 18). Canadian doctors decide whether Indigenous women are fit to be mothers. *CTVNews*. https://www.ctvnews.ca/w5/canadian-doctors-decide-whether-indigenous-women-are-fit-to-be-mothers-1.5787101

Allan, B., & Smylie, J. (2015). *First peoples, second class treatment: The role of racism in the health and well-being of Indigenous Peoples in Canada*. Wellesley Institute.

Anderson, K. (2003). Vital signs: Reading colonialism in contemporary adolescent family planning. In B. Lawrence & K. Anderson (Eds.), *Strong women stories: Native vision and community survival* (pp. 174–191). Sumach Press.

Anderson, K. (2011). *Life stages and Native women: Memory, teachings, and story medicine*. University of Manitoba Press.

Astbury-Ward, E., Parry, O., & Carnwell, R. (2012). Stigma, abortion, and disclosure: Findings from a qualitative study. *Journal of Sexual Medicine*, *9*(12), 3137–3147. https://doi.org/10.1111/j.1743-6109.2011.02604.x

BC Women's Hospital and Health Centre. (n.d.). Abortion Services. http://www.bcwomens.ca/health-info/sexual-reproductive-health/abortion-services

Belfrage, M., Ortíz Ramírez, O., & Sorhaindo, A. (2020). Story circles and abortion stigma in Mexico: A mixed-methods evaluation of a new intervention for reducing individual level abortion stigma. *Culture, Health & Sexuality*, *22*(1), 96–111. https://doi.org/10.1080/13691058.2019.1577493

Burnett, K. (2010). *Taking medicine: Women's healing work and colonial contact in southern Alberta, 1880–1930*. UBC Press.

Burnett, K. (2018). Different histories: Reproduction, colonialism, and Treaty 7 communities in southern Alberta. 1880–1940. In S. Stettner, K. Burnett, & T. Hay (Eds.), *Abortion: History, politics and reproductive justice after Morgentaler* (pp. 676–677). UBC Press.

Cattapan, A., Moore, S., & Lawford, K. (2021, March 1). *Reproductive justice and Indigenous women in Saskatchewan: Overview and recommendations*. https://www.schoolofpublicpolicy.sk.ca/research/publications/policy-brief/reproductive-justice-and-indigenous-women-in-sk.php

Cockrill, K., Upadhyay, U. D., Turan, J., & Foster, D. G. (2013). The stigma of having an abortion: Development of a scale and characteristics of women experiencing abortion stigma. *Perspectives on Sexual and Reproductive Health*, *45*(2), 79–88. http://www.jstor.org/stable/42004174

Coen-Sanchez, K., Idriss-Wheeler, D., Bancroft, X., El-Mowafi, I. M., Yalahow, A., Etowa, J., & Yaya, S. (2022). Reproductive justice in patient care: Tackling systemic racism and health inequities in sexual and reproductive health and rights in Canada. *Reproductive Health*, *19*(44). https://doi.org/10.1186/s12978-022-01328-7

Cohen, M. (2020, April 29). Why the abortion pill is more important than ever during the coronavirus. *Maclean's*. https://www.macleans.ca/opinion/why-the-abortion-pill-is-more-important-than-ever-during-the-coronavirus/

Dyck, E., & Lux, M. (2016). Population control in the "Global North": Canada's response to Indigenous reproductive rights and neo-eugenics. *Canadian Historical Review*, *97*(4), 481–512. http://muse.jhu.edu/article/639431

ekw'í7tl. (n.d.). *Ekw'í7tl*. https://ekwi7tldoulacollective.org/

El-Mowafi, I. M., Yalahow, A., Idriss-Wheeler, D., & Yaya, S. (2021). The politest form of racism: Sexual and reproductive health and rights paradigm in Canada. *Reproductive Health*, *18*(1), 1–5. https://reproductive-health-journal.biomedcentral.com/articles/10.1186/s12978-021-01117-8

Erdman, J. N. (2016). The law of stigma, travel, and the abortion-free island. *Columbia Journal of Gender and Law*, *33*(1), 29. https://link.gale.com/apps/doc/A471000803/LT?u=uvictoria&sid=summon&xid=758f8ec5

Freedman L., Landy, U., Darney, P., & Steinauer, J. (2010). Obstacles to the integration of abortion into obstetrics and gynecology practice. *Perspectives on Sexual and Reproductive Health*, *42*(3), 146–151. https://doi.org/10.1363/4214610

Garcia, J.-L., & Sharif, M. Z. (2015). Black Lives Matter: A commentary on racism and public health. *American Journal of Public Health*, *105*(8), e27–e30. https://ajph.aphapublications.org/doi/10.2105/AJPH.2015.302706

Gilmore, R. (2020, March 30). Canada experiencing shortage of abortion pill amid COVID-19 outbreak. *CTVNews*. https://www.ctvnews.ca/health/coronavirus/canada-experiencing-shortage-of-abortion-pill-amid-covid-19-outbreak-1.4874666

Government of Prince Edward Island. (2021, July 15). *Surgical abortion*. https://www.princeedwardisland.ca/en/information/health-pei/surgical-abortion

Halifax Sexual Health Centre. (n.d.). Pregnancy options. *Halifax Sexual Health Centre*. https://hshc.ca/pregnancy-options/

Hanschmidt, F., Linde, K., Hilbert, A., Riedel- Heller, S. G., & Kersting, A. (2016). Abortion stigma: A systematic review. *Perspectives on Sexual and Reproductive Health*, *48*(4), 169–177. https://doi.org/10.1363/48e8516

Horizon Health Network. (2022). Family Planning Clinic—Abortion Clinic. *Horizon Health Network*. https://horizonnb.ca/services/clinics/family-planning-clinic-abortion-clinic/

International Planned Parenthood Federation. (2016, May 5). *Tackling abortion stigma*. https://www.ippf.org/our-approach/programmes/tackling-abortion-stigma

Ipas. (2018). *Abortion stigma ends here: A toolkit for understanding and action.* https://www.ipas.org/resource/abortion-stigma-ends-here-a-toolkit-for-understanding-and-action/

Kirby, J. (2017, December). A broad vision for reproductive justice. *Briarpatch Magazine.* https://briarpatchmagazine.com/articles/view/broad-vision-reproductive-justice

Koffman, R. L. (n.d.). *Jewish perspectives on reproductive realities.* National Council of Jewish Women. https://www.ncjw.org/wp-content/uploads/2018/02/Jewish-Perspective-on-Reproductive-Realities-FORMATTED11.pdf

Kumar, A., Hessini, L., & Mitchell, E. M. H. (2009). Conceptualizing abortion stigma. *Culture, Health & Sexuality*, *11*(6), 625–639. http://www.jstor.org/stable/27784486

LaRoche, K. J., Wynn, L. L., & Foster, A. M. (2020). "We've got rights and yet we don't have access": Exploring patient experiences accessing medication abortion in Australia. *Contraception*, *101*(4), 256–260. https://doi.org/10.1016/j.contraception.2019.12.008

Lawford, K., & Giles, A. (2012). Marginalization and coercion: Canada's evacuation policy for pregnant First Nations women who live on reserves in rural and remote regions. *Pimatisiwin*, *10*(3), 327–340. https://www.researchgate.net/publication/263305837_Marginalization_and_coercion_Canada's_evacuation_policy_for_pregnant_First_Nations_women_who_live_on_reserves_in_rural_and_remote_regions

LeTourneau, K. (2016). *Abortion stigma around the world: A synthesis of the qualitative literature.* International Network for the Reduction of Abortion Discrimination and Stigma (inroads). https://www.safeabortionwomensright.org/wp-content/uploads/2016/05/AbortionStigmaAroundtheWorld-HR-2.pdf

Loreto, N. (2020, April 1). COVID-19 may limit access to abortions throughout Canada. *Passage: Coronavirus Health.* https://readpassage.com/covid-19-may-limit-access-to-abortions-throughout-canada/

Major, B., & Gramzow, R. H. (1999). Abortion as stigma: Cognitive and emotional implications of concealment. *Journal of Personality and Social Psychology*, *77*(4), 735–745. https://doi.org/10.1037/0022-3514.77.4.735

Mehta, S. (2019, May 21). Still barriers to abortion access on Vancouver Island. *Victoria News.* https://www.vicnews.com/news/still-barriers-to-abortion-access-on-vancouver-island/

Monchalin, R. (2021). Novel coronavirus, access to abortion services, and bridging western and Indigenous knowledges in a postpandemic world. *Women's Health Issues*, *31*(1), 5–8. https://doi.org/10.1016/j.whi.2020.10.004

Monchalin, R., Lesperance, A., Flicker, S., & Native Youth Sexual Health Network. (2015). *Sexy Health Carnival Toolkit: By and for Indigenous youth*. https://static1.squarespace.com/static/5f3550c11c1f590e92ad30eb/t/5f45924d89367a7ca1e8a708/1598394969116/shctoolkit.pdf

Moseson, H., Fix, L., Ragosta, S., Forsberg, H., Hastings, J., Stoeffler, A., Lunn, M. R., Flentje, A., Capriotti, M. R., Lubensky, M. E., & Obedin-Maliver, J. (2021). Abortion experiences and preferences of transgender, nonbinary, and gender-expansive people in the United States. *American Journal of Obstetrics and Gynecology*, *224*(4), 376.e1–376.e11. https://doi.org/10.1016/j.ajog.2020.09.035

Musée de l'Holocauste Montréal. (2019, July 17). *Holocaust Survivor Henry Morgentaler—Abortion rights in Canada* [Video]. YouTube. https://www.youtube.com/watch?v=_GRRhQq8BCU&ab_channel=Mus%C3%A9edel%27HolocausteMontr%C3%A9al

Myran, D., & Bardsley, J. (2018). Abortion remains absent from family medicine training in Canada. *Canadian Family Physician*, *64*(8), 618–619. https://www.ncbi.nlm.nih.gov/pmc/articles/PMC6189888/

National Inquiry into Missing and Murdered Indigenous Women and Girls (Canada). (2019). *Reclaiming power and place: The final report of the National Inquiry into Missing and Murdered Indigenous Women and Girls*. https://www.mmiwg-ffada.ca/final-report/

Northern Manitoba Abortion Support. (n.d.). [Facebook]. https://www.facebook.com/northernmbabortionsupport/

Northern Reproductive Justice Network. (n.d.). [Facebook]. https://www.facebook.com/groups/northernreproductivejusticenetwork

Opal Clinic. (2022). *Abortion*. https://opalyukon.ca/abortion

Planned Parenthood. (2020). *Therapeutic abortion in NL*. https://www.plannedparenthoodnlshc.com/uploads/1/0/0/3/100308324/therapeutic_abortion_in_nl.pdf

Rasmussen, P. (2019). Colonizing racialized bodies. *On Politics*, *13*(1), 18–29. https://journals.uvic.ca/index.php/onpolitics/article/view/19415

Reading, C., & Wien, F. (2009). *Health inequalities and social determinants of Aboriginal peoples' health*. National Collaborating Centre for Aboriginal Health. http://www.nccah-ccnsa.ca/docs/social%20determinates/nccah-loppie-wien_report.pdf

Redvers, N. (2019). Epilogue. In *The science of the sacred: Bridging global Indigenous medicine systems and modern scientific principles* (pp. 215–221). North Atlantic Books.

Ross, L. J. (2017). Reproductive justice as intersectional feminist activism. *Souls*, *19*(3), 286–314. https://doi.org/10.1080/10999949.2017.1389634

Sethna, C., & Doull, M. (2013). Spatial disparities and travel to freestanding abortion clinics in Canada. *Women's Studies International Forum*, *38*, 52–62. https://doi.org/10.1016/j.wsif.2013.02.001

Shaw, D., & Norman, W. V. (2020). When there are no abortion laws: A case study of Canada. *Best Practice & Research Clinical Obstetrics & Gynaecology*, *62*, 49–62. https://doi.org/10.1016/j.bpobgyn.2019.05.010

Shaw, J. (2013). Abortion in Canada as a social justice issue in contemporary Canada. *Critical Social Work*, *14*(2), Article 2. https://doi.org/10.22329/csw.v14i2.5878

Shellenberg, K. M., Moore, A. M., Bankole, A., Juarez, F., Omideyi, A. K., Palomino, N., & Tsui, A. O. (2011). Social stigma and disclosure about induced abortion: Results from an exploratory study. *Global Public Health*, *6*(Suppl 1), S111–125. https://doi.org/10.1080/17441692.2011.594072

Shellenberg, K. M., & Tsui, A. O. (2012). Correlates of perceived and internalized stigma among abortion patients in the USA: An exploration by race and Hispanic ethnicity. *International Journal of Gynecology & Obstetrics*, *118*(S2), S152–S159. https://doi.org/10.1016/S0020-7292(12)60015-0

Shout Your Abortion. (n.d.). *Shout Your Abortion*. https://shoutyourabortion.com/

SisterSong Women of Color Reproductive Justice Collective. (n.d.). Reproductive justice. https://www.sistersong.net/reproductive-justice

Stangl, A. L., Earnshaw, V. A., Logie, C. H., van Brakel, W., C. Simbayi, L., Barré, I., & Dovidio, J. F. (2019). The health stigma and discrimination framework: A global, crosscutting framework to inform research, intervention development, and policy on health-related stigmas. *BMC Medicine*, *17*(1), 31. https://doi.org/10.1186/s12916-019-1271-3

UN Women. (2020, July 1). *Intersectional feminism: What it means and why it matters right now*. https://www.unwomen.org/en/news/stories/2020/6/explainer-intersectional-feminism-what-it-means-and-why-it-matters

CHAPTER 6: DECONSTRUCTING ABLEISM IN HEALTHCARE, BY MAREN B. AKYÜREK AND NATALIE FRANDSEN

Accessible Canada Act (S.C. 2019, c. 10). https://laws-lois.justice.gc.ca/eng/acts/A-0.6/

Aguayo-Romero, R. A. (2021). (Re)centering black feminism into intersectionality research. *American Journal of Public Health*, *111*(1), 101–103. https://doi.org/10.2105/AJPH.2020.306005

Ahmedani, B. K. (2011). Mental health stigma: Society, individuals, and the profession. *Journal of Social Work Values and Ethics*, *8*, 1–4.

Al-Azawei, A., Serenelli, F., & Lundqvist, K. (2016). Universal design for learning (UDL): A content analysis of peer-reviewed journal papers from 2012 to 2015. *Journal of the Scholarship of Teaching and Learning*, *16*(3), 39–56.

Alberta Human Rights Commission (2010). *Duty to accommodate students with disabilities in post-secondary educational institutions: Interpretive bulletin.* https://www.albertahumanrights.ab.ca/publications/bulletins_sheets_booklets/bulletins/Pages/duty_to_accommodate_students.aspx#What%20is%20accommodation

Aldridge, S. (2008). The regulation of health professionals: An overview of the British Columbia experience. *Journal of Medical Imaging and Radiation Sciences*, *39*(1), 4–10. https://doi.org/10.1016/j.jmir.2008.01.001

Allan, L., Hatala, A., Ijaz, S., Courchene, E. D., & Bushie, E. B. (2020). Indigenous-led health care partnerships in Canada. *CMAJ*, *192*(9), E208–E216. https://doi.org/10.1503/cmaj.190728

Arim, R. (2015). *A profile of persons with disabilities among Canadians aged 15 years or older, 2012.* (Catalogue no. 89-654-X). Statistics Canada. https://www150.statcan.gc.ca/n1/pub/89-654-x/89-654-x2015001-eng.pdf

Bailey, M., & Mobley, I. A. (2019). Work in the intersections: A Black feminist disability framework. *Gender and Society*, *33*(1), 19–40. https://doi.org/10.1177/0891243218801523

British Columbia Human Rights Code, R.S.B.C. (1996). c. 210.

Brown, N. (2021). *Lived experiences of ableism in academia: Strategies for inclusion in higher education*. Policy Press.

Bulk, L. Y., Tikhonova, J., Gagnon, J. M., Battalova, A., Mayer, Y., Krupa, T., Lee, M., Nimmon, L., & Jarus, T. (2020). Disabled healthcare professionals' diverse, embodied, and socially embedded experiences. *Advances in Health Sciences Education: Theory and Practice*, *25*(1), 111–129. https://doi.org/10.1007/s10459-019-09912-6

Canadian Charter of Rights and Freedoms, Part I of the Constitution Act, 1982, being Schedule B to the Canada Act 1982 (UK), c. 11.

Canadian Encyclopedia. (2022). *Timeline: Women's suffrage.* https://www.thecanadianencyclopedia.ca/en/timeline/womens-suffrage

Canadian Human Rights Act (RSC 1985, c H-6).

Canadian Human Rights Commission (CHRC). (2010). *Your guide to understanding the Canadian Human Rights Act.* Minister of Public Works and

Government Services. https://www.chrc-ccdp.gc.ca/sites/default/files/2020-07/chra_guide_lcdp-eng.pdf

Canadian Human Rights Commission (CHRC). (2017). *Left out: Challenges faced by persons with disabilities in Canadian schools.* https://www.chrc-ccdp.gc.ca/eng/content/left-out-challenges-faced-persons-disabilities-canadas-schools

Canadian Mental Health Association (CMHA). (2017). *A guide to peer support programs on post-secondary campuses.* https://healthycampuses.ca/wp-content/uploads/2017/09/HMHC-A-guide-to-peer-support-programs-on-post-secondary-campuses.pdf

Canadian Standards Association. (2020). *National Standard of Canada: Mental health and well-being for post-secondary students.* CSA Group.

Capp, M. J. (2017). The effectiveness of universal design for learning: A meta-analysis of literature between 2013 and 2016. *International Journal of Inclusive Education*, *21*(8), 791–807. https://doi.org/10.1080/13603116.2017.1325074

Carleton University. (2022). *How to become a doctor.* https://admissions.carleton.ca/programs-of-study/how-to-choose-a-major/professional-degrees/how-to-become-a-doctor/

Cohen, J. J., Gabriel, B. A., & Terrell, G. (2002). The case for diversity in the health care workforce. *Health Affairs*, *21*, 5, 90–102. https://doi.org/10.1377/hlthaff.21.5.90

Collins, P. H. (2019). *Intersectionality as critical social theory.* Duke University Press.

Condra, M., Dineen, M., Gauthier, S., Gills, H., & Jack-Davies, A. (2015). Academic accommodations for postsecondary students with mental health disabilities in Ontario, Canada: Review of the literature and reflections on emerging issues. *Journal of Postsecondary Education and Disability*, *28*(3), 277–291.

Corrigan, P. W., & Rao, D. (2012). On the self-stigma of mental illness: Stages, disclosure, and strategies for change. *Canadian Journal of Psychiatry*, *57*(8), 464–469.

Cox, D. H., & Klas, L. D. (1996). Students with learning disabilities in Canadian colleges and universities: A primer for service provision. *Journal of Learning Disabilities*, *29*(1), 93–97. https://doi.org/10.1177/002221949602900111

Crooks, V. A., Agarwal, G., & Harrison, A. (2012). Chronically ill Canadians' experiences of being unattached to a family doctor: A qualitative study of marginalized patients in British Columbia. *BMC Family Practice*, *13*(69), https://doi.org/10.1186/1471-2296-13-69

Crow, L. (2010). Including all of our lives: Renewing the social model of disability. In C. Walsh, K. Sheehy, K. Simmons, M. Nind, & J. Rix (Eds.), *Equality, participation and inclusion* (pp. 124–140). Routledge.

Dolmage, J. (2017). *Academic ableism*. University of Michigan Press. https://doi.org/10.3998/mpub.9708722

Dunn, D. S. (2019). Outsider privileges can lead to insider disadvantages: Some psychosocial aspects of ableism. *Journal of Social Issues*, *75*(3), 665–682. https://doi.org/10.1111/josi.12331

Employment and Social Development Canada. (2020). *Summary of the Accessible Canada Act*. Government of Canada. https://www.canada.ca/en/employment-social-development/programs/accessible-people-disabilities/act-summary.html

Epstein, I., Khanlou, N., Ermel, R. E., Sherk, M., Simmonds, K. K., Balaquiao, L., & Chang, K.-Y. (2021). Students who identify with a disability and instructors' experiences in nursing practice: A scoping review. *International Journal of Mental Health and Addiction*, *19*(1), 91–118.

Furrie, A. D. (2017). *Post-secondary: Their experience—past and present final report*. National Educational Association of Disabled Students. https://www.neads.ca/en/about/media/Final%20reportCSD2012AdeleFurrie2-3.pdf

Galtung, J., & Fischer, D. (2013). *Johan Galtung: Pioneer of peace research*. Springer Berlin Heidelberg. https://doi.org/10.1007/978-3-642-32481-9

Garland-Thomson, R. (2002). Integrating disability, transforming feminist theory. *NWSA Journal*, *14*(3), 1–32. https://doi.org/10.1353/nwsa.2003.0005

Garland-Thomson, R. (2005). Feminist disability studies. *Signs: Journal of Women in Culture and Society*, *30*(2), 1557–1587. https://doi.org/10.1086/423352

Goering, S. (2015). Rethinking disability: The social model of disability and chronic disease. *Current Reviews in Musculoskeletal Medicine*, *8*(2), 134–138. https://doi.org/10.1007/s12178-015-9273-z

Goethals, T., Schauwer, E. D., & Hove, G. V. (2015). Weaving intersectionality into disability studies research: Inclusion, reflexivity and anti-essentialism. *Journal of Diversity and Gender Studies*, *2*(1–2), 75–94. https://doi.org/10.11116/jdivegendstud.2.1-2.0075

Goodley, D. (2014). *Dis/ability studies: Theorising disablism and ableism*. Routledge.

Grech, S. (2015). Decolonising Eurocentric disability studies: Why colonialism matters in the disability and Global South debate. *Social Identities*, *21*(1), 6–21. https://doi.org/10.1080/13504630.2014.995347

Hahmann, T., Badets, N., & Hughes, J. (2019). *Indigenous people with disabilities in Canada: First Nations people living off reserve, Métis and Inuit aged 15 years and older.* (Catalogue no. 89-653-X2019005). Statistics Canada. https://www150.statcan.gc.ca/n1/en/pub/89-653-x/89-653-x2019005-eng.pdf?st=kXf-0t3E

Hall, T. E., Meyer, A., & Rose, D. H. (Eds.). (2012). *Universal design for learning in the classroom: Practical applications.* Guilford Press.

Hammarström, A. (1999). Why feminism in public health? *Scandinavian Journal of Public Health, 27*(4), 241–244. https://doi.org/10.1177/14034948990270040601

Hyman, I., Vahabi, M., Bailey, A., Patel, S., Guruge, S., Wilson-Mitchell, K., & Wong, J. P. (2016). Taking action on violence through research, policy, and practice. *Global Health Research and Policy, 1*(1), 6. https://doi.org/10.1186/s41256-016-0006-7

Inegbedion, H., Sunday, E., Asaleye, A., Lawal, A., & Adebanji, A. (2020). Managing diversity for organizational efficiency. *SAGE Open, 10*(1), 215824401990017. https://doi.org/10.1177/2158244019900173

Kattari, S. K., Olzman, M., & Hanna, M. D. (2018). "You look fine!": Ableist experiences by people with invisible disabilities. *Affilia, 33*(4), 477–492. https://doi.org/10.1177/0886109918778073

Kimpson, S. A. (2021). *Basic income, gender & disability.* Women's Legal Education & Action Fund. https://www.leaf.ca/wp-content/uploads/2021/09/Basic-Income-Gender-Disability-Full-Report-Final.pdf

Kumari Campbell, F. A. (2008). Exploring internalized ableism using critical race theory. *Disability & Society, 23*(2), 151–162. https://doi.org/10.1080/09687590701841190

Lett, K., Tamaian, A., & Klest, B. (2020). Impact of ableist microaggressions on university students with self-identified disabilities. *Disability & Society, 35*(9), 1441–1456. https://doi.org/10.1080/09687599.2019.1680344

Lindsay, S., Cagliostro. E., & Carafa, G. (2018). A systematic review of barriers and facilitators of disability disclosure and accommodations for youth in post-secondary education. *International Journal of Disability, Development and Education, 65*(5), 526–556. https://doi.org/10.1080/1034912X.2018.1430352

McSpadden, E. (2022). I'm not crazy or anything: Exploring culture, mental health stigma, and mental health service use among urban community college students. *Community College Journal of Research and Practice, 46*(3), 202–214. https://doi.org/10.1080/10668926.2021.1922321

Meeks, L. M., Case, B., Plegue, M., Moreland, C. J., Jain, S., & Taylor, N. (2020). National prevalence of disability and clinical accommodations in medical education. *Journal of Medical Education and Curricular Development*, *7*, 1–4. https://doi.org/10.1177/2382120520965249

Mickahail, B. A. & Andrews, K. A. (2017). Embracing people with special needs and disabilities. In C. T. E. de Aquino & R. W. Robertson (Eds.), *Diversity and inclusion in the global workplace: Aligning initiatives with strategic business goals* (pp. 139–152). Springer International Publishing.

Moroz, N., Moroz, I., & D'Angelo, M. S. (2020). Mental health services in Canada: Barriers and cost-effective solutions to increase access. *Healthcare Management Forum*, *33*(6), 282–287.

Morris, S., Fawcett, G., Laurent, B., & Hughes, J. (2018). *Canadian Survey on Disability: A demographic, employment and income profile of Canadians with disabilities aged 15 years and over, 2017.* (Catalogue no. 89-654-X2018002). Statistics Canada. https://www150.statcan.gc.ca/n1/en/pub/89-654-x/89-654-x2018002-eng.pdf?st=QisLCefA

Mullins, L., & Preyde, M. (2013). The lived experience of students with an invisible disability at a Canadian university. *Disability & Society*, *28*(2), 147–160.

Mulvany, J. (2000). Disability, impairment or illness? The relevance of the social model of disability to the study of mental disorder. *Sociology of Health & Illness*, *22*(5), 582–601.

Nancekivell, S. E., Shah, P., & Gelman, S. A. (2020). Maybe they're born with it, or maybe it's experience: Toward a deeper understanding of the learning style myth. *Journal of Educational Psychology*, *112*(2), 221–235.

Nario-Redmond, M. R., Kemerling, A. A., & Silverman, A. (2019). Hostile, benevolent, and ambivalent ableism: Contemporary manifestations. *Journal of Social Issues*, *75*(3), 726–756. https://doi.org/10.1111/josi.12337

National Collaborating Centre on Healthy Public Policy. (2015). *Health inequalities and intersectionality*. https://www.ncchpp.ca/docs/2015_Ineg_Ineq_Intersectionnalite_En.pdf

NEADS. (2018). *Landscape of accessibility and accommodation in post-secondary education for students with disabilities.* https://www.neads.ca/en/about/media/AccessibilityandAccommodation%202018-5landscapereport.pdf

Oliver, M. (2013). The social model of disability: Thirty years on. *Disability & Society*, *28*(7), 1024–1026. https://doi.org/10.1080/09687599.2013.818773

Oliver, M., Sapey, B., & Thomas, P. (2006). *Social work with disabled people* (3rd ed.). Palgrave Macmillan.

Ontario Human Rights Commission. (n.d.). *Main barriers to education for students with disabilities.* https://www.ohrc.on.ca/en/main-barriers-education-students-disabilities-fact-sheet

Ontario Universities Accessible Campus (2017). *Educator's accessibility toolkit.* https://accessiblecampus.ca/tools-resources/educators-tool-kit/introduction-accessible-education/

Owens, J. (2015), Exploring the critiques of the social model of disability: The transformative possibility of Arendt's notion of power. *Sociology of Health and Illness*, *37*, 385–403. https://doi.org/10.1111/1467-9566.12199

Pashler, H., McDaniel, M., Rohrer, D., & Bjork, R. (2009). Learning styles: Concepts and evidence. *Psychological Science in the Public Interest*, *9*(3), 105–119. https://doi.org/10.1111/j.1539-6053.2009.01038.x

Peruzzo, F. (2020). I am not disabled: Difference, ethics, critique and refusal of neoliberal academic selves. In N. Brown & J. Leigh (Eds.), *Ableism in academia* (pp. 31–50). UCL Press.

Pickard, B. (2020). *Challenging deficit-based discourse in higher education through a social connection model of responsibility: A critical disability studies perspective* [Doctoral dissertation]. University of South Wales/ Prifysgol De Cymru. https://pure.southwales.ac.uk/ws/portalfiles/portal/5591861/Beth_Pickard_PhD_by_Portfolio_FINAL_Volumes_1_3.pdf

Public Health Agency of Canada (2019). *Social determinants of health and health inequalities.* https://www.canada.ca/en/public-health/services/health-promotion/population-health/what-determines-health.html

Queen's University. (2016). *Policy: Academic accommodations for students with disabilities.* https://www.queensu.ca/secretariat/sites/uslcwww/files/uploaded_files/policies/senateandtrustees/ACADACCOMMPOLICY2016.pdf

Reaume, G. (2014). Understanding critical disability studies. *CMAJ*, *186*(16), 1248–1249. https://doi.org/10.1503/cmaj.141236

Richie, C. S. (2019). Not sick: Liberal, trans, and crip feminist critiques of medicalization. *Journal of Bioethical Inquiry*, *16*(3), 375–387.

Rios, D., Magasi, S., Novak, C., & Harniss, M. (2016). Conducting accessible research: Including people with disabilities in public health, epidemiological, and outcomes studies. *American Journal of Public Health (1971)*, *106*(12), 2137–2144. https://doi.org/10.2105/AJPH.2016.303448

Saddler, N., Adams, S., Robinson, L. A., & Okafor, I. (2021). Taking initiative in addressing diversity in medicine. *Canadian Journal of Science, Mathematics and Technology Education*, *21*(2), 309–320. https://doi.org/10.1007/s42330-021-00154-6

Schalk, S. (2017). Critical disability studies as methodology. *Lateral*, *6*(1). https://csalateral.org/issue/6-1/forum-alt-humanities-critical-disability-studies-methodology-schalk/

Schalk, S., & Kim, J. B. (2020). Integrating race, transforming feminist disability studies. *Signs: Journal of Women in Culture and Society*, *46*(1), 31–55. https://doi.org/10.1086/709213

Shakespeare, T. (2018). *Disability: The basics*. Routledge.

Shakespeare, T., & Watson, N. (2010). Beyond models: Understanding the complexity of disabled people's lives. In G. Scrambler & S. Scrambler (Eds.), *New directions in the sociology of chronic and disabling conditions* (pp. 57–76). Palgrave Macmillan.

Simon Fraser University. (n.d.). *Determining accommodations*. https://www.sfu.ca/students/accessible-learning/establishing-accommodations/accommodation.html

Statistics Canada. (2015). *A profile of persons with disabilities among Canadians aged 15 years or older, 2012*. https://www150.statcan.gc.ca/n1/en/pub/89-654-x/89-654-x2015001-eng.pdf?st=MEVJnTmE

Statistics Canada. (2022). *Measuring disability in Canada* [Infographic] (No. 11-627-M). https://www150.statcan.gc.ca/n1/en/pub/11-627-m/11-627-m2022062-eng.pdf?st=R85d0z6z

United Nations (UN). (2006). *Convention on the rights of persons with disabilities*. https://www.un.org/development/desa/disabilities/convention-on-the-rights-of-persons-with-disabilities.html

United Nations Human Rights (UN Human Rights). (2014). *The convention on the rights of persons with disabilities: Training guide*. Professional training series No. 19. https://www.ohchr.org/sites/default/files/Documents/Publications/CRPD_TrainingGuide_PTS19_EN_Accessible.pdf

United Nations Treaty Collection (UN Treaty Collection). (2011). *Treaty series: Treaties and international agreements registered or filed and recorded with the Secretariat of the United Nations* [Vol. 2515]. https://treaties.un.org/doc/Publication/UNTS/Volume%202515/v2515.pdf

Vancouver Community College. (2022). *Dental hygiene*. https://www.vcc.ca/programs/dental-hygiene/

World Health Organization (WHO). (2022). *Disability*. https://www.who.int/health-topics/disability#tab=tab_1

Wolforth, J. (2016). Students with disabilities. In C. C. Strange & D. H. Cox (Eds.), *Serving diverse students in Canadian higher education* (pp. 128–144). McGill-Queen's University Press.

Wright, E. (2019, September 30). Pretending to be something you are not: Passing, disability, and identity. *Medium*. https://medium.com/@elizabeth_87041/pretending-to-be-something-you-are-not-passing-disability-and-identity-c6b0c766b503

Xiao, H., Carney, D. M., Youn, S. J., Janis, R. A., Castonguay, L. G., Hayes, J. A., & Locke, B. D. (2017). Are we in crisis? National mental health and treatment trends in college counseling centers. *Psychological Services*, *14*(4), 407–415. https://doi.org/10.1037/ser0000130

CHAPTER 7: QUEER AND TRANS PERSPECTIVES ON OBSTETRIC AND GYNECOLOGICAL VIOLENCE: CENTRING THOSE AT THE MARGINS TO CAPTURE THE INTERSECTIONAL EFFECTS OF THE PHENOMENON, BY MYLÈNE SHANKLAND AND IVY LYNN BOURGEAULT

Birth Monopoly. (2022). *Obstetric violence*. https://birthmonopoly.com/obstetric-violence/

Bohren, M. A., Vogel, J. P., Hunter, E. C., Lutsiv, O., Makh, S. K., Souza, J. P., Aguiar, C., Coneglian, F. S., Diniz, A. L. A., Tunçalp, Ö., Javadi, D., Oladapo, O. T., Khosla, R., Hindin, M. J., & Gülmezoglu, A. M. (2015). The mistreatment of women during childbirth in health facilities globally: A mixed-methods systematic review. *PLoS Medicine*, *12*(6), e1001847. https://doi.org/10.1371/journal.pmed.1001847

Bowser, D., & Hill, K. (2010). *Exploring evidence for disrespect and abuse in facility-based childbirth: Report of a landscape analysis*. Traction Project. http://www.tractionproject.org/sites/default/files/Respectful_Care_at_Birth_9-20-101_Final.pdf

Briceño Morales, X., Enciso Chaves, L. V., & Yepes Delgado, C. E. (2018). Neither medicine nor health care staff members are violent by nature: Obstetric violence from an interactionist perspective. *Qualitative Health Research*, *28*(8), 1308–1319. https://doi.org/10.1177/1049732318763351

Burrow, S., Goldberg, L., Searle, J., & Aston, M. (2018). Vulnerability, harm, and compromised ethics revealed by the experiences of queer birthing women in rural healthcare. *Journal of Bioethical Inquiry*, *15*(4), 511–524. https://doi.org/10.1007/s11673-018-9882-5

Chadwick, R. (2020). Practices of silencing. Birth, marginality and epistemic violence. In C. Pickles & J. Herring (Eds.), *Childbirth, vulnerability and law. Exploring issues of violence and control* (pp. 30–48). Routledge.

Colen, S. (1986). "With respect and feelings": Voices of West Indian child care and domestic workers in New York City. In J. Cole (Ed.), *All American women: Ties that bind* (pp. 46–70). The Free Press.

Colen, S. (1995) "Like a mother to them": Stratified reproduction and West Indian childcare workers and employers in New York. In F. D. Ginsburg and R. Rapp (Eds.), *Conceiving the new world order: The global politics of reproduction* (pp. 78–102). University of California Press.

Dean, M. A., Victor, E., & Guidry Grimes, L. (2016). Inhospitable healthcare space: Why diversity training on LGBTQIA issues is not enough. *Bioethical Inquiry*, *13*, 557–570. https://doi.org/10.1007/s11673-016-9738-9

Dutton, L., Koenig, K., & Kristopher, F. (2008). Gynecologic care of the female-to-male transgender man. *Journal of Midwifery & Women's Health*, *53*(4), 331–337. https://doi.org/10.1016/j.jmwh.2008.02.003

Garcia, L. M. (2020). A concept analysis of obstetric violence in the United States of America. *Nursing Forum*, *55*(4), 654–663. https://doi.org/10.1111/nuf.12482

Greenfield, M., & Darwin, Z. (2021). Trans and non-binary pregnancy, traumatic birth, and perinatal mental health: A scoping review. *International Journal of Transgender Health*, *22*(1–2), 203–216. https://doi.org/10.1080/26895269.2020.1841057

Hill, N. (2019). Understanding obstetric violence as violence against mothers through the lens of matricentric feminism. *Journal of the Motherhood Initiative*, *10*(1–2), 233–243. https://jarm.journals.yorku.ca/index.php/jarm/article/view/40566

Hodnett, E. D. (2002). Pain and women's satisfaction with the experience of childbirth: A systematic review. *American Journal of Obstetrics and Gynaecology*, *186*, 160–172. https://doi.org/10.1067/mob.2002.121141

Hoffkling, A., Obedin-Maliver, J., & Sevelius, J. (2017). From erasure to opportunity: A qualitative study of the experiences of transgender men around pregnancy and recommendations for providers. *BMC Pregnancy and Childbirth*, *17*, 8–20. https://doi.org/10.1186/s12884-017-1491-5

Jardim, D. M. B., & Modena, C. M. (2018). Obstetric violence in the daily routine of care and its characteristics. *Revista Latino-Americana De Enfermagem*, *26*, e3069. https://doi.org/10.1590/1518-8345.2450.3069

Katz, L., Amorim, M. M., Giordano, J. C., Bastos, M. H., & Brilhante, A. V. M. (2020). Who is afraid of obstetric violence? *Brazilian Journal of Mother and Child Health, 20*(2), 623–626.

Lévesque, S., & Ferron-Parayre, A. (2021). To use or not to use the term "obstetric violence": Commentary on the article by Swartz and Lappeman. *Violence Against Women, 27*(8), 1009–1018. https://doi.org/10.1177/107780122199645

Light, A. D., Zimbrunes, S. E., & Gomez-Lobo, V. (2017). Reproductive and obstetrical care for transgender patients. *Current Obstetrics and Gynecology Reports, 6*(2), 149–155.

Love, H. (2014). Queer. *Transgender Studies Quarterly, 1*(1–2), 172–176.

MacDonald, T. K., Walks, M., Biener, M., & Kibbe, A. (2021). Disrupting the norms: Reproduction, gender identity, gender dysphoria, and intersectionality. *International Journal of Transgender Health,* 22(1–2), 18–29. https://doi.org/10.1080/26895269.2020.1848692

Michel, C., & Squires, C. (2018). Entre vécu de l'accouchement et réalité médiale: Les violences obstétricales. *Carnet PSY,* 22–33.

Moseson, H., Zazanis, N., Goldberg, E., Fix, L., Durden, M., Stoeffler, A., Hastings, J., Cudlitz, L., Lesser-Lee, B., Letcher, L., Reyes, A., & Obedin-Maliver, J. (2020). The imperative for transgender and gender nonbinary inclusion: Beyond women's health. *Obstetrics & Gynecology, 135*(5), 1059–1068. https://doi.org/10.1097/AOG.0000000000003816

Olde, E., van der Hart, O., Kleber, R., & van Son, M. (2006). Posttraumatic stress following childbirth: A review. *Clinical Psychology Review, 26,* 1–16. https://doi.org/10.1016/j.cpr.2005.07.002

Pérez D'Gregorio, R. (2010). Obstetric violence: A new legal term introduced in Venezuela. *International Journal of Gynecology & Obstetrics, 111*(3), 201–202. https://doi.org/10.1016/j.ijgo.2010.09.002

Puar, J. K. (2007). *Terrorist assemblages: Homonationalism in queer times.* Duke University Press.

Pyne, J. (2012). *Transforming family: Trans parents and their struggles strategies, and strengths.* LGBTQ Parenting Network, Sherbourne Health Centre.

Quattrocchi, P. (2019). Obstetric violence observatory: Contributions of Argentina to the international debate. *Medical Anthropology, 38*(8), 762–776. https://doi.org/10.1080/01459740.2019.1609471

Regroupement Naissance-Renaissance. (2019). *Avis sur les mauvais traitements et les violences envers les femmes dans les services de soins de santé reproductive avec attention particulière sur l'accouchement.* https://www.ohchr.org/Documents/Issues/Women/SR/ReproductiveHealthCare/Regroupement%20Naissance-Renaissance%20Canada.pdf

Rice, J. G., Bjargardóttir, H. B., & Sigurjónsdóttir, H. B. (2020). Child protection, disability and obstetric violence: Three case studies from Iceland. *International Journal of Environmental Research and Public Health*, *18*(1). https://doi.org/10.3390/ijerph18010158

Richardson, B., Price, S., & Campbell-Yeo, M. (2018). Redefining perinatal experience: A philosophical exploration of a hypothetical case of gender diversity in labour and birth. *Journal of Clinical Nursing*, *28*(3–4), 703–710. https://doi.org/10.1111/jocn.14521

Riggs, D. W., & Bartholomaeus, C. (2020). Toward trans reproductive justice: A qualitative analysis of views on fertility preservation for Australian transgender and non-binary people. *Journal of Social Issues*, *76*(2), 314–337. https://doi.org/10.1111/josi.12364

Rodríguez-Almagro, J., Hernández-Martínez, A., Rodríguez-Almagro, D., Quirós-García, J. M., Martínez-Galiano, J. M., & Gómez-Salgado, J. (2019). Women's perceptions of living a traumatic childbirth experience and factors related to a birth experience. *International Journal of Environmental Research and Public Health*, *16*(9), 1654. https://doi.org/10.3390/ijerph16091654

Sadler, M., Santos, M. J., Ruiz-Berdún, D., Rojas, G. L., Skoko, E., Gillen, P., & Clausen, J. A. (2016). Moving beyond disrespect and abuse: Addressing the structural dimensions of obstetric violence. *Reproductive Health Matters*, *24*(47), 47–55. https://doi.org/10.1016/j.rhm.2016.04.002

Savage, V., & Castro, A. (2017). Measuring mistreatment of women during childbirth: A review of terminology and methodological approaches. *Reproductive Health*, *14*(138). https://doi.org/10.1186/s12978-017-0403-5

Schroll, A.-M., Kjaergaard, H., & Migtgaard, J. (2013). Encountering abuse in health care: Lifetime experiences in postnatal women—A qualitative study. *BMC Pregnancy and Childbirth*, *13*(74), 1–11. http://www.biomedcentral.com/1471-2393/13/74

Shabot, S. C. (2016). Making loud bodies "feminine": A feminist-phenomenological analysis of obstetric violence. *Human Studies*, *39*(2), 231–247. https://doi.org/10.1007/s10746-015-9369-x

Shabot, S. C. (2021). We birth with others: Towards a Beauvoirian understanding of obstetric violence. *European Journal of Women's Studies*, *28*(2), 1–16. https://doi-org/10.1177/1350506820919474

Shabot, S. C., & Korem, K. (2018). Domesticating bodies: The role of shame in obstetric violence. *Hypatia*, *33*(3), 384–401. https://doi.org/10.1111/hypa.12428

Shankland, M., & Abergel, É. (2022). La reconnaissance sociale intersubjective de l'expérience de la grossesse chez les hommes trans: Étude de cas multiples. *Recherches féministes, 34*(1), 181–200. https://doi.org./10.7202/1085248ar

Swartz, L., & Lappeman, M. (2021). Making care better in the context of violence: The limits of blame. *Violence Against Women, 27*(8), 1028–1034. https://doi.org/10.1177/1077801221996468

Vedam, S., Stoll, K., Taiwo, T. K., Rubashkin, N., Cheyney, M., Strauss, N., McLemore, M., Cadena, M., Nethery, E., Rushton, E., Schummers, L., Declercq, E., & the GVtM-US Steering Council. (2019). The Giving Voice to Mothers study: Inequity and mistreatment during pregnancy and childbirth in the United States. *Reproductive Health, 16*(77), 1–18. https://doi.org/10.1186/s12978-019-0729-2

Walks, M. (2005). Womb is womb, but is birth birth? A look at the queer interaction of medical services, social context and identity understandings in Canadian birthing experiences. *Canadian Woman Studies/Les Cahiers de la femme*, 24(1), 68–73.

Walks, M. (2014). Stratified reproduction: Making the case for butch lesbian's, transmen's and genderqueer individual's experiences in British Columbia. In S. Paterson, F. Scale, & M. K. Sokolon (Eds.), *Fertile Ground. Exploring Reproduction in Canada* (pp. 74–93). McGill-Queen's University Press.

Walks, M. (2017). The gender of pregnancy. In G. T. Bonifacio (Ed.), *Global Currents in Gender and Feminisms* (pp. 181–194). Emerald Publishing Limited. https://doi.org/10.1108/978-1-78714-483-520171017

Warner, L., Kurtiş, T., & Adya, A. (2020). Navigating criticism of intersectional approaches: Reclaiming intersectionality for global social justice and well-being. *Women & Therapy, 43*(3–4), 262–277. https://doi.org./10.1080/02703149.2020.1729477

Wingo, E., Ingraham, N., & Roberts, S. C. M. (2018). Reproductive health care priorities and barriers to effective care for LGBTQ people assigned female at birth: A qualitative study. *Women's Health Issues, 28*(4), 350–357. https://doi.org/10.1016/j.whi.2018.03.002

World Health Organization (WHO). (2015). *The prevention and elimination of disrespect and abuse during facility-based childbirth: WHO statement.* https://apps.who.int/iris/bitstream/handle/10665/134588/WHO_RHR_14.23_eng.pdf

CHAPTER 8: BLACK FEMINISM IN CRITICAL PUBLIC HEALTH RESEARCH, POLICY, AND PROGRAMMING: THEORY AND PRACTICE FOR PROMOTING THE HEALTH AND WELL-BEING OF BLACK WOMEN, BY TOLA MBULAHENI, FIQIR WORKU, FALAN BENNETT, NAKIA LEE-FOON, AND KIMBERLY ROBINSON

Ahmed, R., Jamal, O., Ishak, W., Nabi, K., & Mustafa, N. (2021). Racial equity in the fight against COVID-19: A qualitative study examining the importance of collecting race-based data in the Canadian context. *Tropical Diseases, Travel Medicine and Vaccines*, 7(1), 1–6.

Baeten, J. M., Donnell, D., Ndase, P., Mugo, N. R., Campbell, J. D., Wangisi, J., Tappero, J. W., Bukusi, E. A., Cohen, C. R., Katabira, E., Ronald, A., Tumwesigye, E., Were, E., Fife, K. H., Kiarie, J., Farquhar, C., John-Stewart, G., Kakia, A., Odoyo, J., ... & Celum, C. (2012). Antiretroviral prophylaxis for HIV prevention in heterosexual men and women. *New England Journal of Medicine*, *367*(5), 399–410.

Block, S., Galabuzi-Grace, E., & Tranjan, R. (2019). *Canada's colour coded income inequality*. Canadian Centre for Policy Alternatives.

Canadian Women's Foundation, Canadian Centre for Policy Alternatives, Ontario Nonprofit Network, & Faraday, F. (2020). *Resetting normal: Women, decent work and Canada's fractured care economy*.

CATIE. (2016). Pre-exposure prophylaxis (PrEP): Fact sheet. https://www.catie.ca/sites/default/files/PrEP%20EN%202019%2012%2016.pdf

Cénat, J. M., McIntee, S.-E., Mukunzi, J. N., & Noorishad, P.-G. (2021). Overrepresentation of Black children in the child welfare system: A systematic review to understand and better act. *Children and Youth Services Review*, *120*, 105714.

Chiu, M., Maclagan, L. C., Tu, J. V., & Shah, B. R. (2015). Temporal trends in cardiovascular disease risk factors among white, South Asian, Chinese and Black groups in Ontario, Canada, 2001 to 2012: A population-based study. *BMJ Open*, *5*(8), e007232.

Collins, P. H. (2002). *Black feminist thought: Knowledge, consciousness, and the politics of empowerment*. Routledge.

Combahee River Collective. (1983). The Combahee River Collective statement. *Home Girls: A Black Feminist Anthology*, *1*, 264–274.

Cooper, A. (2007). Acts of resistance: Black men and women engage slavery in Upper Canada, 1793–1803. *Ontario History, 99*(1), 5.

Creese, G., & Wiebe, B. (2012). "Survival employment": Gender and deskilling among African immigrants in Canada. *International Migration, 50*(5), 56–76.

Crenshaw, K. (1989). Demarginalizing the intersection of race and sex: A Black feminist critique of antidiscrimination doctrine, feminist theory and antiracist politics. *University of Chicago Legal Forum, 1989*(1), 139–167.

Dudley, Rachel. (2016). *Haunted hospital: J. Marion Sims and the legacies of enslaved women* [Doctoral dissertation]. Emory University. https://etd.library.emory.edu/concern/etds/qj72p792f?locale=en

Elgersman Lee, M. (2013). *Unyielding spirits: Black women and slavery in early Canada and Jamaica*. Routledge.

Foster, J. (2021). Tracking precarity: Employment pathways of precarious status migrant workers in Canada. *Canadian Journal of Sociology, 46*(3), 257–278.

Gilman, S. L. (1985). Black bodies, white bodies: Toward an iconography of female sexuality in late nineteenth-century art, medicine, and literature. *Critical Inquiry, 12*(1), 204–242.

Guttmann A., Gandhi, S., Wanigaratne S., Lu, H., Ferreira-Legere, L. E., Paul, J., Gozdyra, P., Campbell, T., Chung, H., Fung, K., Chen, B., Kwong, J. C., Rosella, L., Shah, B. R., Saunders, N., Paterson, J. M., Bronskill, S. E., Azimaee, M., Vermeulen, M. J., & Schull, M. J. (2020). *COVID-19 in immigrants, refugees and other newcomers in Ontario: Characteristics of those tested and those confirmed positive, as of June 13, 2020*. IC/ES. https://www.ices.on.ca/Publications/Atlases-and-Reports/2020/COVID-19-in-Immigrants-Refugees-and-Other-Newcomers-in-Ontario

Haddad, A. C., Weeks, A., Robert, A., & Totten, S. (2021). HIV in Canada—surveillance report, 2019. *Canada Communicable Disease Report, 47*(1), 77–86.

Hapsari, A. P., Ho, J. W., Meaney, C., Avery, L., Hassen, N., Jetha, A., Lay, A. M., Rotondi, M., Zuberi, Z., & Pinto, A. (2022). The working conditions for personal support workers in the Greater Toronto Area during the COVID-19 pandemic: A mixed-methods study. *Canadian Journal of Public Health, 113*(6), 817–833.

Henry, F. (1968). The West Indian Domestic Scheme in Canada. *Social and Economic Studies, 17*(1), 83–91.

Hill, D. G. (1992). *The freedom-seekers: Blacks in early Canada*. Stoddart.

Hogarth, R. A. (2017). *Medicalizing Blackness: Making racial difference in the Atlantic world, 1780–1840*. UNC Press Books.

Human Rights Council. (2017). *Report of the Working Group of Experts on People of African Descent on its mission to Canada*.

International Labour Organization. (2022, February 9). *Decent work indicators.* https://www.ilo.org/integration/themes/mdw/WCMS_189392/lang--en/index.htm

Katshunga, J., & Massaquoi, N. (2019). *Black women and girls.* Canadian Centre for Policy Alternatives.

Kelley, N., & Trebilcock, M. J. (2000). *The making of the mosaic: A history of Canadian immigration policy.* University of Toronto Press.

King, B., Fallon, B., Boyd, R., Black, T., Antwi-Boasiako, K., & O'Connor, C. (2017). Factors associated with racial differences in child welfare investigative decision-making in Ontario, Canada. *Child Abuse & Neglect, 73,* 89–105.

Lawson, E. (2013). The gendered working lives of seven Jamaican women in Canada: A story about "here" and "there" in a transnational economy. *Feminist Formations, 25*(1), 138–156.

Leah, R., & Morgan, G. (1979). Immigrant women fight back: The case of the seven Jamaican women. *Resources for Feminist Research, 7*(3), 23–24.

Logie, C. H. (2015). (Where) do queer women belong? Theorizing intersectional and compulsory heterosexism in HIV research. *Critical Public Health, 25*(5), 527–538.

Logie, C. H., & Gibson, M. F. (2013). A mark that is no mark? Queer women and violence in HIV discourse. *Culture, Health & Sexuality, 15*(1), 29–43.

Logie, C. H., James, L., Tharao, W., & Loutfy, M. R. (2011). HIV, gender, race, sexual orientation, and sex work: A qualitative study of intersectional stigma experienced by HIV-positive women in Ontario, Canada. *PLoS medicine, 8*(11), e1001124.

Logie, C. H., Okumu, M., Ryan, S., Yehdego, D. M., & Lee-Foon, N. (2018). Adapting and pilot testing the Healthy Love HIV and sexually transmitted infection prevention intervention with African, Caribbean and Black women in community-based settings in Toronto, Canada. *International Journal of STD & AIDS, 29*(8), 751–759.

Lum, J. M., Ying, A., & Sladek, J. (2015). *Ontario personal support workers in home and community care: CRNCC/PSNO survey results.* Canadian Research Network for Care in the Community.

Massaquoi, N., Mbulaheni, T., & Habanyama, M. (2021, March 24). Opinion: Black women face three pandemics. *Healthing.* https://www.healthing.ca/opinion/opinion-black-women-face-three-pandemics.

Massaquoi, N., & Wane, N. N. (Eds.). (2007). *Theorizing empowerment: Canadian perspectives on Black feminist thought.* Inanna Publications & Education Incorporated.

Maynard, R. (2017). *Policing Black lives: State violence in Canada from slavery to the present*. Fernwood Publishing.

McKinnon, B., Yang, S., Kramer, M. S., Bushnik, T., Sheppard, A. J., & Kaufman, J. S. (2016). Comparison of Black–white disparities in preterm birth between Canada and the United States. *CMAJ*, *188*(1), E19–E26.

Mianda, G. (2020, December 4). Black humanity: Bearing witness to COVID-19 [The original sin of anti-Black racism]. APA 2019 Antipode intervention symposium, Toronto, ON. https://antipodeonline.org/wp-content/uploads/2020/12/2.-Mianda.pdf

Mooten, N. (2021). *Racism, discrimination and migrant workers in Canada: Evidence from the literature*. Government of Canada. https://www.canada.ca/en/immigration-refugees-citizenship/corporate/reports-statistics/research/racism-discrimination-migrant-workers-canada-evidence-literature.html

Neeganagwedgin, E. (2013). Narratives from within: Black women and schooling in the Canadian context. *Alberta Journal of Educational Research*, *59*(2), 226–246.

Nelson, L. E., James, L., Coleman, T., Etowa, J., Husbands, W., Lofters, A., Mitchell, M. O., Nguemo, J. D., Nnorom, O., Oraka, C., Rana, J., Siddiqi, A., & Wilson, C. L. (2019). A recipe for increasing racial and gender disparities in HIV infection: A critical analysis of the Canadian guideline on pre-exposure prophylaxis and non-occupational post-exposure prophylaxis' responsiveness to the HIV epidemics among women and Black communities. *Canadian Journal of Human Sexuality*, *28*(1), 1–4.

Ontario Human Rights Commission. (2018). *Interrupted childhoods: Over-representation of Indigenous and Black children in Ontario welfare system*. https://cwrp.ca/sites/default/files/publications/en/interrupted_childhoods_over-representation_of_indigenous_and_black_children_in_ontario_child_welfare_accessible.pdf

Owens, D. C., & Fett, S. M. (2019). Black maternal and infant health: Historical legacies of slavery. *American Journal of Public Health*, *109*(10), 1342–1345.

Parks Canada. (2022). *West Indian Domestic Scheme (1955–1967) national historic event*. https://parks.canada.ca/culture/designation/evenement-event/domestiques-domestic

Perritt, J. (2020). #WhiteCoatsForBlackLives—addressing physicians' complicity in criminalizing communities. *New England Journal of Medicine*, *383*(19), 1804–1806.

Pinto, A. D., Hapsari, A. P., Ho, J., Meaney, C., Avery, L., Hassen, N., Jetha, A., Lay, A. M., Rotondi, M., & Zuberi, D. (2022). Precarious work among personal support workers in the Greater Toronto Area: A respondent-driven sampling study. *CMAJ*, *10*(2), E527–E538.

Public Safety Canada Portfolio Corrections Statistics Committee (2022). *2020 corrections and conditional release statistical overview*. https://www.publicsafety.gc.ca/cnt/rsrcs/pblctns/ccrso-2020/ccrso-2020-en.pdf

Richie, B. E. (2012). *Arrested justice: Black women, violence, and America's prison nation*. New York University Press.

Ross, L., & Solinger, R. (2017). *Reproductive justice: An introduction*. University of California Press.

Sathiyamoorthy, T. (2020, May 7). *Supporting support workers: PSWs need increased protections during COVID-19*. Wellesley Institute. https://www.wellesleyinstitute.com/work-health/supporting-support-workers-psws-need-increased-protections-during-covid-19/

Siddiqi, A., Shahidi, F. V., Ramraj, C., & Williams, D. R. (2017). Associations between race, discrimination and risk for chronic disease in a population-based sample from Canada. *Social Science & Medicine*, *194*, 135–141.

Stapleton, J. (2019). *The working poor in the Toronto region: A closer look at the increasing numbers*. Metcalf Foundation.

Statistics Canada. (2017). *Immigration and ethnocultural diversity: Key results from the 2016 census* (No. 89-657-X). https://www150.statcan.gc.ca/n1/daily-quotidien/171025/dq171025b-eng.htm

Statistics Canada. (2019). *Diversity of the Black population in Canada: An overview* (No. 89-657-X) https://www150.statcan.gc.ca/n1/pub/89-657-x/89-657-x2019002-eng.htm

Statistics Canada. (2020a). *Diversity of the Black population in Canada: An overview* (No. 89-657-X). https://www150.statcan.gc.ca/n1/pub/89-657-x/89-657-x2020001-eng.htm

Statistics Canada. (2020b). *Changes in the socioeconomic situation of Canada's Black population, 2001–2016* (No. 89-657-X). https://www150.statcan.gc.ca/n1/pub/89-657-x/89-657-x2020001-eng.htm

Statistics Canada. (2022). *The Canadian census: A rich portrait of the country's religious and ethnocultural diversity* (No. 98-316-X2016001). https://www150.statcan.gc.ca/n1/daily-quotidien/221026/dq221026b-eng.htm

Stettner, S., Burnett, K., & Hay, T. (Eds.). (2017). *Abortion: History, politics, and reproductive justice after Morgentaler*. UBC Press.

Tan, D. H., Hull, M. W., Yoong, D., Tremblay, C., O'Byrne, P., Thomas, R., Kille, J., Baril, J.-G., Cox, J., Giguere, P., Harris, M., Hughes, C., MacPherson, P., O'Donnell, S., Reimer, J., Singh, A., Barrett, L., Bogoch, I., Jollimore, J., & Shafran, S. (2017). Canadian guideline on HIV pre-exposure prophylaxis and nonoccupational postexposure prophylaxis. *CMAJ*, *189*(47), E1448–E1458.

Tharao, E., & Massaquoi, N. (2001). Black women and HIV/AIDS: Contextualizing their realities, their silence, and proposed solutions. *Canadian Woman Studies*, *21*(2), 72–80.

Tharao, W. E., Calzavara, L., Bullock, S., Daftary, A., Ryan, S., Kaul, R., Loutfy, M., Luyombya, H., Arnold, K., Godoy, S., Burchell, A., Yehdego, M., & Leonard, L. (2018, April 26–29). Factors influencing HIV acquisition among African, Caribbean and Black women infected with HIV post-migration [Conference presentation]. CAHR Conference, Vancouver, BC.

Turner, T. (2016). *One voice, one vision: Changing the Ontario child welfare system to better serve African Canadians—Practice framework Part 1: Research report.* Ontario Association of Children's Aid Societies. http://www.oacas.org/wp-content/uploads/2016/09/One-Vision-One-Voice-Part-1_digital_english-May-2019.pdf

United Nations Committee on the Rights of the Child (2022). *Concluding observations on the combined fifth and sixth reports of Canada.* https://tbinternet.ohchr.org/Treaties/CRC/Shared%20Documents/CAN/CRC_C_CAN_CO_5-6_48911_E.pdf

Veenstra, G., & Patterson, A. C. (2016). Black-white health inequalities in Canada. *Journal of Immigrant and Minority Health*, *18*(1), 51–57.

Vernon, K. (Ed.). (2020). *The Black prairie archives: An anthology*. Wilfrid Laurier University Press.

Walker, J. W. S. G. (1992). *The Black Loyalists: The search for a promised land in Nova Scotia and Sierra Leone, 1783–1870*. University of Toronto Press.

Williams, C. C., Newman, P. A., Sakamoto, I., & Massaquoi, N. A. (2009). HIV prevention risks for Black women in Canada. *Social Science & Medicine*, *68*(1), 12–20.

Winks, R. W. (1997). *The Blacks in Canada: A history* (2nd ed.). McGill-Queen's University Press.

Workers Action Center (2020). *Implementing 10 days of paid sick leave: What workers need.* https://workersactioncentre.org/wp-content/uploads/2020/05/Implementing-10-days-of-paid-sick-leave-May-2020.pdf

CHAPTER 9: TAKING A REPRODUCTIVE JUSTICE LENS IN PUBLIC HEALTH POLICY: A CASE STUDY ON FAMILY LAW FOR 2SLGBTQIA+ PARENTS AND FAMILIES, BY MICHELLE W. Y. TAM AND LORI E. ROSS

Acevedo-Garcia, D., Rosenfeld, L. E., Hardy, E., McArdle, N., & Osypuk, T. L. (2013). Future directions in research on institutional and interpersonal discrimination and children's health. *American Journal of Public Health*, *103*(10), 1754–1763.

Action Canada. (2021, April 20). *Canada's 2021 federal budget: Analysis.* https://www.actioncanadashr.org/news/2021-04-20-canadas-2021-federal-budget-analysis

Alaazi, D. A., Ahola, A. N., Okeke-Ihejirika, P., Yohani, S., Vallianatos, H., & Salami, B. (2021). Immigrants and the Western media: A critical discourse analysis of newspaper framings of African immigrant parenting in Canada. *Journal of Ethnic and Migration Studies*, *47*(19), 4478–4496.

Asian Communities for Reproductive Justice. (2005). *A new vision for advancing our movement for reproductive health, reproductive rights and reproductive justice.*

Berkowitz, D. (2020). Gay men and surrogacy. In A. E. Goldberg & K. R. Allen (Eds.), *LGBTQ-parent families* (pp. 143–160). Springer.

Bjork-James, S. (2020). White sexual politics: The patriarchal family in white nationalism and the religious right. *Transforming Anthropology*, 28(1), 58–73.

Chiweshe, M., Mavuso, J., & Macleod, C. (2017). Reproductive justice in context: South African and Zimbabwean women's narratives of their abortion decision. *Feminism & Psychology*, 27(2), 203–224.

Cohen, C. (1997). Punks, bulldaggers, and welfare queens: The radical potential of queer politics? *GLQ: A Journal of Lesbian and Gay Studies*, *3*(4), 437–465.

Cohen, C. (2019). The radical potential of queer? Twenty years later. *GLQ: A Journal of Lesbian and Gay Studies*, 25(1), 140–144.

Combahee River Collective. (1977). *A Black feminist statement.* Kitchen Table, Women of Colour Press.

Crenshaw, K. (1989). Mapping the margins: Intersectionality, identity politics, and violence against women of color. *Stanford Law Review*, *43*(6), 1241–1299.

Davis, A. (1982). Racism, birth control and reproductive rights. In A. Davis (Ed.), *Women, race and class* (202–271). Women's Press.

Dixon, M., Librach, C., & Gandhi, S. (2019, April). Cultural sensitivities in third party assisted reproduction [Webinar].

Fantus, S., & Newman, P. A. (2019). Motivations to pursue surrogacy for gay fathers in Canada: A qualitative investigation. *Journal of GLBT Family Studies*, *15*(4), 342–356.

Global Affairs Canada. (2017, March 8). *Canada announces support for sexual and reproductive health and rights* [Press release]. https://www.canada.ca/en/global-affairs/news/2017/03/canada_announcessupportforsexualandreproductivehealthandrights.html

Goldberg, A. E., & Smith, J. Z. (2011). Stigma, social context, and mental health: Lesbian and gay couples across the transition to adoptive parenthood. *Journal of Counseling Psychology*, *58*, 139–150.

Green, D., Tarasoff, L. A., & Epstein, R. (2012). *Meeting the assisted human reproduction (AHR) needs of lesbian, gay, bisexual, trans and queer (LGBTQ) people in Canada: A fact sheet for AHR service providers.* LGBTQ Parenting Network.

Hunter, A. (2015). Lesbian mommy blogging in Canada: Documenting subtle homophobia in Canadian society and building community online. *Journal of Lesbian Studies, 19*(2), 212–229.

Kirby, J. (2017, December 22). *A broad vision for reproductive justice.* Action Canada for Sexual Health and Rights. https://www.actioncanadashr.org/news/2017-12-22-broad-vision-reproductive-justice

Kite, M. E., & Bryant-Lees, K. B. (2016). Historical and contemporary attitudes toward homosexuality. *Teaching of Psychology, 43*(2), 164–170.

Lick, D. J., Tornello, S. L., Riskind, R. G., Schmidt, K. M., & Patterson, C. J. (2012). Social climate for sexual minorities predicts well-being among heterosexual offspring of lesbian and gay parents. *Sexuality Research and Social Policy, 9*, 99–112.

Macleod, C. I., Beynon-Jones, S., & Toerien, M. (2017). Articulating reproductive justice through reparative justice: Case studies of abortion in Great Britain and South Africa. *Culture, Health & Sexuality, 19*(5), 601–615.

Morrison, M. A., Morrison, T. G., Harriman, R. L., & Jewell, L. M. (2008). Old-fashioned and modern prejudice toward Aboriginals in Canada. In M. A. Morrison & T. G. Morrison (Eds.), *The psychology of modern prejudice* (pp. 277–305). Nova Science Publishers.

M.R.L.P. and S.A.T. v. The Attorney General of Canada, the Government of Saskatchewan, Saskatchewan Health Authority, Dr. Kristine Mytopher, Dr. Ahmed Ezzat, Dr. Ian Lund, John Doe and Jane Doe, 2017 Sask QB 1485.

Murphy, M. (2012). *Seizing the means of reproduction.* Duke University Press.

Norton, A. T., & Herek, G. M. (2013). Heterosexuals' attitudes toward transgender people: Findings from a national probability sample of US adults. *Sex Roles, 68*(11), 738–753.

Patterson, C. J. (2013). Sexual orientation and family lives. In C. J. Patterson & A. R. D'Augelli (Eds.), *Handbook of psychology and sexual orientation* (pp. 223–236). Oxford University Press.

Pfeffer, C. A., & Jones, K. B. (2020). Transgender-parent families. In A. E. Goldberg & K. R. Allen (Eds.), *LGBTQ-parent families* (pp. 199–214). Springer.

Pollitt, A. M., Reczek, C., & Umberson, D. (2020). LGBTQ-parent families and health. In A. E. Goldberg & K. R. Allen (Eds.), *LGBTQ-parent families* (pp. 125–140). Springer.

Ross, L. (2006). Understanding reproductive justice: Transforming the pro-choice movement. *Off Our Backs, 36*(4), 14–19.

Ross, L., & Solinger, R. (2017). *Reproductive justice: An introduction* (Vol. 1). University of California Press.

Ross, L. E., Epstein, R., Anderson, S., & Eady, A. (2009). Policy, practice, and personal narratives: Experiences of LGBTQ people with adoption in Ontario, Canada. *Adoption Quarterly, 12*(3–4), 272–293.

Ross, L. E., Steele, L., & Sapiro, B. (2005). Perceptions of predisposing and protective factors for perinatal depression in same-sex parents. *Journal of Midwifery & Women's Health, 50*(6), e65–70.

Ross, L. J. (2017). Reproductive justice as intersectional feminist activism. *Souls, 19*(3), 286–314.

Senate of Canada. (2019, May 15). Parliament. House of Commons. Standing Committee on Human Rights. Evidence of Proceedings. Meeting No. 42, 42nd Parl., 1st Session (Online). https://sencanada.ca/en/Content/SEN/Committee/421/ridr/42cv-e

Shapiro, J. (2020). The law governing LGBTQ-parent families in the United States. In A. E. Goldberg & K. R. Allen (Eds.), *LGBTQ-parent families* (pp. 365–382). Springer.

SisterSong Women of Color Reproductive Justice Collective. (n.d.). *Reproductive justice.* https://www.sistersong.net/reproductive-justice/

Snow, D. (2016). Measuring parentage policy in the Canadian provinces: A comparative framework. *Canadian Public Administration, 59*(1), 5–25.

Women's Earth Alliance & Native Youth Sexual Health Network. (2016). *Violence on the land, violence on our bodies: Building an Indigenous response to environmental violence.*

CHAPTER 10: STRANGERS IN OUR HOMELAND: THE IMPACT OF RACISM ACROSS HEALTHCARE POLICY AND DELIVERY FOR INDIGENOUS PEOPLES IN CANADA, BY MIKAELA D. GABRIEL

Absolon, K. (2010). Indigenous wholistic theory: A knowledge set for practice. *First Peoples Child & Family Review, 5*(2), 74–87.

Absolon, K. E. (2016). Wholistic and ethical: Social inclusion with Indigenous Peoples. *Social Inclusion, 4*(1), 44–56.

Akena, F. A. (2012). Critical analysis of the production of Western knowledge and its implications for Indigenous knowledge and decolonization. *Journal of Black Studies, 43*(6), 599–619.

Allan, B., & Smylie, J. (2015). *First Peoples, second class treatment: The role of racism in the health and well-being of Indigenous Peoples in Canada*. Wellesley Institute.

Anderson, I., Baum, F., & Bentley, M. (Eds.). (2007). *Beyond bandaids: Exploring the underlying social determinants of Aboriginal health*. CRC for Aboriginal Health.

Barnett, L., & Kendall, E. (2011). Culturally appropriate methods for enhancing the participation of Aboriginal Australians in health-promoting programs. *Health Promotion Journal of Australia, 22*(1), 27–32.

Barwin, L. (2012). *Places of tradition, places of research: The evaluation of traditional medicine workshops using culturally and locally relevant methods* [Dissertation]. University of Ottawa.

Black, K., & McBean, E. (2016). Increased Indigenous participation in environmental decision-making: A policy analysis for the improvement of Indigenous health. *International Indigenous Policy Journal*, *7*(4), 5.

Boot, G. R., & Lowell, A. (2019). Acknowledging and promoting Indigenous knowledges, paradigms, and practices within health-literacy related policy and practice documents across Australia, Canada, and New Zealand. *International Indigenous Policy Journal*, *10*(3).

Brady, M. (1995). Culture in treatment, culture as treatment. A critical appraisal of developments in addictions programs for Indigenous North Americans and Australians. *Social Science & Medicine, 41*(11), 1487–1498.

Browne, A. J. (2017). Moving beyond description: Closing the health equity gap by redressing racism impacting Indigenous populations. *Social Science & Medicine*, *184*, 23–26.

Browne, J., de Leeuw, E., Gleeson, D., Adams, K., Atkinson, P., & Hayes, R. (2017). A network approach to policy framing: A case study of the National Aboriginal and Torres Strait Islander Health Plan. *Social Science & Medicine, 172,* 10–18.

Cooper, D. (2011). Closing the gap in cultural understanding: Social determinants of health in Indigenous policy in Australia. AMSANT.

de Leeuw, S., Lindsay, N., & Greenwood, M. (2015). Introduction: Rethinking determinants of Indigenous Peoples' health in Canada. In M. Greenwood, S. de Leeuw, N. Lindsay, & C. Reading (Eds.), *Determinants of Indigenous Peoples' health in Canada*. Canadian Scholars.

Eby, D. K. (2007). Primary care at the Alaska Native Medical Centre: A fully deployed "new model" of primary care. *International Journal of Circumpolar Health*, *66*(Suppl 1), 4–13.

Eshet, D. (2015). *Stolen lives: The Indigenous Peoples of Canada and the Indian residential schools*. Facing History and Ourselves, Centre for Social Innovation.

Fisher, M., Battams, S., McDermott, D., Baum, F., & MacDougall, C. (2018). How the social determinants of Indigenous health became policy reality for Australia's National Aboriginal and Torres Strait Islander Health Plan. *Journal of Social Policy, 48*(1), 1–21.

Fohlich, K. L., Ross, N., & Richmond, C. (2006). Health disparities in Canada today: Some evidence and a theoretical framework. *Health Policy, 79*(2–3), 132–143.

Gabriel, M. D. (2015). *Indigenous homelessness and traditional knowledge: Stories of Elders and outreach support* [Master's thesis]. University of Toronto.

Gabriel, M. D. (2021). *Employment and education pathways: Exploring traditional knowledge supports for transitions out of homelessness for Indigenous Peoples* [Doctoral dissertation]. University of Toronto.

George, E., Mackean, T., Baum, F., & Fisher, M. (2019). Social determinants of Indigenous health and Indigenous rights in policy: A scoping review and analysis of problem representation. *International Indigenous Policy Journal, 10*(2).

Henderson, R., Montesanti, S., Crowshoe, L., & Leduc, C. (2018). Advancing Indigenous primary health care policy in Alberta, Canada. *Health Policy, 122*, 638–644.

Hill, D. M. (2003). *Traditional medicine in contemporary contexts: Protecting and respecting Indigenous knowledge and medicine.* National Aboriginal Health Organization (NAHO).

Indian Act (R.S., 1985, c. I–5), Canada (1985).

Josewski, V. (2012). Analysing "cultural safety" in mental health policy reform: Lessons from British Columbia, Canada. *Critical Public Health, 22*(2), 223–234.

Lambert, M., Luke, J., Downey, B., Crengle, S., Kelaher, M., Reid, S., & Smylie, J. (2014). Health literacy: Health professionals' understandings and their perceptions of barriers that Indigenous patients encounter. *BMC Health Services Research, 14*(1), 614.

Lavoie, J. G. (2013). Policy silences: Why Canada needs a national First Nation, Inuit, and Métis health policy. *International Journal of Circumpolar Health, 72*, 22690.

Lavoie, J. G., Browne, A. J., Varcoe, C., Wong, S., & Fridkin, A. (2015). Missing pathways to self-governance: Aboriginal health policy in British Columbia. *International Indigenous Policy Journal, 6*(1), 1–21. https://doi.org/10.18584/iipj.2015.6.1.2

McCallum, M. J., & Perry, A.(2018). *Structures of indifference: An Indigenous life and death in a Canadian city*. University of Manitoba Press.

Mitchell, T., & MacLeod, T. (2014). Aboriginal social policy: A critical community mental health issue. *CJCMH, 33*(1), 109–122.

National Aboriginal Health Organization (NAHO). (2003). *What First Nations people think about their health and health care: National Aboriginal Health Organization's public opinion poll on Aboriginal health and health care in Canada.*

National Archives of Canada. (n.d.). Record Group 10, vol. 6810, file 470-2-3, vol. 7, 55 (L-3), and 63 (N-3).

Priest, N., MacKean, T., Davis, E., Briggs, L., & Waters, E. (2012). Aboriginal perspectives of child health and wellbeing in an urban setting: Developing a conceptual framework. *Health Sociology Review, 21*(2), 180–195.

Reading, C. (2015). Structural determinants of Aboriginal Peoples' health. In M. Greenwood, S. de Leeuw, N. Lindsay, & C. Reading (Eds.), *Determinants of Indigenous Peoples' health in Canada* (pp. 3–15). Canadian Scholars.

Robbins, J. A., & Dewar, J. (2011). Traditional Indigenous approaches to healing and the modern welfare of traditional knowledge, spirituality and lands: A critical reflection on practices and policies taken from the Canadian Indigenous example. *International Indigenous Policy Journal, 2*(4).

Royal Commission on Aboriginal Peoples. (1996). *Report of the Royal Commission on Aboriginal Peoples.* Minister of Supply and Services Canada.

Sherwood, J. (2013). Colonisation—it's bad for your health: The context of Aboriginal health. *Contemporary Nurse, 46*(1), 28–40.

Smylie, J., Williams, L., & Cooper, N. (2006). Culture-based literacy and Aboriginal health. *Canadian Journal of Public Health, 9*(Suppl 2), S21–S25.

Statistics Canada. (2016). *Aboriginal peoples and Aboriginal languages in Canada: 2016 Census.*

Struthers, R., Eschiti, V. S., & Patchell, B. (2004). Traditional Indigenous healing: Part 1. *CTNM, 10*(3), 141–149.

Thistle, J. (2017). *Indigenous definition of homelessness in Canada.* Canadian Observatory on Homelessness Press.

Truth and Reconciliation Commission of Canada. (2015). *Truth and Reconciliation Commission of Canada: Calls to Action.* https://www2.gov.bc.ca/assets/gov/british-columbians-our-governments/indigenous-people/aboriginal-peoples-documents/calls_to_action_english2.pdf

Vass, A., Mitchell, A., & Dhurrkay, Y. (2011). Health literacy and Australian Indigenous Peoples: An analysis of the role of language and worldview. *Health Promotion Journal of Australia, 22*(1), 33–37.

Woolford, A. (2009). Ontological destruction: Genocide and Canadian Aboriginal Peoples. *GSP*, *4*(1), 81–97.

Wylie, L., McConkey, S., & Corrado, A. M. (2019). Colonial legacies and collaborative action: Improving Indigenous Peoples' health care in Canada. *International Indigenous Policy Journal*, *10*(5).

CHAPTER 11: THE CRITICAL IMPORTANCE OF ADDRESSING GENDER AND RACIAL INEQUITIES IN THE PUBLIC HEALTH SYSTEM, BY CHRISTINA SALMON AND ANDREA TRICCO

Amano-Patiño, N., Faraglia, E., Giannitsarou, C., & Hasna, Z. (2020). Who is doing new research in the time of COVID-19? Not the female economists. *VoxEU*. https://voxeu.org/article/who-doing-new-research-time-covid-19-not-female-economists

Andersen, J. P., Nielsen, M. W., Simone, N. L., Lewiss, R. E., & Jagsi, R. (2020). COVID-19 medical papers have fewer women first authors than expected. *Elife*, *9*, e58807. https://doi.org/10.7554/eLife.58807

Associated Press. (2020, July 18). From Rep. John Lewis, quotes in a long life of activism. *Washington Post*. https://www.washingtonpost.com/national/from-rep-john-lewis-quotes-in-a-long-life-of-activism/2020/07/18/7ee684d8-c8b0-11ea-a825-8722004e4150_story.html

Bethune, R., Absher, N., Obiagwu, M., Qarmout, T., Steeves, M., Yaghoubi, M., Tikoo, R., Szafron, M., Dell, C., & Farag, M. (2019). Social determinants of self-reported health for Canada's Indigenous peoples: A public health approach. *Public Health*, *176*, 172–180. https://doi.org/10.1016/j.puhe.2018.03.007

Cohen, P., & Gavett, G. (2019, November 18). The day-to-day work of diversity and inclusion. *Harvard Business Review*.

Crenshaw, K. (1989). Demarginalizing the intersection of race and sex: A Black feminist critique of antidiscrimination doctrine, feminist theory and antiracist politics. *University of Chicago Legal Forum*, *1989*(1), 139–167.

Crenshaw, K. (1991). Mapping the margins: Intersectionality, identity politics, and violence against women of color. *Stanford Law Review*, *43*(6), 1241–1299.

Dryden, O., & Nnorom, O. (2021). Time to dismantle systemic anti-Black racism in medicine in Canada. *CMAJ*, *193*(2), E55–E57. https://doi.org/10.1503/cmaj.201579

Fazackerley, A. (2020, May 12). Women's research plummets during lockdown—but articles from men increase. *The Guardian*. https://www.theguardian.com/education/2020/may/12/womens-research-plummets-during-lockdown-but-articles-from-men-increase

Franke, R. (2018). *What is structural racism? Some thoughts for anti-racist activists.* Michigan State University. https://msuweb.montclair.edu/~franker/FrankeWhatIsStructuralRacism.pdf

Frederickson, M. (2020). *COVID-19's gendered impact on academic productivity.* GitHub. https://github.com/drfreder/pandemic-pub-bias

Gabster, B. P., van Daalen, K., Dhatt, R., & Barry, M. (2020). Challenges for the female academic during the COVID-19 pandemic. *The Lancet, 395*(10242), 1968–1970. https://doi.org/10.1016/S0140-6736(20)31412-4

Glass, C., & Cook, A. (2020). Performative contortions: How white women and people of colour navigate elite leadership roles. *Gender, Work & Organization, 27*(6), 1232–1252. https://doi.org/https://doi.org/10.1111/gwao.12463

Government of Manitoba. (2021, March 21). *COVID-19 infections in Manitoba.* https://www.gov.mb.ca/health/publichealth/surveillance/docs/rei_external.pdf

Hammarström, A. (1999). Why feminism in public health? *Scandinavian Journal of Public Health, 27*(4), 241–244. https://www.ncbi.nlm.nih.gov/pubmed/10724464

Hirshfield, L. E., & Joseph, T. D. (2012). "We need a woman, we need a black woman": Gender, race, and identity taxation in the academy. *Gender and Education, 24*(2), 213–227. https://doi.org/10.1080/09540253.2011.606208

Hogenboom, M. (2022). The hidden load: How "thinking of everything" holds mums back. *BBC.* https://www.bbc.com/worklife/article/20210518-the-hidden-load-how-thinking-of-everything-holds-mums-back

Hou, F., & Schimmele, C. (2020). *Adults with a health education but not working in health occupations.* Statistics Canada. https://www150.statcan.gc.ca/n1/pub/45-28-0001/2020001/article/00004-eng.htm

MacDougall, A., Valley, J., & Jeffrey, J. (2021). *Diversity disclosure practices.* https://www.osler.com/osler/media/Osler/reports/corporate-governance/Osler-Diversity-Disclosure-Practices-report-2021.pdf

McKinsey & Company. (2020, July 15). *COVID-19 and gender equality: Countering the regressive effects.* https://www.mckinsey.com/featured-insights/future-of-work/covid-19-and-gender-equality-countering-the-regressive-effects

McKinsey & Company. (2021, September 27). *Women in the workplace 2021.* https://www.mckinsey.com/featured-insights/diversity-and-inclusion/women-in-the-workplace

McLean, S. (2018). *"We built a life from nothing": White settler colonialism and the myth of meritocracy.* Canadian Centre for Policy Alternatives. https://policyalternatives.ca/sites/default/files/uploads/publications/National%20Office/2017/12/McLean.pdf

Minello, A. (2020). The pandemic and the female academic. *Nature.* https://www.nature.com/articles/d41586-020-01135-9

Morgan, K. P. (1996). Describing the emperor's new clothes: Three myths of educational (in)equality. In A. Diller, B. Houston, K. P. Morgan, & M. Ayim (Eds.), *The gender question in education: Theory, pedagogy, and politics.* Routledge.

Nixon, S. A. (2019). The coin model of privilege and critical allyship: Implications for health. *BMC Public Health, 19*(1), 1637. https://doi.org/10.1186/s12889-019-7884-9

Rajan, D., Koch, K., Rohrer, K., Bajnoczki, C., Socha, A., Voss, M., Nicod, M., Ridde, V., & Koonin, J. (2020). Governance of the COVID-19 response: A call for more inclusive and transparent decision-making. *BMJ Global Health, 5*(5). https://doi.org/10.1136/bmjgh-2020-002655

Richardson, L., & Murphy, T. (2018). *Bringing reconciliation to healthcare in Canada: Wise practices for healthcare leaders.* HealthcareCAN. https://www.healthcarecan.ca/wp-content/themes/camyno/assets/document/Reports/2018/HCC/EN/TRCC_EN.pdf

Rogers, W. A. (2006). Feminism and public health ethics. *Journal of Medical Ethics, 32*(6), 351–354. https://doi.org/10.1136/jme.2005.013466

Sergeant, A., Saha, S., Lalwani, A., Sergeant, A., McNair, A., Larrazabal, E., Yang, K., Bogler, O., Dhoot, A., Werb, D., Maghsoudi, N., Richardson, L., Hawker, G., Siddiqi, A., Verma, A., & Razak, F. (2022). Diversity among health care leaders in Canada: A cross-sectional study of perceived gender and race. *CMAJ, 194*(10), E371–E377. https://doi.org/10.1503/cmaj.211340

Shamseer, L., Bourgeault, I., Grunfeld, E., Moore, A., Peer, N., Straus, S. E., & Tricco, A. C. (2021). Will COVID-19 result in a giant step backwards for women in academic science? *Journal of Clinical Epidemiology, 134,* 160–166. https://doi.org/10.1016/j.jclinepi.2021.03.004

Sidanius, J., & Pratto, F. (1999). Social dominance theory: A new synthesis. In J. Sidanius & J. Jost (Eds.), *Social dominance: An intergroup theory of social hierarchy and oppression.* (pp. 31–58). University of Cambridge Press.

Sinclair, M. (2010). *Truth and Reconciliation Commission of Canada, 9th Session of the United Nations Permanent Forum on Indigenous Issues.* United Nations, New York. http://www.classactionservices.ca/irs/documents/TRC_UN_Speech_CMS_FINAL_April_27_2010_000.pdf

Sriharan, A., Ratnapalan, S., Tricco, A. C., Lupea, D., Ayala, A. P., Pang, H., & Lee, D. D. (2020). Occupational stress, burnout, and depression in women in healthcare during COVID-19 pandemic: Rapid scoping review.

Frontiers in Global Women's Health, *1*, 596690. https://doi.org/10.3389/fgwh.2020.596690

Tucker, J. (2022). *Men have now recouped their pandemic related labour force losses while women lag behind*. National Women's Law Center. https://nwlc.org/wp-content/uploads/2022/02/January-Jobs-Day-updated.pdf

United Nations. (2020). *How COVID-19 impacts women and girls*. (2020). https://interactive.unwomen.org/multimedia/explainer/covid19/en/index.html?gclid=CjwKCAiAg8OBBhA8EiwAlKw3kuPnCbzEUOBCef1ZJj6eIVNtv9TEs0HqTvAk7EjgiSp8MgKwlx8R2RoCiKAQAvD_BwE

US Bureau of Labour Statistics. (2022a). *Table A-1. Employment status of the civilian population by sex and age*. https://www.bls.gov/news.release/empsit.t01.htm

US Bureau of Labour Statistics. (2022b). *Table A-2. Employment status of the civilian population by race, sex, and age*. https://www.bls.gov/news.release/empsit.t02.htm

US Bureau of Labour Statistics. (2022c). *Table A-3. Employment status of the Hispanic or Latino population by sex and age*. https://www.bls.gov/news.release/empsit.t03.htm

Viglione, G. (2020). Are women publishing less during the pandemic? Here's what the data say. *Nature*, *581*(7809), 365–366. https://doi.org/10.1038/d41586-020-01294-9

Williams, D. R., Lawrence, J. A., & Davis, B. A. (2019). Racism and health: Evidence and needed research. *Annual Review of Public Health*, *40*, 105–125. https://doi.org/10.1146/annurev-publhealth-040218-043750

World Health Organization. (n.d.). *Gender and health*. www.who.int/health-topics/gender#tab=tab_1

Yu, P. T., Parsa, P. V., Hassanein, O., Rogers, S. O., & Chang, D. C. (2013). Minorities struggle to advance in academic medicine: A 12-y review of diversity at the highest levels of America's teaching institutions. *Journal of Surgical Research*, *182*(2), 212–218. https://doi.org/10.1016/j.jss.2012.06.049

CHAPTER 12: RECLAMATION OF MATRIARCHY AND KINSHIP SYSTEMS, BY MIRANDA LESPERANCE

Allan, B., Smylie, J., & Wellesley Institute. (2015). *First Peoples, second class treatment: The role of racism in the health and well-being of Indigenous Peoples in Canada*. Wellesley Institute.

Alston-O'Connor, E. (2019). The Sixties Scoop. *Critical Social Work*, *11*(1). https://doi.org/10.22329/csw.v11i1.5816

Anderson, K., & Lavell-Harvard, D. M. (2014). *Mothers of the nations: Indigenous mothering as global resistance, reclaiming and recovering*. Demeter Press.

Black, K. A., Rich, R., & Felske-Durksen, C. (2021). Forced and coerced sterilization of Indigenous Peoples: Considerations for health care providers. *Journal of Obstetrics and Gynaecology Canada*, *43*(9), 1090–1093. https://doi.org/10.1016/j.jogc.2021.04.006

Blackstock, C. (2015). Should governments be above the law? The Canadian Human Rights Tribunal on First Nations child welfare. *Children Australia*, *40*(2), 95–103. https://doi.org/10.1017/cha.2015.6

Canadian Research Knowledge Network. (n.d.). The Jesuit relations and allied documents. *Canadiana Online*. https://www.canadiana.ca/view/oocihm.07535/34?r=0&s=1

Crenshaw, K. (1991). Mapping the margins: Intersectionality, identity politics, and violence against women of color. *Stanford Law Review*, *43*(6), 1241–1299. https://doi.org/10.2307/1229039

Daoud, N., Smylie, J., Urquia, M., Allan, B., & O'Campo, P. (2013). The contribution of socio-economic position to the excesses of violence and intimate partner violence among Aboriginal versus non-Aboriginal women in Canada. *Canadian Journal of Public Health*, *104*(4), e278–e283. https://doi.org/10.17269/cjph.104.3724

Dyck, E. (2013). *Facing eugenics: Reproduction, sterilization, and the politics of choice*. University of Toronto Press.

First Nations Information Governance Centre. (2020). *Strengths-based approaches to Indigenous research and the development of well-being indicators*. https://fnigc.ca/wp-content/uploads/2021/05/FNIGC-Research-Series-SBA_v04.pdf

Garner, R., Guimond, E., & Senécal, S. (2013). The socio-economic characteristics of First Nation teen mothers. *International Indigenous Policy Journal*, *4*(1). https://doi.org/10.18584/iipj.2013.4.1.9

Greenwood, M., de Leeuw, S., & Lindsay, N. (2018). Challenges in health equity for Indigenous Peoples in Canada. *The Lancet*, *391*(10131), 1645–1648. https://doi.org/10.1016/s0140-6736(18)30177-6

Guèvremont, A., & Kohen, D. (2013). The physical and mental health of off-reserve First Nations children of teen mothers. *International Indigenous Policy Journal*, *4*(1). https://doi.org/10.18584/iipj.2013.4.1.2

Hay, T., Blackstock, C., & Kirlew, M. (2020). Dr. Peter Bryce (1853–1932): Whistleblower on residential schools. *CMAJ*, *192*(9), E223–E224. https://doi.org/10.1503/cmaj.190862

Hull, J. (2013). Potential barriers to Aboriginal teenaged mothers' access to maternal and parental benefits. *International Indigenous Policy Journal, 4*(1). https://doi.org/10.18584/iipj.2013.4.1.5

Kirmayer, L. J., Dandeneau, S., Marshall, E., Phillips, M. K., & Williamson, K. J. (2011). Rethinking resilience from Indigenous perspectives. *Canadian Journal of Psychiatry, 56*(2), 84–91. https://doi.org/10.1177/070674371105600203

Lavell, J. C., & Lavell-Harvard, D. M. (2006). *"Until our hearts are on the ground": Aboriginal mothering, oppression, resistance and rebirth.* Demeter Press.

Legacy of Hope. (2017). *Bi-Giwen: Truth telling from the Sixties Scoop.* https://legacyofhope.ca/bigiwen/

Lesperance, M. L. (2022). *We are stories, not labels: Anishinaabekweg childrearing experiences* [Doctoral dissertation]. University of Toronto, TSpace Repository. https://tspace.library.utoronto.ca/bitstream/1807/125400/2/Lesperance_Miranda_Leigh_202211_PhD_thesis.pdf

Minthorn, R. S. (2022). *Indigenous motherhood in the academy.* Rutgers University Press.

Minthorn, R. Z. (2018). Indigenous motherhood in the academy, building our children to be good relatives. *Wicazo Sa Review, 33*(2), 62. https://doi.org/10.5749/wicazosareview.33.2.0062

Muir, N., & Bohr, Y. (2019). Contemporary practice of traditional Aboriginal child rearing: A review. *First Peoples Child & Family Review, 14*(1), 153–165. https://fpcfr.com/index.php/FPCFR/article/view/378

Nichols, J., & Nyholm, E. (1995). *A concise dictionary of Minnesota Ojibwe.* University of Minnesota Press.

O'Driscoll, T., Payne, L., Kelly, L., Cromarty, H., Pierre-Hansen, N. S., & Terry, C. (2011). Traditional First Nations birthing practices: Interviews with Elders in northwestern Ontario. *Journal of Obstetrics and Gynaecology Canada, 33*(1), 24–29. https://doi.org/10.1016/s1701-2163(16)34768-5

Ryan, S. D., Hinterlong, J., Hegar, R. L., & Johnson, L. B. (2010). Kin adopting kin: In the best interest of the children? *Children and Youth Services Review, 32*(12), 1631–1639. https://doi.org/10.1016/j.childyouth.2010.06.013

Senate of Canada. (2019, April 3). Proceeding of the Standing Senate Committee on Human Rights. Issue No. 40—Evidence. https://sencanada.ca/en/Content/Sen/Committee/421/RIDR/40ev-54643-e

Sharma, S., Kolahdooz, F., Launier, K., Nader, F., June Yi, K., Baker, P., McHugh, T. L., & Vallianatos, H. (2016). Canadian Indigenous Women's perspectives of maternal health and health care services: A systematic review. *Diversity & Equality in Health and Care, 13*(5). https://doi.org/10.21767/2049-5471.100073

Statistics Canada. (2016). *First Nations, Métis and Inuit women*. https://www150.statcan.gc.ca/n1/pub/89-503-x/2015001/article/14313-eng.htm

Trocmé, N., Knoke, D., & Blackstock, C. (2004). Pathways to the overrepresentation of Aboriginal children in Canada's child welfare system. *Social Service Review*, *78*(4), 577–600. https://doi.org/10.1086/424545

Truth and Reconciliation Commission of Canada. (2016). *A knock on the door: The essential history of residential schools from the Truth and Reconciliation Commission of Canada*. University of Manitoba Press.

Van Herk, K. A., Smith, D., & Andrew, C. (2011). Identity matters: Aboriginal mothers' experiences of accessing health care. *Contemporary Nurse*, *37*(1), 57–68. https://doi.org/10.5172/conu.2011.37.1.057

Walls, M. L., & Whitbeck, L. B. (2012). The intergenerational effects of relocation policies on Indigenous families. *Journal of Family Issues*, *33*(9), 1272–1293. https://doi.org/10.1177/0192513x12447178

Webstad, P. (2021). *Beyond the orange shirt story: A collection of stories from family and friends of Phyllis Webstad before, during, and after their residential school experiences*. Medicine Wheel Education.

Wildcat, M. (2019). Wahkohtowin in action. *Constitutional Forum/Forum Constitutionnel*, *27*(1), 13. https://doi.org/10.21991/cf29370

Wright, L., Dell, C. A., & First Nations Information Governance Centre. (2020). Tobacco smoking among First Nations youth living on-reserve and in northern communities: A mixed methods study. *International Indigenous Policy Journal*, *11*(4), 1–30. https://doi.org/10.18584/iipj.2020.11.4.13369

CHAPTER 13: ENGENDERING A FEMINIST ETHIC OF CARE TO TRAINING A NEW GENERATION OF PUBLIC HEALTH RESEARCHERS: REFLECTING ON 4THERECORD, BY SARAH FLICKER, NADHA HASSEN, JESSICA FIELDS, AND 4THERECORD RESEARCH TEAM, WITH AMANDA GALUSHA, ANJALEE SRINIVASAN, CAITLIN ARIZALA, EMILY SUTTON, JESSICA J. MENCIA, JULIA FERGUSON, KETHMI EGODAGE, KEZIA ARINKA, NADIA BEVAN, REECE RABANAL, SEVENTY HALL, VAISHNAVY PUVIPALAN, AND ZARIN TASNIM

Ahmed, S. (2017). *Living a feminist life*. Duke University Press.

Bay-Cheng, L. Y. (2009). Beyond trickle-down benefits to research participants. *Social Work Research*, *33*(4), 243–247.

Bay-Cheng, L. Y. (2017). Seeing how far I've come: The impact of the digital sexual life history calendar on young adult research participants. *Journal of Sex Research*, *54*(3), 284–295.

Beckman, L. J. (2014). Training in feminist research methodology: Doing research on the margins. *Women & Therapy*, *37*(1–2), 164–177. https://doi.org/10.1080/02703149.2014.850347

Blakely, K. (2007). Reflections on the role of emotion in feminist research. *International Journal of Qualitative Methods*, *6*(2), 59–68.

Finlay, L. (2002). Negotiating the swamp: The opportunity and challenge of reflexivity in research practice. *Qualitative Research*, *2*(2), 209–230.

Gilligan, C. (1993). *In a different voice: Psychological theory and women's development.* Harvard University Press.

Gringeri, C. E., Wahab, S., & Anderson-Nathe, B. (2010). What makes it feminist?: Mapping the landscape of feminist social work research. *Affilia*, *25*(4), 390–405.

Harding, S. (1987). Introduction. In S. Harding (Ed.), *Feminism and methodology* (pp. 1–14). Indiana University Press.

hooks, b. (2014). *Feminism is for everybody: Passionate politics* (2nd ed.). Routledge.

Liboiron, M., Ammendolia, J., Winsor, K., Zahara, A., Bradshaw, H., Melvin, J., Mather, C., Dawe, N., Wells, E., Liboiron, F., Fürst, B., Coyle, C., Saturno, J., Novacefski, M., Westscott, S., & Liboiron, F. (2017). Equity in author order: A feminist laboratory's approach. *Catalyst: Feminism, Theory, Technoscience*, *3*(2), 1–17.

Mauthner, N. S., & Edwards, R. (2010). Feminist research management in higher education in Britain: Possibilities and practices. *Gender, Work & Organization*, *17*(5), 481–502.

McKittrick, K. (2021). Dear science. In K. McKittrick (Ed.), *Dear science and other stories* (pp. 186–188). Duke University Press.

Moss, P., DeBres, K. J., Cravey, A., Hyndman, J., Hirschboeck, K. K., & Masucci, M. (1999). Toward mentoring as feminist praxis: Strategies for ourselves and others. *Journal of Geography in Higher Education*, *23*(3), 413–427.

Noddings, N. (2013). Caring : A relational approach to ethics and moral education (2nd ed.). University of California Press.

Piepzna-Samarasinha, L. L. (2018). *Care work: Dreaming disability justice.* Arsenal Pulp Press.

Salmon, R., & Steinberg, D. M. (2007). Staying in the mess: Teaching students and practitioners to work effectively in the swamp of important problems. *Social Work with Groups*, *30*(4), 79–94.

Tuhiwai Smith, L. (2012). *Decolonizing methodologies* (2nd ed.). Zed Books.
Wilson, C. L., Singh, A. K., Beals, A. M., Sharma, R., Hunt, B., Furman, E., Darko, N. A., Fante-Coleman, T., Liu, V., & Kivell, N. (2021). Dialogues of disruption: Confronting oppression in the academy. *Global Journal of Community Psychology Practice*, *12*(3).

CHAPTER 14: CHRONICLES OF PUBLIC HEALTH DOCTORAL STUDENTS: OVERCOMING THE IVORY TOWER THROUGH A REVOLUTION OF "SELF-CARE" FOR A BETTER FUTURE, BY COREY MCAULIFFE, IFRAH ABDILLAHI, KARIMA JOY, ASTRID ESCRIG-PINOL, APONDI J. ODHIAMBO, AND RENÉE MONCHALIN

Absolon, K. E. (2011). *Kaandossiwin: How we come to know*. Fernwood Publishing.
Allan, B., & Smylie, J. (2015). *First Peoples, second class treatment: The role of racism in the health and well-being of Indigenous Peoples in Canada*. Wellesley Institute.
Canadian Public Health Association. (2020). *Public health: A conceptual framework*. https://www.cpha.ca/what-public-health
DeAngelo, L., Schuster, M. T., & Lachaud, Q. A. (2021). The faculty role in grooming and gatekeeping students' of color potential along the professoriate pipeline. *Review of Higher Education*, *44*(4), 493–521. https://doi.org/10.1353/RHE.2021.0010
Dryden, O. S., & Nnorom, O. (2021). Time to dismantle systemic anti-Black racism in medicine in Canada. *CMAJ*, *193*(2), E55–E57. https://doi.org/10.1503/cmaj.201579
Gaudry, A., & Lorenz, D. (2018a). Indigenization as inclusion, reconciliation, and decolonization: Navigating the different visions for indigenizing the Canadian academy. *AlterNative: An International Journal of Indigenous Peoples*, *14*(3), 218–227.
Gaudry, A., & Lorenz, D. (2018b). Decolonization for the masses?: Indigenous content requirements in the changing Canadian post-secondary environment. In L. Smith, E. Tuck, & K. Yang, *Indigenous and decolonizing studies in education: Mapping the long view* (pp. 159–174). Routledge.
Grande, S. (2018). Refusing the university. In E. Tuck & K. W. Yang (Eds.), *Toward what justice? Describing diverse dreams of justice in education* (pp. 47–65). Routledge.

Grimes, K. (2018). Let Black people be: A plea for racial specificity in the afterlife of Africanized slavery. *Journal of Religious Ethics*, *46*(3), 496–520. https://doi.org/10.1111/jore.12229

Hankivsky, O. (2014). Rethinking care ethics: On the promise and potential of an intersectional analysis. *American Political Science Review*, *108*(2), 252–264.

Heleta, S. (2016). Decolonisation of higher education: Dismantling epistemic violence and Eurocentrism in South Africa. *Transformation in Higher Education*, *1*, a9. https://doi.org/10.4102/the.v1i1.9

Jee-Lyn García, J., & Sharif, M. Z. (2015). Black lives matter: A commentary on racism and public health. *American Journal of Public Health*, 105, e27–e30.

Kelley, R. D. (2016, March 1). Black study, Black struggle. *Boston Review*. https://bostonreview.net/forum/robin-kelley-black-struggle-campus-protest/

Kielsgard, R., & Brown, L. (2021). Trans, autistic and BIPOC: Living at the intersections of autism, race and gender diversity. In M. Kourti (Ed.), *Working with autistic transgender and non-binary people: Research, practice and experience* (pp. 71–88). Jessica Kingsley Publishers.

King, T. L., Navarro, J., & Smith, A. (2020). Beyond incommensurability: Toward an otherwise stance on Black and Indigenous relationality. In T. L. King, J. Navarro, & A. Smith, *Otherwise worlds* (pp. 1–23). https://doi.org/10.1215/9781478012023-001

Knotek, S. E., Foley-Nicpon, M., Kozbelt, A., Olszewski-Kubilius, P., Portenga, S., Subotnik, R. F., & Worrell, F. C. (2020). Gatekeeping in high-performance settings. *Review of General Psychology*, *24*(3), 254–267. https://doi.org/10.1177/1089268020905578

Kuokkanen, R. (2008). What is hospitality in the academy? Epistemic ignorance and the (im)possible gift. *Review of Education, Pedagogy, and Cultural Studies*, *30*(1), 60–82.

Lawson, E. S. (2020). Anti-Black racism on the sidelines: The limits of "listening sessions" to address institutional racism at Canadian universities. *Canadian Review of Sociology*, *57*(3), 491–494. https://doi.org/10.1111/cars.12296

Liaschenko, J., & Peter, E. (2006). Feminist ethics: A way of doing ethics. In A. Davis, V. Tschudin, & L. de Raeve (Eds.), *Essentials of teaching and learning in nursing ethics: Content and methods* (pp. 181–190). Elsevier.

Lindemann, H. (2006). *An invitation to feminist ethics*. McGraw-Hill.

Ribbens McCarthy, J. (2012). Caring after death: Issues of embodiment and relationality. In C. Rogers & S. Weller (Eds.), *Critical approaches to care: Understanding caring relations, identities and cultures* (pp. 183–194). Routledge.

Robinson, F. (2015). Care ethics, political theory, and the future of feminism. In D. Engster & M. Hamington (Eds.), *Care ethics and political theory* (pp. 293–312). Oxford University Press.

Rodríguez, D. (2012). Racial/colonial genocide and the "neoliberal academy": In excess of a problematic. *American Quarterly*, *64*(4), 809–813.

Sharpe, B. (2020, March 27). How universal health care fails queer communities. *The Walrus*. https://thewalrus.ca/how-universal-health-care-fails-queer-communities/

Tronto, J. (1993). *Moral boundaries: A political argument for an ethic of care*. Routledge.

Tuck, E., & Yang, W. K. (2012). Decolonization is not a metaphor. *Decolonization: Indigeneity, Education & Society*, *1*(1), 1–40.

Tuhiwai Smith, L. (2012). *Decolonizing methodologies* (2nd ed.). Zed Books.

Walker, M. U. (2007). The subject of moral philosophy, with postscript. In M. U. Walker (Ed.), *Moral understandings: A feminist study in ethics*. Oxford University Press.

Wolfe, P. (2006). Settler colonialism and the elimination of the Native. *Journal of Genocide Research*, *8*(4), 387–409.

Yakubovich, A. R., & Maki, K. (2021). Preventing gender-based homelessness in Canada during the COVID-19 pandemic and beyond: The need to account for violence against women. *Violence Against Women*, 28(10), 2587–2599.

CHAPTER 15: PUBLIC HEALTH FEMINISM AND HOUSING: STATUS QUO OR TRANSFORMATIONAL? BY MELISSA PERRI AND PATRICIA O'CAMPO

Adams, C. (2021, March 26). Evanston is the first US city to issue slavery reparations. Experts say it's a noble start. *NBC News*. https://www.nbcnews.com/news/nbcblk/evanston-s-reparations-plan-noble-start-complicated-process-experts-say-n1262096

Akbar, P. A., Li, S., Shertzer, A., & Walsh, R. P. (2019). *Racial segregation in housing markets and the erosion of Black wealth*. National Bureau of Economic Research.

Arvin, M., & Morrill, E. (2013). Decolonizing feminism: Challenging connections between settler colonialism and heteropatriarchy. *Feminist Formations*, *25*(1), 8–34.

Bell, S. E. (1987). Changing ideas: The medicalization of menopause. *Social Science and Medicine*, *24*(6), 535–542.

Bell, S. E., & Figert, A. E. (2010). Gender and the medicalization of healthcare. In E. Kuhlmann (Ed.), *The Palgrave handbook of gender and healthcare* (2nd ed.). Palgrave.

Bell, S. E., & Figert, A. E. (2012). Medicalization and pharmaceuticalization at the intersections: Looking backward, sideways and forward. *Social Science and Medicine*, *75*(5), 775–783.

Braveman, P. A., Kumanyika, S., Fielding, J., LaVeist, T., Borrell, L. N., Manerscheid, R., & Troutman, A. (2011). Health disparities and health equity: The issue is justice. *American Journal of Public Health*, *101*(1), S149–S155.

Brisbois, B., O'Campo, P., & Kamalanathan, J. (2018). Inequities in cities and in urban health. In S. Galea & D. Vlahoy (Eds.), *Urban health* (pp. 73–81). Oxford University Press.

Cheng, P., Lin, Z., & Liu, Y. (2015). Racial discrepancy in mortgage interest rates. *Journal of Real Estate Finance and Economics*, *51*, 101–120.

Cho, S., Crenshaw, K., & McCall, L. (2013). Toward a field of intersectionality studies: Theory, applications, and praxis. *Intersectionality: Theorizing Power, Empowering Theory*, *38*(4), 1–26.

Clarke, C. (1981). Lesbianism: An act of resistance. In C. R. McCann, S. K. Kim, & E. Ergun (Eds.), *Feminist theory reader: Local and global perspectives* (5th ed., pp. 54–59). Routledge.

Collins, P. H. (1989). The social construction of Black feminist thought. *University of Chicago Press Journals*, *14*(4), 745–773.

Collins, P. H. (2015). Intersectionality's definitional dilemmas. *Annual Review of Sociology*, *41*, 1–20.

Collins, P. H. (2019). *Intersectionality as critical social theory*. Duke University Press

Collins, P. H., & Bilge, S. (2020). *Intersectionality* (2nd ed.). Polity Press.

Combahee River Collective. (1981). *A Black feminist statement*. Kitchen Table, Women of Colour Press.

Conrad, P. (1975). The discovery of hyperkinesis: Notes on the medicalization of deviant behavior. *Social Problems*, *23*(1), 12–21.

Conrad, P. (1992). Medicalization and social control. *Annual Review of Sociology*, *16*, 209–232.

Conrad, P., & Scheider, J. W. (1980). Looking at levels of medicalization: A comment on Strong's critique of the thesis of medical imperialism. *Social Science and Medicine*, *14A*, 75–79.

Crenshaw, K. (1989). Demarginalizing the intersection of race and sex: A Black feminist critique of antidiscrimination doctrine, feminist theory and antiracist politics. *University of Chicago Legal Forum*, *1989*(1), 139–167.

Crenshaw, K. (1991). Mapping the margins: Intersectionality, identity politics, and violence against women of color. *Stanford Law Review*, *43*(6), 1241–1299.

Crotty, M. (1998). Constructionism: The making of meaning. In *The foundations of social research: Meaning and perspective* (pp. 1–24). SAGE.

CSDH. (2008). *Closing the gap in a generation: Health equity through action on the social determinants of health. Final Report of the Commission on Social Determinants of Health.* World Health Organization.

Edley, N. (2001). Unravelling social constructionism. *Theory & Psychology*, *11*(2), 433–441.

Gaetz, S., Dej, E., Richter, T., & Redman, M. (2016). *The state of homelessness in Canada 2016*. Canadian Observatory on Homelessness. https://homelesshub.ca/sites/default/files/SOHC16_final_20Oct2016.pdf

Grande, S. (2003). Whitestream feminism and the colonialist project: A review of contemporary feminist pedagogy and praxis. *Educational Theory*, *53*(3), 1–19.

Hansen, H. (2017). Assisted technologies of social reproduction: Pharmaceutical prothesis or gender, race, and class in the white opioid "crisis." *Contemporary Drug Problems*, *44*(4), 321–338.

Hansen, H., & Roberts, S. K. (2012). Two tiers of biomedicalization: Methadone buprenorphine and the racial politics of addiction treatment. *Critical Perspectives on Addiction*, *14*, 79–102.

Kandiyoti, D. (1988). Bargaining with patriarchy. In C. R. McCann, S. K. Kim, & E. Ergun (Eds.), *Feminist theory reader: Local and global perspectives* (5th ed., pp. 60–65). Routledge.

Lykes, M. B. (1985). Gender and individualistic vs. collective bases of social individuality. *Journal of Personality Psychology*, *53*, 357–383.

Maluf, S. W. (2011). Brazilian feminisms: Central and peripheral issues. *Feminist Review Conference Proceedings*, *98*(Suppl 1), e36–51.

Mama, A. (2011). What does it mean to do feminist research in African contexts? *Feminist Review Conference Proceedings*, *98*(Suppl 1), e4–e20.

Mawani, F. N. (2018). *Conceptualization, measurement, and association of underemployment to mental health inequities between immigrant and Canadian-born labour force participants* [Doctoral thesis]. University of Toronto, TSpace Repository. http://hdl.handle.net/1807/89809

McGibbon, E. (Ed.). (2021). *Oppression: A social determinant of health*. Fernwood Publishing.

Milevska, S. (2011). Solidarity and intersectionality: What can transnational feminist theory learn from regional feminist activism. *Feminist Review Conference Proceedings*, *98*(Suppl 1), e52–e61.

Mitra, N. (2011). Domestic violence research: Expanding understandings but limited perspective. *Feminist Review Conference Proceedings*, *98*(Suppl 1), e62–e78.

Murphy, J., Vallieres, F., Bentall, R. P., Shevlin, M., McBride, O., Hartman, T. K., McKay, R., Bennett, K., Mason, L., Gibson-Miller, J., Levita, L., Martinez, A. P., Stocks, T. V. A., Karatzias, T., & Hyland, P. (2021). Psychological characteristics associated with COVID-19 vaccine hesitancy and resistance in Ireland and the United Kingdom. *Nature Communications*, *12*(29), 1–15.

Nash, J. C. (2008). Re-thinking intersectionality. In C. R. McCann, S. K. Kim, & E. Ergun (Eds.), *Feminist theory reader: Local and global perspectives* (5th ed., pp. 117–123). Routledge.

Perri, M., Metheny, N., Matheson, F. L., Potvin, K., & O'Campo, P. (2021). Finding opportunity in the COVID-19 crisis: Prioritizing gender in the design of social protection policies *Health Promotion International*, *37*(1), 1–11.

Perri, M., & O'Campo, P. (2021). A gap in knowledge surrounding urban housing interventions: A call for gender redistribution. *Health Promotion Internal*, *36*(4), 908–912.

Phelan, J. C., Link, B. G., & Tehranifar, P. (2010). Social conditions as fundamental causes of health inequalities: Theory, evidence, and policy implications. *Journal of Health and Social Behaviour*, *51*, S28–40.

Phillips, S. P. (2005). Defining and measuring gender: A social determinant of health whose time has come. *International Journal for Equity in Health*, *4*(11).

Phipps, A. (2021). White tears, white rage: Victimhood and (as) violence in mainstream feminism. *European Journal of Cultural Studies*, *24*(1), 81–93.

Pirtle, W. N. L. (2022). "White people still come out on top": The persistence of white supremacy in shaping coloured South Africans' perceptions of racial hierarchy and experiences of racism in post-Apartheid South Africa. *Social Sciences*, *11*(70), 1–14.

Premji, S. (2018). "It's totally destroyed our life": Exploring the pathways and mechanisms between precarious employment and health and well-being among immigrant men and women in Toronto. *International Journal of Health Services*, *48*, 106–127.

Riessman, C. K. (1983). Women and medicalization: A new perspective. *Social Policy*, *14*, 3–18.

Roberts, A., & Zulfiqar, G. M. (2019). The political economy of women's entrepreneurship initiatives in Pakistan: Reflections on gender, class, and "development." *Review of International Political Economy, 26*(3), 410–435.

Rolfe, S., Garnham, L., Godwin, J., Anderson, I., Seaman, P., & Donaldson, C. (2020). Housing as a social determinant of health and wellbeing: Developing an empirically informed realist theoretical framework. *BMC Public Health, 20*(1138), 1–19.

Roseman, S. R., Barber, P. G., & Neis, B. (2015). Towards a feminist political economy framework for analyzing employment-related geographical mobility. *Studies in Political Economy, 95*, 175–203.

Schwan, K., Vaccaro, M., Reid, L., Ali, N., & Baig, K. (2021). *The Pan-Canadian Women's Housing & Homelessness survey.* https://womenshomelessness.ca/wp-content/uploads/EN-Pan-Canadian-Womens-Housing-Homelessness-Survey-FINAL-28-Sept-2021.pdf

Schwan, K., Versteegh, A., Perri, M., Caplan, R., Baig, K., Dej, E., Jenkinson, J., Brais, H., Eiboff, F., & Chaleshtari, T. P. (2020). *The state of women's housing need & homelessness in Canada: Literature review* (A. Hache, A. Nelson, E. Kratochvil, & J. Malenfant, Eds.). Canadian Observatory on Homelessness Press.

Sharkey, P. (2013). *Stuck in place: Urban neighborhoods and the end of progress toward racial equality.* University of Chicago Press.

Short, S. E., Yang, Y. C., & Jenkins, T. M. (2013). Sex, gender, genetics, and health. *American Journal of Public Health, 103*(1), S93–101.

Silverstein, J. (2017). Intersectionality, resistance, and history-making: A conversation between Carolyn D'Cruz, Ruth DeSouza, Samia Khatun, and Crystal McKinnon. *Lilith: A Feminist History Journal, 23*, 15–22.

Singh, A., Daniel, L., Baker, E., & Bentley, R. (2019). Housing disadvantage and poor mental health: A systematic review. *American Journal of Preventative Medicine, 57*(2), 262–272.

Smith, P. M., & Mustard, C. A. (2010). The unequal distribution of occupational health and safety risks among immigrants to Canada compared to Canadian-born labour market participants: 1993–2005. *Safety Science, 48*, 1296–1303.

Syed, I. U. (2021). Feminist political economy of health: Current perspectives and future directions. *Healthcare, 9*(2), 1–15.

Tuck, E., & Yang, K. W. (2012). Decolonization is not a metaphor. *Decolonization: Indigeneity, Education, & Society, 1*(1), 1–40.

Tyson, C. (2003). Research, race, and an epistemology of emancipation. *Counterpoints, 195*, 19–28.

Upadhyay, N. (2021). Coloniality of white feminism and its transphobia: A comment on Burt. *Feminist Criminology, 16*(4), 539–544.

van Hagen, L. J., Muntinga, M., Appelman, Y., & Verdonk, P. (2020). Sex- and gender-sensitive public health research: An analysis of research proposals in a research institute in the Netherlands. *Women & Health, 61*(1), 109–119.

Vosko, L. F. (2002). The pasts (and futures) of feminist political economy in Canada: Reviving the debate. *Studies in Political Economy, 68*(1), 55–83.

CHAPTER 16: PUBLIC HEALTH FEMINIST FUTURES AND MOVING FORWARD, BY RENÉE MONCHALIN

Canadian Public Health Association. (2020). *What is public health?* https://www.cpha.ca/what-public-health

Freire, P. ([1970] 2007). *Pedagogy of the oppressed* (M. B. Ramos, Trans.). Continuum.

FSC
www.fsc.org
MIX
Papier | Fördert gute Waldnutzung
FSC® C083411

Kolibri 360 GmbH
Ferdinand-Jühlke-Straße 7
99095 Erfurt, Deutschland
produktsicherheit@kolibri360.de